Practical Emergency Resuscitation and Critical Care

T0295281

Practical Emergency Resuscitation and Critical Care

Second Edition

EDITED BY

Kaushal Shah

Weill Cornell Medical Center, New York

Jarone Lee

Massachusetts General Hospital, Boston

Clark G. Owyang

Weill Cornell Medical Center, New York

Benjamin Christian Renne

Massachusetts General Hospital, Boston

ASSISTANT EDITORS

Shuhan He

Massachusetts General Hospital, Boston

Adi Balk

Ben Gurion University of the Negev, Be'er Sheva, Israel

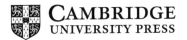

CAMBRIDGE
UNIVERSITY PRESS

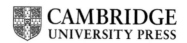

Shaftesbury Road, Cambridge CB2 8EA, United Kingdom

One Liberty Plaza, 20th Floor, New York, NY 10006, USA

477 Williamstown Road, Port Melbourne, VIC 3207, Australia

314–321, 3rd Floor, Plot 3, Splendor Forum, Jasola District Centre, New Delhi – 110025, India

103 Penang Road, #05-06/07, Visioncrest Commercial, Singapore 238467

Cambridge University Press is part of Cambridge University Press & Assessment, a department of the University of Cambridge.

We share the University's mission to contribute to society through the pursuit of education, learning and research at the highest international levels of excellence.

www.cambridge.org
Information on this title: www.cambridge.org/9781009055628

DOI: 10.1017/9781009052566

First Edition 2013
Second Edition 2024

Printed in the United Kingdom by TJ Books Limited, Padstow Cornwall

A catalogue record for this publication is available from the British Library.

Library of Congress Cataloging-in-Publication Data
Names: Shah, Kaushal, editor. | Lee, Jarone, editor. | Owyang, Clark G., editor. | Renne, Benjamin Christian, editor.
Title: Practical emergency resuscitation and critical care / edited by Kaushal Shah, Jarone Lee, Clark G. Owyang, Benjamin Christian Renne.
Description: Second edition. | Cambridge, United Kingdom ; New York, NY : Cambridge University Press, 2023. | Includes bibliographical references and index.
Identifiers: LCCN 2023003020 (print) | LCCN 2023003021 (ebook) | ISBN 9781009055628 (paperback) | ISBN 9781009052566 (epub)
Subjects: MESH: Critical Care | Emergency Medical Services | Resuscitation | Handbook
Classification: LCC RC86.7 (print) | LCC RC86.7 (ebook) | NLM WX 39 | DDC 616.02/8–dc23/eng/20230518
LC record available at https://lccn.loc.gov/2023003020
LC ebook record available at https://lccn.loc.gov/2023003021

ISBN 978-1-009-05562-8 Paperback

Contents

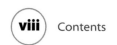

Contributors

Editors

Jarone Lee
Massachusetts General Hospital, Boston, MA, US

Kaushal Shah
Weill Cornell Medical Center, New York, NY, US

Associate Editors

Clark G. Owyang
Weill Cornell Medical Center, New York, NY, US

Benjamin Christian Renne
Massachusetts General Hospital, Boston, MA, US

Assistant Editors

Adi Balk
Ben Gurion University of the Nege, Beersheva, Israel

Shuhan He
Massachusetts General Hospital, Boston, MA, US

Section Editors

Mark Andreae
Critical Care and Emergency Medicine Physician, Icahn School of Medicine at Mount Sinai, New York City, NY, US

Jason M. Block

Intensivist, Abbott Northwestern Hospital, Community instructor, Emergency medicine and Critical Care Medicine, University of Minnesota Minneapolis, MN, US

Michael N. Cocchi

Associate Chief Medical Officer, Beth Israel Deaconess Medical Center, Boston, MA, US

Cassidy Dahn

Assistant Professor, Emergency Medicine, Clinical, Attending, Critical Care and Emergency Medicine, NYU Langone Health, New York, NY, US

Brandon Godbout

Assistant Professor, Emergency Medicine, Zucker School of Medicine at Hofstra/Northwell, Emergency Medicine, Manhasset, NY, US

Kari Gorder

Cardiovascular Critical Care, The Christ Hospital, Cincinnati, OH, US

Annette M. Ilg

Emergency Medicine and Critical Care, Brigham and Women's Hospital, Boston, MA, US

Ashley Shreves

Emergency Medicine and Hospice and Palliative Care Physician, Ochsner Health, New Orleans, LA, US

Todd Siegel

Emergency Medicine Physician, Beth Israel Deaconess Medical Center, Boston, MA, US

Susan Wilcox

Medical Director, ICU Lahey Hospital & Medical Center, Burlington, MA, US

Julie Winkle

Associate Professor, Anesthesia Critical Care, University of Colorado School of Medicine, Aurora, CO, US

Contributors

Robert Adams

Virginia Commonwealth University School of Medicine, Richmond, VA, US

John Arbo
Department of Emergency Medicine, UT Health Science Center at San Antonio, Joe R and Teresa Lozano Long School of Medicine, San Antonio, TX, US

Christopher Allison
Department of Medicine, Brown University, Providence, RI, US

Abeer Almasary
Department of Emergency Medicine, Baylor College of Medicine, Houston, TX, US

Kenneth R. L. Bernard
UVA Community Health, Prince William Medical Center, Manassas, Virginia, US

Lauren Becker
Department of Medicine, Division of Critical Care, University of Maryland, Baltimore, MD, US

Amy Caggiula
George Washington University Medical Center, Washington DC, US

Jennifer Carnell
Department of Emergency Medicine, Baylor College of Medicine, Houston, TX, US

Christine K. Chan
Montefiore Medical Center - Albert Einstein College of Medicine, Bronx, NY, US

Jayaram Chelluri
Division of Critical care, St Mary Medical Center, Langhorne, PA, US

Erica Chimelski
Department of Medicine, Stanford Health Care, Stanford, CA, US

David Convissar
Massachusetts General Hospital, Boston, MA, US

Cristal Cristia
Department of Emergency Medicine, Baptist Hospital System, San Antonio, TX, US

Peter G. Czarnecki
Beth Israel Deaconess Medical Center Harvard Medical School, Boston, MA, US

Vishal Demla
Division of Critical Care, UTHealth, Houston, TX, US

Amar Deshwar
Massachusetts General Hospital & Brigham and Women's Hospital, Boston, MA, US

Katie Dickerson
Massachusetts General Hospital & Brigham and Women's Hospital, Boston, MA, US

Amanda Doodlesack
Beth Israel Lahey Health Department of Emergency Medicine, Harvard Medical School, Boston, MA, US

Yves Duroseau
Department of Emergency Medicine, Donald & Barbara Zucker School of Medicine at Hofstra/Northwell, NY, US

Daniel Herbert-Cohen
Ronald O. Perelman Department of Emergency Medicine, NYU Grossman School of Medicine, New York City, NY, US

Sarah Fisher
The University of Texas MD Anderson Cancer Center, Houston, TX, US

Brian C. Geyer
Banner Estrella Medical Center, University of Arizona, Phoenix, AZ, US

Paul Ginart
Massachusetts General Hospital & Brigham and Women's Hospital, Boston, MA, US

Adam L. Gottula
University of Michigan, Department of Emergency Medicine and Department of Anesthesiology, Ann Arbor, MI, US

Carla Haack
The University of Texas MD Anderson Cancer Center, Houston, TX, US

Katrina Harper-Kirksey
Smidt Heart Institute, Cedars Sinai Medical Center, Los Angeles, CA, US

Gregory Hayward
Northwest Permanente Physicians and Surgeons, Portland, OR, US

Nadine Himelfarb
Department of Emergency Medicine, Alpert Medical School of Brown University, Providence, RI, US

Raymond Hou
Department of Emergency Medicine, Donald & Barbara Zucker School of Medicine at Hofstra/Northwell, NY, US

Jake Hoyne
Beth Israel Lahey Health Department of Emergency Medicine, Harvard Medical School, Boston, MA, US

Calvin E. Hwang
Department of Orthopaedic Surgery/Sports Medicine, Stanford University School of Medicine, Stanford, CA, US

Jacob D. Isserman
Department of Emergency Medicine, Medstar Washington Hospital Center, Georgetown University School of Medicine, Washington, DC, US

Imikomobong Ibia
Massachusetts General Hospital & Brigham and Women's Hospital, Boston, MA, US

Ermias Jirru
Department of Medicine, Texas A&M Health Science Center College of Medicine, Baylor University Medical Center, Dallas, TX, US

Joshua W. Joseph
Department of Emergency Medicine, Beth Israel Deaconess Medical Center, Harvard Medical School, Boston, MA, US

Elena Kapilovich
University of Rochester Medical Center, Rochester, NY, US

Feras Khan
Henrico Doctors' Hospital, HCA Virginia - ICC Healthcare, Richmond, VA, US

Joshua Kolikoff
Beth Israel Lahey Health Department of Emergency Medicine, Harvard Medical School, Boston, MA, US

Sothivin Lanh
Emory University School of Medicine, Atlanta, GA, US

Calvin Lee
Beth Israel Lahey Health Primary Care, Winchester, MA, US

Stefi Lee
Department of Medicine, Brigham and Women's Hospital, Boston, MA, US

Charles Lei
Department of Emergency Medicine, Vanderbilt University Medical Center, Nashville, TN, US

Elisabeth Lessenich
Emergency Department, Hospital Group Bretagne Sud, Lorient, France

Jai Madhok
Department of Anesthesiology, Perioperative and Pain Medicine, Stanford University School of Medicine, Stanford, CA, US

Brandon Maughan
Department of Emergency Medicine, Oregon Health & Science University, Portland, OR, US

Rmaah Memon
Massachusetts General Hospital & Brigham and Women's Hospital, Boston, MA, US

Payal Modi
University of Massachusetts Medical School, Worchester, MA, US

Shan Modi
University of Pittsburgh Medical Center, Pittsburgh, PA, US

Joel Moll
Virginia Commonwealth University School of Medicine, Richmond, VA, US

Kathryn Oskar
Massachusetts General Hospital & Brigham and Women's Hospital, Boston, MA, US

Nathaniel Oz
Emergency Medicine, Brown University, Providence, RI, US

Di Pan
Division of Pulmonary and Critical Care Medicine, Weill Cornell Medical College, New York, NY, US

Jeffrey Pepin
Department of Anesthesiology, Divison of Critical Care, Washington University School of Medicine, St. Louis, MO, US

Zubaid Rafique
Department of Emergency Medicine, Baylor College of Medicine, Houston, TX, US

Chanu Rhee
Brigham and Women's Hospital, Harvard Medical School, Boston, MA, US

Desiree Rogers
Emory Healthcare, Atlanta, GA, US

Daniel Rolston
Department of Emergency Medicine, Donald & Barbara Zucker School of Medicine at Hofstra/Northwell, NY, US

Steven C. Rougas
Department of Emergency Medicine, Alpert Medical School of Brown University, Providence, RI, US

John Rozehnal
Department of Emergency Medicine, Mount Sinai Health System, New York, NY, US

Benjamin Schnapp
BerbeeWalsh Department of Emergency Medicine, University of Wisconsin School of Medicine and Public Health, Madison, WI, US

Navdeep Sekhon
Department of Emergency Medicine, Baylor College of Medicine, Houston, TX, US

Aqsa Shakoor
NYU Langone Health, New York, NY, US

Christopher Shaw
Oregon Health and Science University Hospital, Portland, OR, US

Robert L. Sherwin
Detroit Medical Center, Wayne State University, Department of Emergency Medicine, Detroit, MI, US

Ashley Shreves
Department of Emergency Medicine and Department of Palliative Care, Ochsner Medical Center, New Orleans, LA, US

Jeffrey N. Siegelman
Emory University School of Medicine, Atlanta, GA, US

Liza Gonen Smith
Department of Emergency Medicine, UMass Chan Medical School, Worcester, MA, US and Department of Emergency Medicine, Tufts University School of Medicine, Boston, MA, US

Aaron Surrey
Department of Emergency Medicine, University of Michigan Medical School, Ann Abor, MI, US

Robert David Tidwell
Emergency Medicine, University of Arizona College of Medicine, Tuscon, AZ, US

Melissa Villars
Department of Emergency Medicine, Mount Sinai Health System, New York, NY, US

Danielle Walsh
NYU Langone Health, New York, NY, US

Matthew L. Wong
Department of Emergency Medicine, Beth Israel Deaconess Medical Center, Harvard Medical School, Boston, MA, US PC Clackamas, OR, US

Benjamin Zabar
Fire Department City of New York, New York, NY, US

Preface

Every day more and more critically ill patients arrive at the emergency department (ED) requiring both rapid stabilization and the full spectrum of treatments that are normally delivered in intensive care units (ICU). This book's content is unique in that it was written, researched, and edited by physicians with training in both emergency medicine and critical care from leading medical institutions throughout the world. It describes the initial steps in the stabilization of acutely ill patients, and also details the management if they continue to further decompensate. This book fills an important niche by providing concise, evidence-based summaries of key material and concepts. It will surely help practitioners at all levels of experience better manage their critically ill patients. Not only does it provide key points and details of well-established and evidence-based interventions in bullet point format, but it is easy to read and portable – ideal for the busy clinician at the bedside.

SECTION 1

General Critical Care

ANNETTE ILG

Shock

KENNETH R. L. BERNARD

Introduction

- **Shock** is a pathological state resulting from **inadequate delivery, increased demand, or poor utilization** of **metabolic substrates** (i.e., oxygen and glucose) which leads to **cellular dysfunction and cell death**. This leads to progressive acidosis, endothelial dysfunction, and inflammatory cascade that results in **end-organ injury**.
- Early in the course of shock, compensatory mechanisms may attempt to augment **cardiac output (CO)** and/or **systemic vascular resistance (SVR)** in an effort to improve tissue perfusion.
- Without treatment, those compensatory mechanisms are overwhelmed, leading to decompensated shock, multiorgan failure (MOF) and death.
- Shock can be conceptualized as a derangement of the three components of the circulatory system:
  - **the pump (the heart)**
  - **the fluid (intravascular volume)**
  - **the tank (blood vessels)**

Table 1.1 Categories of shock and differential diagnosis

Distributive	Severe inflammatory response syndrome (SIRS) and sepsis, neurogenic, anaphylaxis, adrenal insufficiency/Addisonian crisis, drug or toxin reaction, hepatic failure
Hypovolemic	Hemorrhage (trauma, GI bleed, ruptured AAA), GI losses (diarrhea, vomiting, fistula), insensible losses, third spacing (pancreatitis, burns)
Cardiogenic	Myocardial infarction, myocarditis, arrhythmia, cardiac contusion, valve dysfunction, thyrotoxicosis, end-stage cardiomyopathy
Obstructive	Tension pneumothorax, cardiac tamponade, pulmonary embolism (PE), constrictive pericarditis, abdominal compartment syndrome

- Conventional mechanisms of shock are in turn classified as:
  - **cardiogenic/obstructive** (pump failure or outflow obstruction)
  - **hypovolemic** (fluid/blood loss)
  - **distributive** (tank malfunction) (Table 1.1).
- Shock may be multifactorial, encompassing more than one category (e.g., septic shock can also result in septic cardiomyopathy, adding a cardiogenic component to the shock state).

Presentation

- Shock can present in a variety of ways and, especially in the **early stages**, patients may report **very subtle, vague** or **generalized symptoms** such as restlessness, anxiety, fatigue, or slight confusion. In these early stages, patients may be in **compensated shock**.
- Without rapid intervention, patients quickly progress to the critical state of **decompensated** or **refractory shock** and will appear **in distress, pale, diaphoretic, tachypneic, tachycardic, hypotensive, and encephalopathic**. At this point, **MOF** and **irreversible tissue injury** is likely present.
- Subtle clues from the patient's history – including past medical conditions, preceding events, and appearance – can help clinicians categorize a patient's shock state (Table 1.2).

Table 1.2 Presentations of shock

Category	History	Past medical history	Appearance
Distributive	Fever, chills, headache, dyspnea, wheezes, stridor, meningismus, malaise, myalgias, cough, dysuria, diarrhea	Immunocompromised, allergies, adrenal insufficiency	Diaphoretic, distressed, flushed, warm skin
Hypovolemic	Poor intake, excessive vomiting or diarrhea, GI bleed or evidence of trauma	Coagulopathy (acquired or inherited), upper or lower GI bleed	Rapid and weak pulse, cool skin, delayed capillary refill, tachypneic, dry mucous membranes, poor skin turgor
Cardiogenic	Syncope, dyspnea, chest pain, palpitations	Coronary artery disease, myocardial infarction, dysrhythmia, congestive heart failure	Tachypneic, jugular venous distension, new murmur, delayed capillary refill, wheezes, rales, cool skin, murmur
Obstructive	Trauma, dyspnea	COPD, connective tissue disorder, malignancy	JVD, muffled heart sounds, asymmetric breath sounds, tracheal deviation

- A commonly held misbelief that often leads to delayed treatment and poorer outcomes is that **shock necessitates hypotension**. Not all patients with shock are hypotensive, and not all hypotensive patients are in shock.

Diagnosis and Evaluation

Epidemiology

- In all comers, etiology of shock from most to least common:
  - Septic $>>>$ Hypovolemic $>$ Cardiogenic/Obstructive

Vital Signs

- No single vital sign in isolation is sufficient to diagnose or identify the possible etiology of shock.
  - Tachycardia, hypotension, tachypnea, fever should all raise suspicion for shock.
- Multiple **qSOFA (quick SOFA) criteria** predict poor outcomes and mortality in critically ill patients.
  - Altered mental status (GCS $<$ 15)
  - Respiratory rate $\geq$ 22
  - Systolic BP $\leq$ 100

Clinical Signs

- Shock should be suspected when patients present with a **constellation** of signs including **ill-appearance, confusion, tachycardia, tachypnea, hypotension, and poor urine output**.
- Warm extremities caused by vasodilation suggest distributive shock.
- Cold extremities caused by vasoconstriction suggest hypovolemic or cardiogenic shock.
- Jugular venous distention is usually present with cardiogenic/obstructive shock.
- A narrow pulse pressure (systolic BP - diastolic BP) suggests hypovolemic or cardiogenic shock.
- Dry mucous membranes, poor skin turgor, pallor, and low jugular venous pressure, are suggestive of hypovolemic shock.
- Tachypnea and Kussmaul breathing are often present with significant acidosis.
- Encephalopathy is often present with poor cerebral blood flow, renal failure, liver failure, hypoxia, and acidemia caused by shock states.
- Urticaria, facial or lip swelling, stridor and wheeze suggest anaphylaxis.

Laboratory Tests

- A complete blood count will identify leukocytosis or bandemia. It will also identify anemia (Hct $<$ 30% or Hgb $<$ 10). However, a normal value may be misleading in the acute stage of blood loss.

- Serum chemistry will assess renal function, hydration status, and detect electrolyte derangements.
- Cardiac biomarkers can identify myocardial injury.
- Lactate and base deficits may reflect tissue hypoperfusion (though are not specific for this); these markers are most useful as markers of effectiveness of a resuscitation.
- Arterial or venous blood gases will identify oxygenation or ventilation disorders and severe acid–base disturbances.
- Coagulation studies can identify coagulopathy associated with hemorrhagic shock and/or shock-related hepatic synthetic dysfunction.
- Urine or serum human chorionic gonadotropin (hCG) should be obtained in female patients of childbearing age for pregnancy.

Electrocardiogram (ECG)

- Key to identify and diagnose acute coronary syndromes, malignant arrhythmias, or electrolyte disturbances.

Imaging

- Chest radiography may show edema, effusion, consolidation, pneumothorax, or an enlarged mediastinum and cardiac silhouette.
- Pelvic radiography as a screening tool in trauma may reveal a clinically significant pelvic fracture as a source of hemodynamic instability.
- Point-of-care ultrasonography (US) is a cheap, readily available bedside tool that can be very useful in the identification and management of undifferentiated shock.
  - Several protocols such as: The Focused Assessment with Sonography in Trauma (FAST), Rapid Ultrasound in Shock and Hypotension (RUSH), and the Abdominal and Cardiac Evaluation (ACES) protocols were developed to assist in the bedside diagnosis of shock to identify organ dysfunction, fluid responsiveness, and potentially guide specific interventions e.g., pericardiocentesis. The standard anatomical views are described below:
    - Cardiac views can reveal pericardial effusion, assess ventricular function, and identify valvular dysfunction or tamponade physiology.

- Views of the inferior vena cava (IVC) can assess volume responsiveness.
- Lung views can quickly identify pneumothorax, consolidation, presence of pulmonary edema or effusions.
- Abdominal views will identify free fluid.
- Views of the thoracic and abdominal aorta can identify dissection or aneurysm.
- Lower extremity vascular ultrasound can identify deep venous thrombosis suggesting coagulopathy and increasing suspicion of pulmonary embolism.

- Computed tomography (CT) scanning may be helpful in identifying the source of **undifferentiated shock**, identifying etiologies such as pulmonary embolism, aortic dissection, intra-abdominal sepsis, or trauma.

Invasive Hemodynamic Monitoring

- An arterial line, central venous catheter, or pulmonary artery catheter can further differentiate shock by determining myriad hemodynamic variables.
- A central venous catheter placed into a central vein allows for the administration of vasoactive medications and measurements of a central venous pressure (CVP) and central venous oxygen saturation ($ScvO_2$).
- An arterial catheter allows for accurate, real-time measurement of pulse pressure and mean arterial pressure (MAP).
- A pulmonary artery catheter (PAC) is an invasive catheter placed in the pulmonary artery that allows a clinician to directly measure PCWP (surrogate for left atrial pressure), pulmonary artery pressure, CO, CI, and SVR. Together, these data can help differentiate the underlying shock profile (Table 1.3). However, the use of a PAC is controversial and rarely performed in the emergency department.

Critical Management

Brief Summary Checklist

- ☑ ABCs
- ☑ Fluids or blood as indicated

Table 1.3 Differentiating categories of shock

	CVP	ScvO$_2$	CI	SVR
Distributive	↓	↑ or ↓	↑ or ↓	↓
Hypovolemic	↓	↓	↓	↑
Cardiogenic	↑	↓	↓	↑
Obstructive	↑	↓	↓	↑

☑ Vasopressors if concern for shock and MAP < 65

☑ Labs

☑ Imaging (US, XR, or CT) to investigate cause

☑ Targeted interventions

Principles of shock management are **focused on restoring and maintaining adequate tissue perfusion** and providing specific interventions to **reverse the underlying cause**.

General approach with the ABCs (airway, breathing, circulation):

- **Airway**
  - ☐ Airway maneuvers such as repositioning, shoulder roll, and jaw thrust.
  - ☐ Airway adjuncts (nasal pharyngeal/oral airway), supraglottic device, or intubation to secure airway if necessary.
- **Breathing**
  - ☐ Administer supplementary oxygen with goal Sp02 > 90%.
  - ☐ Positive pressure support to decrease work of breathing and improve ventilation as necessary.
- **Circulation**
  - ☐ Assess peripheral pulses and telemetry heart rate: provide pacing, cardioversion, defibrillation as necessary.
  - ☐ Obtain peripheral IV (PIV), central IV, or interosseous (IO) access immediately.
  - ☐ If hypovolemic or hemorrhagic shock is suspected, administer **20–30 mL/kg of isotonic crystalloid** and/or blood products (as applicable).
  - ☐ Consider **inotrope/pressor** support for distributive or cardiogenic/obstructive shock or undifferentiated but volume-unresponsive patients (Table 1.4):

Table 1.4 Vasopressors and Inotropes

Agent	Receptors	Mechanism of action	Effective dose
Vasopressors			
Epinephrine	α, β	Vasoconstriction, inotropy, chronotropy	1–10 micrograms/minute
Norepinephrine	$α_1 > β_1$	Vasoconstriction, mild inotropy, and chronotropy	2–30 micrograms/minute
Phenylephrine	$α_1$	Vasoconstriction	10–300 micrograms/minute
Vasopressin	V_1	Vasoconstriction	0.01–0.04 U/minute
Dopamine	D, α, β	Inotropy and chronotropy at lower doses, vasoconstriction at high doses	2–20 micrograms/kg/minute
Inotropes			
Dobutamine	$β_1 = β_2$	Inotropy, chronotropy, vasodilation at high doses	2–20 micrograms/kg per minute
Milrinone	Phosphodiesterase-inhibitor	Inotropy, chronotropy, vasodilation at high doses	0.25–0.75 micrograms/kg per minute

○ Target a MAP ≥ 65 mmHg to ensure proper perfusion of the vital organs.
○ **Norepinephrine**, an inopressor, is the agent of choice in septic shock.
○ Vasopressin, a pure vasopressor, can be added in cases of refractory septic shock.
○ Dobutamine, an inodilator, is the preferred agent in decompensated heart failure in patients who are normotensive or mildly hypotensive. It may need to be given in conjunction with vasopressors due to its mechanism as an inodilator.
○ Epinephrine, an inopressor with higher inotropic properties than norepinephrine, may be preferable to dobutamine in suspected mixed septic and cardiogenic shock. Consider as primary vasopressor in pediatric cases.

- Consider systemic glucocorticoids (e.g., hydrocortisone 50 mg every 6 hours), in cases of shock not responding to volume resuscitation and/or multiple vasopressors.

Targeted Interventions

- Antibiotics and source control for suspected sepsis.
- Needle decompression or tube thoracostomy for tension pneumothorax.
- Pericardiocentesis for cardiac tamponade.
- Hemorrhage control, e.g., tourniquet, direct pressure, Resuscitative Endovascular Balloon Occlusion of the Aorta (REBOA), pelvic binder.
- Resuscitative thoracotomy in trauma.
- Systemic thrombolytics for suspected massive pulmonary embolism.
- Advanced cardiac life support (ACLS) protocols for unstable arrhythmia management.
- Revascularization procedure for acute coronary syndrome.
- IM Epinephrine, albuterol, antihistamines, glucocorticoid for anaphylaxis.
- Systemic glucocorticoid for suspected adrenal crisis.
- Antipyretics for fever control.

Assessing Resuscitation Efforts

- After the initial resuscitation phase or specific intervention is administered, it is important to continually assess resuscitation efforts and maintain a structured approach to reassessing the patient.
- Physiologic responses suggesting effective resuscitation are improvement in heart rate, urine output, mental status, and pulse pressure, though in isolation none of these is a reliable surrogate for volume status.
- Be aware that static markers such as CVP have limited validity and utility in assessing volume status.
- One well-validated method to assess the adequacy of volume resuscitation is the **passive leg raise maneuver.** With an arterial line in place to reliably indicate pulse pressure (SBP-DBP), transition the patient from head elevated 45°and legs flat to head flat and legs 45° elevated; an increase in pulse pressure of 10 mmHg with this change in position

suggests volume responsiveness and may indicate further crystalloid or blood product resuscitation as is applicable.

- Improving lactate and base deficit levels suggest appropriate response to resuscitation in hemorrhagic shock.

Sudden Deterioration

- Be alert for changes in mental status, loss of pulse oximetry plethysmographic waveform, or unobtainable blood pressures; suspect cardiovascular collapse, check peripheral and central pulses, and consider early inotrope/pressor support until stabilized.
- Refractory shock requiring multiple vasopressor agents should prompt a systematic consideration of causes:
  - **Correct?** Is the blood pressure correct? Are vasopressor agents correctly infusing?
  - **Control?** Is there a need for urgent septic or hemorrhagic source control?
  - **Confounders?** Are certain medications (e.g., sedatives) worsening hypotension?
  - **Cortisol?** Is the patient adrenally insufficient and requiring stress dose steroids?
  - **Cardiac?** Is there a missed cardiac etiology such as massive pericardial tamponade?
  - **Calcium?** Is the ionized calcium low (a frequent occurrence during hemorrhagic shock resuscitation)?
  - **Compartment?** Is there abdominal compartment syndrome causing IVC compression?

Special Circumstances

Pediatric Patients

- Recognition of shock is challenging due to variations in age-dependent vital signs, difficulty in assessing mental status, and the nonspecific symptoms such as irritability and poor feeding.

- Shock should be suspected in children presenting with delayed capillary refill, dry mucous membranes, absent tears, or somnolence, which suggest poor perfusion.
- Children have strong compensatory mechanisms and by the time they are hypotensive, may already be in an irreversible state of shock.

Pregnant Patients

- Management is made more difficult due to changes in maternal physiology and due to the considerations for both maternal and fetal wellbeing.
- Shock may be caused by pregnancy-specific diagnoses such as peripartum hemorrhage, pulmonary embolism, peripartum cardiomyopathy, or supine hypotensive syndrome.
- Usual monitoring modalities are still employed in addition to cardiotocographic monitoring of the fetus.
- The first resuscitative maneuver, while securing the ABCs, is to have the patient in the **left lateral decubitus position**. This alleviates pressure on the IVC, allowing increased venous return to the heart.

Geriatric Patients

- Elderly patients experience significantly more morbidity and mortality from all causes of shock due to their limited ability to augment cardiac output and maintain vascular tone.
- They often have multiple comorbidities that distort the diagnosis and management of shock.
- Due to numerous comorbidities, they are also very high risk for **polypharmacy:** on multiple hemodynamically significant medications (e.g., beta blockers, calcium channel blockers, etc.). Always consider these medications as a cause for their shock, either accidental overdose or accumulation of renally cleared medications due to acute kidney injury.

BIBLIOGRAPHY

Vincent J-L, & De Backer D. Circulatory shock. *New Engl J Med* 2013;369(18):1726–1734.

De Backer D, Biston P, Devriendt J, et al. Comparison of dopamine and norepinephrine in the treatment of shock. *New Engl J Med* 2010;362(9):779–789.

Gamper G, Havel C, Arrich J, et al. Vasopressors for hypotensive shock. *Cochrane Database Syst Rev* 2016;2.

Rhodes, A, Evans L, Alhazzani W, et al. Surviving sepsis campaign: International guidelines for management of sepsis and septic shock: 2016. *Intensive Care Med* 2017;43(3):304–377.

2

Airway Management

AMANDA DOODLESACK

Chapter 2:
Airway Management

  Key to Airway Success

Recognize failure early and implement contingency plan

Consider NIV

- Can provide 100% FiO_2, PEEP, and pressure support.
- Appropriate for patients who can maintain a patent airway.
- Avoids risk associated with intubation.

Consider Intubation

- Expected hemodynamic deterioration.
- Need to decrease patient's metabolic demand (i.e., work of breathing).
- Secures patent airway.

 NIV

 Intubation

Remember This

- Includes use of CPAP/BiPAP.
- Can drastically increase oxygenation in the appropriate patient.

Remember This

- Position to optimize glottis view.
- Perform sufficient pre-oxygenation.
- Use a bougie introducer or external laryngeal manipulation if necessary.
- Confirm placement with end tidal capnography.

RSI Drugs

Sedatives
Consider lower sedative doses in the hemodynamically unstable patient.

- Etomidate (0.3 mg/kg)
- Ketamine (1.5–2 mg/kg)
- Propofol (1.5–2 mg/kg)
- Midazolam (0.3 mg/kg)

Paralytics

- Succinylcholine (1.5–2 mg/kg)
- Rocuronium (1.2 mg/kg)

Difficult Airways and Unique Circumstances

- ❗ Have a double setup ready.
- ❗ Sedative and paralytic create optimal conditions.
- ❗ Beware of hemodynamic collapse; have a pressor drip ready.

Introduction

- Airway management is one of the core fundamental skills of the emergency medicine and critical care physician.
- Airway management is time-critical and can literally mean the difference between life and death.
- Airway management encompasses the overlapping management of oxygenation, ventilation, and airway protection.

Airway Principles

See Table 2.1.

- Top priorities are planning, backup planning, recognizing failure, and decision-making.
- Staying calm permits proper decision-making, while undue haste can be detrimental.
- Each aspect of airway management is modular. Components can be mixed as needed (e.g., video laryngoscopy with a bougie; awake intubation after preoxygenation with noninvasive ventilation).

Recognizing Failure

See Figure 2.1.

- When first-line techniques fail to result in intubation, early identification of failure is paramount.
- If unsuccessful, laryngoscopy should be abandoned and oxygen restored with mask ventilation.

Table 2.1 Principles for safe emergency airway management

Judicious use of rapid sequence intubation (RSI) versus awake technique
Back-up planning
Prioritization of oxygenation
Early recognition of failure
Early use of surgical technique if necessary
Avoidance of ED intubation if necessary

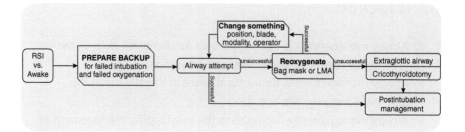

Figure 2.1

Adapted from Strayer R. Emergency Department Intubation Checklist v13. 2012. © Reuben Strayer & emupdates.com, used with permission. Available from: http://emupdates.com/2012/07/08/emergency-department-intubation-checklist-v13/ [last accessed February 14, 2023].

- Extraglottic airways (EGA) can be placed quickly and may provide better ventilation than bag-mask ventilation.
- If an intubation attempt fails *and* reoxygenation fails (despite use of an EGA), this is known as a **"can't intubate, can't oxygenate" scenario** and a cricothyrotomy must be performed immediately.
- Failure to recognize a "can't intubate, can't oxygenate" scenario will result in the patient's death.

Decision to Intubate

See Table 2.2.

Many factors at play must be balanced, including:

- Early management of a sick patient needing hemodynamic resuscitation.
- Potential danger of paralyzing a patient (e.g., difficult airways).
- Limited clinical evaluation of an intubated patient.
- Anticipated clinical course.

Noninvasive Ventilation

- In patients protecting their airway, noninvasive ventilation (NIV) may be appropriate.
- Many patients will improve dramatically with NIV and avoid intubation.

Table 2.2 Indications for intubation

Indication	Rationale	Comments
Ventilation	The patient is not safely breathing on their own	Circumstances make it difficult to match the patient's inherent drive (e.g., salicylate toxicity)
Oxygenation	Intubation allows high FiO_2 and positive end-expiratory pressure protection	Noninvasive ventilation may suffice for many patients
Protection	Alterations in mental status may blunt protective airway reflexes, and conditions such as vomiting may result in aspiration	Obstructive processes (e.g., expanding hematoma) may threaten tracheal patency
Expected course	A presently stable patient may be expected to deteriorate	Early intubation is often safer prior to deterioration
Metabolic demand	Decrease work of breathing in critically ill patients (e.g., severe sepsis)	Oxygen consumption from respiration alone can rise from baseline of 5% to 50%

- NIV provides:
  - Up to 100% FiO_2.
  - Pressure-support, decreasing the work of breathing.
  - PEEP, overcoming shunt physiology (e.g., severe pneumonia, acute pulmonary edema).
- Although alteration in mental status is a traditional relative contraindication to NIV, critically ill emergency department (ED) patients can be closely monitored on NIV by experienced airway operators.
- NIV can be used to achieve two simultaneous goals:
  - It can potentially improve the patient sufficiently to obviate the need for intubation.
  - Barring sufficient improvement, NIV will optimize preoxygenation if intubation is necessary.

Oxygenation

- Oxygenation is the primary concern in airway management.
- As hemoglobin and oxygen bind cooperatively, desaturation is slow above SpO_2 90%.

- Below 90%, hemoglobin molecules quickly lose bound oxygen, and critical hypoxia can occur in seconds.
- Due to the technical aspects of pulse oximetry, there is the phenomenon of **pulse oximeter lag** – in which the reported SpO_2 may lag up to 2 minutes behind the actual SpO_2. Therefore, a reading in the 80–90% range may indicate that the actual SpO_2 is much lower.
- Laryngoscopy should be paused when SpO_2 reads 90% in order for the patient to be reoxygenated.

Laryngoscopy and Intubation

- The following steps are necessary to place an endotracheal tube (or an EGA):
  - Positioning
  - Oxygenation
  - Equipment and discussion of back-up plan
  - Medication administration
  - Laryngoscopy and intubation (or EGA placement)
  - Postintubation management

Positioning

- Proper positioning is essential for laryngoscopy.
- The same positioning principles will aid in preoxygenation and mask ventilation.
- Proper positioning lifts the anterior pharyngeal structures off the posterior pharynx and optimizes glottis view.
- Prior to direct laryngoscopy, place the patient in the **ear-to-sternal-notch position:** the patient's head should be elevated for the external auditory meatus to be at the same level as the manubrium, in a plane parallel to the ceiling (Figure 2.2a).
- Positioning for video laryngoscopy (VL):
  - VL with conventional blades: positioning is unchanged.

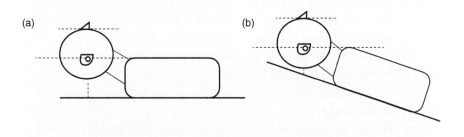

Figure 2.2 Patient positioning.

- ○ VL with an angulated blade: completely neutral head and neck position, with the head flat on the bed and the face plane parallel to the ceiling.
- ○ Note that VL hand positioning and technique could be different from traditional direct laryngoscopy (e.g., Glidescope)
- ○ Most patients (but especially the obese, volume overloaded, or those at risk for vomiting) will benefit from elevating the head of the bed to 30 degrees while maintaining the same positioning principles (Figure 2.2b).

Preoxygenation

- The goal of **preoxygenation** is not merely to achieve an SpO_2 of 100%, but also to perform **denitrogenation**, i.e., completely filling the lungs with oxygen to act as an oxygen reservoir during laryngoscopy.
- Preoxygenate with high-flow oxygen, such as a non-rebreather mask (NRB), set to 15 liters per minute or higher, for at least 3 minutes.
- If hypoxemia persists despite high-flow oxygen, the patient is likely shunting and will likely benefit from PEEP delivered via NIV prior to intubation.
- Obtunded hypoxemic patients, if still ventilating on their own, may be safer to ventilate with NIV under close supervision than with bag-mask ventilation.

- In the apneic patient, bag-mask ventilation (BMV) should be performed.
  - Two-operator technique will provide a better mask seal as one operator can use both hands to secure the mask to the patient's face.
  - Nasal trumpets and oral airways, if tolerated, can be invaluable in maintaining pharyngeal patency.
  - Use slow, smooth, controlled breaths of only half the volume of a standard bag.
  - Patients obtunded due to severe metabolic acidosis will require a much faster respiratory rate, and must be ventilated during the apneic period to avoid cardiac arrest.
  - Most bags accept a **PEEP valve**, which should always be used when available to help address against shunt physiology and maintain lung recruitment.
  - Ventilators can be attached to masks, allowing for control of tidal volumes, respiratory rate, and PEEP if needed.
- Fully obtunded and apneic patients oxygenate better with the rapid placement of an EGA.

Apneic Oxygenation

- The preoxygenation device (NRB or NIV) should be left in place during the apneic period following induction.
- During laryngoscopy, a nasal cannula set to 15 LPM or a high-flow nasal cannula device may be used to augment oxygenation during laryngoscopy.
- If there are insufficient oxygen wall adaptors to provide three sources of oxygen (bag-mask, NRB, and nasal cannula), place a portable oxygen tank under the bed to provide a third source.

Extraglottic Airways

- Numerous EGA options exist, primarily laryngeal tubes (mainly used in the pre-hospital setting) and laryngeal masks.
- EGA are typically used as rescue devices when it is difficult to provide BMV and are critical in addressing hypoxemia between intubation attempts that does not respond to BMV.

- Laryngeal masks do not fully "secure" the airway, as vomit may dislodge them.
- Many second-generation laryngeal masks permit intubation through the mask.

Laryngoscopy

- Principles of laryngoscopy are identical for direct and video laryngoscopy, with the exception of different positioning.
  - ○ Suction should be available under the patient's right shoulder. Two or more Yankauer suction tips may be necessary if blood, vomit, or copious secretions are expected.
  - ○ Various devices exist for video laryngoscopy.
    - ▪ Many devices use traditional curved blades and may be used either with the video monitor or for direct laryngoscopy.
    - ▪ Devices with angulated or indirect blades are operated similarly but do not allow for direct visualization.
    - ▪ Angulated blades will often insert too far; if the glottis cannot be seen, withdraw slowly.
    - ▪ Lifting the handle straight toward the ceiling may also improve the view.
    - ▪ Video devices improve views but may be defeated by blood, mucus, or vomit.
    - ▪ Tube delivery may be more difficult with angulated blades as the angle of approach to the trachea is steeper.
      - ☐ Once a view of the glottis is obtained, it can be helpful to withdraw the video laryngoscope slightly to give yourself more space to manipulate the tube into the trachea; think of this colloquially as a **"cheap seats view"**
  - ○ Stylets vastly improve tube control and delivery and should be shaped straight to the cuff, then angled to 35 degrees.
  - ○ Deliver the tube from the side (3-o'clock) to ensure the tube will not obscure the glottic view.
  - ○ Glottic view is categorized by the **Cormack-Lehane system** (Figure 2.3)
    - ▪ Grade I: the entire glottis opening is visualized.
    - ▪ Grade II: only the posterior aspect of the glottis opening is visualized.
    - ▪ Grade III: only the tip of the epiglottis is visualized.
    - ▪ Grade IV: only the soft palate is visualized.

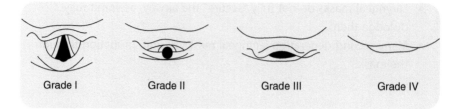

Figure 2.3 Cormack-Lehane glottic view.

- A partial glottic (Grade 2) view is sufficient if the tube can be directed above the posterior cartilages.
- Tube delivery with angulated VL is often facilitated with malleable stylets shaped similarly to the blade, or with proprietary stylets.

Bimanual Laryngoscopy

- Bimanual laryngoscopy is essential to optimizing difficult views and includes both **external laryngeal manipulation (ELM)** and **head mobilization**.
- Any glottic view other than a perfect grade 1 will benefit from bimanual laryngoscopy.
- ELM involves using the right hand to manipulate the external larynx in multiple different directions until the glottic view is improved.
- Head mobilization is performed by using the right hand to mobilize the head by lifting the occiput upward.
- If the view is improved, ask an assistant to help maintain the position of the larynx or head and place the endotracheal tube with your right hand.
- ELM is not cricoid pressure; cricoid pressure occludes the esophagus to avoid passive regurgitation. It is unlikely to work and may worsen the glottic view.

Bougie Introducer

- The bougie introducer, also known as an Eschmann stylet, is a valuable adjunct in poor glottic views.
- The bougie is threaded through the glottis and the tube is delivered "over the wire."

- Upon advancement of the bougie, the trachea's cartilaginous rings can often be felt (although not always).
- If difficulty passing the bougie into the glottic opening is encountered, rotate the bougie counterclockwise 90°.

Confirmation of Placement

- Traditional indicators such as chest rise, auscultation, humidity (fogging) in the tube, chest radiography, and SpO_2 are helpful but unreliable.
- The preferred method for confirmation of endotracheal intubation is capnography.
- Colorimetric capnography: disposable litmus-paper devices that change color from purple to yellow.
  - Only accurate *if color change persists over 6 breaths*.
  - Inaccurate if the airway is soiled by vomit.
- Waveform capnography is nearly 100% accurate; end-tidal capnography is near gold-standard.
- Capnography should also be used to confirm ventilation with EGA.

Rapid Sequence Intubation

- Rapid sequence intubation (RSI) is the rapid administration of an induction and paralytic agent.
- The overwhelming majority of ED intubations use RSI.
- Adequate preoxygenation is a prerequisite for safe RSI.
- One goal of RSI is to avoid positive-pressure ventilation during the apneic period to minimize the risk of vomiting due to gastric insufflation (*Remember: most ED patients are not NPO*).
- RSI has been proven to be safe and effective as paralysis optimizes intubating conditions.

Rapid Sequence Intubation Medications

See Table 2.3.

- The cornerstone of RSI is the simultaneous use of a potent sedative and fast-acting paralytic.

Table 2.3 Rapid sequence intubation medications

Sedative agents	Dose	Properties
Etomidate	0.3 mg/kg	Linked to adrenal suppression of unclear clinical importance
Ketamine	1.5–2 mg/kg	Releases endogenous catecholamines; bronchodilator
Propofol	1.5–2 mg/kg	Antiepileptic; bronchodilator
Midazolam	0.3 mg/kg	Antiepileptic
Paralytic agents	**Dose**	**Properties**
Succinylcholine	1.5–2 mg/kg	May precipitate hyperkalemia in vulnerable patients (e.g., neuromuscular disorders)
Rocuronium	1.2 mg/kg	Time of onset and intubating conditions identical to succinylcholine if dosed 1.2 mg/kg

- Every induction agent (including ketamine) will cause hypotension when used at full dose in shocked patients due to the phenomenon of **sympatholysis** (i.e., blunting of endogenous catecholamines by high-dose sedation).
- Earlier concerns about use of ketamine in elevated intracranial pressure are unfounded.
- Onset of paralysis is 30–45 seconds with either succinylcholine or appropriately dosed rocuronium ($\geq$ 1.2 mg/kg)
- Succinylcholine is widely used but may precipitate hyperkalemia. At-risk populations include:
  - Neuromuscular disorders (acquired and congenital).
  - Sepsis, burns (> *24 hrs old*), and crush injuries (generally only vulnerable > 3 days after onset).
  - Preexisting hyperkalemia (dialysis/renal failure patients).
- Traditionally, succinylcholine was favored over rocuronium due to its short duration of action (8–10 minutes) and the thought that a difficult airway will be salvaged by the patient regaining spontaneous breathing; this point is moot and dogmatic for several reasons:
  - Sugammadex is potentially available as a reversal agent for rocuronium.

- ○ Most patients in "can't intubate, can't ventilate" situations will critically desaturate well prior to return of muscle tone.
- ○ Most difficult airways will only become *more difficult* as a patient spontaneously breathes against positive pressure breaths and a true "can't intubate, can't oxygenate" is most appropriately managed by an emergent cricothyroidotomy.

Assessing Airway Difficulty

See Table 2.4.

- Predicting the difficult airway is – unto itself – difficult.
- The gestalt of an experienced physician is likely equal to or superior to specific rules, and is usually informed by similar elements.
- Features that potentially increase intubation difficulty include:
  - ○ Obesity
  - ○ Short neck
  - ○ Decreased neck mobility
  - ○ Small mouth opening
  - ○ Recessed chin
- Most patients are safe for RSI.
- Some patients with predicted difficult airways may be too unstable for an awake intubation; they will benefit from a **double setup:**
  - ○ Fully prepared for cricothyroidotomy.
  - ○ Equipment open at the bedside.
  - ○ Cricothyroid membrane marked.
  - ○ Neck sterilized.

Table 2.4 Technique for increasing levels of risk

Risk scale	Technique	Example
Low risk	RSI	Most patients
Possible difficulty, stable	Awake	Obese patient with short neck
Possible difficulty, unstable	Double setup	Expanding neck hematoma
Likely difficulty, stable	OR	Ludwig's angina, epiglottitis

- ○ While one physician is ready to immediately perform the surgical airway if needed, a separate physician takes a single attempt at RSI.
- A double setup will help overcome the cognitive burden of identifying the need for surgical airway if necessary.
- If time allows, some patients may benefit from techniques not possible in the ED and should be considered for definitive control in the operating room (OR).
- Sedative-only intubation, while seemingly attractive, is potentially dangerous.
  - ○ Intubating without paralysis means conditions are not optimized.
  - ○ The dose of sedative often necessary for the patient to tolerate laryngoscopy will obliterate respiratory drive, eliminating the benefit of avoiding paralysis.
  - ○ Sedation alone is unlikely to diminish airway reflexes; the risk of vomiting and aspiration caused by laryngoscopy is high.
  - ○ Accordingly, all ED patients undergoing intubation should receive sedation and either paralytics or **topicalization.**

Special Circumstances

Awake Intubatiation

- Awake intubation refers to the use of topical anesthetic instead of paralytic agents to facilitate intubation, while maintaining the patient's respiratory drive and protective airway reflexes.
- "Awake intubation" is a misnomer, as patients require some level of sedation.
- While maintaining the patient's respiratory drive confers a clear level of safety, without paralysis, intubating conditions are not optimized.
- Most ED intubations utilize RSI, so comfort and skill with awake technique may be limited.
- Awake attempt takes minimal amount of time, and if unsuccessful, can be easily converted to RSI.
- Ketamine, ketofol, or dexmedetomidine are optimal agents as they maintain respiratory drive and airway reflexes.
- Video laryngoscopy should be used if available, as the intubating conditions will not be optimized via paralysis.

Hemodynamically Unstable Intubation

- Both induction and mechanical ventilation may cause hypotension even in hemodynamically stable patients; these effects are amplified in shocked patients.
- The underlying cause of shock should be addressed to the extent possible prior to intubation (e.g., blood product resuscitation for hemorrhagic shock).
- For any hemodynamically tenuous intubation, have a vasopressor drip ready if not running prior to induction.
- The **sympatholysis** caused by even normal doses of induction agents can lead to postintubation hemodynamic collapse or death.
- For intubating patients in shock, consider using reduced (e.g., 0.5–0.75 mg/kg) dose of ketamine; this should mitigate awareness without fully blunting the sympathetic drive. Provide more generous sedation after intubation as able.
- Mechanical ventilation unto itself entails a shift from physiological negative-pressure ventilation to positive-pressure ventilation in turn decreasing preload; anticipate this effect to increase as patients are ventilated with higher levels of **positive-end-expiratory-pressure (PEEP)**

Metabolic Acidosis Intubation

- While intubation is often thought as a strategy to improve respiratory compensation for a metabolic acidosis, it can be quite risky for two major reasons:
  - The ventilator (and endotracheal tube) may often not compensate as well as a spontaneously breathing patient.
  - The apneic period often associated with induction can significantly lower pH.
- For these acidotic patients, assess whether intubation can be avoided or is truly necessary (e.g., poor mental status, respiratory failure).
- Ventilate (gently) during the apneic period at a rate similar to the patient's neural ventilatory rate prior to paralysis.
- After intubation, set the ventilator.

Delayed Sequence Intubation

- Hypoxemic patients may not tolerate preoxygenation due to delirium or agitation.
- Under close monitoring, these patients may benefit from delayed sequence intubation: the use of a respiratory-sparing sedative to allow for proper preoxygenation, followed by paralysis and intubation.
- Sedative dosing should be adjusted to maintain the patient's airway reflexes and respiratory drive.
- Ketamine is the first-line agent for delayed sequence intubation (DSI) as it will not blunt airway reflexes or respiratory drive.

BIBLIOGRAPHY

Aguilar SA, Davis DP. Latency of pulse oximetry signal with use of digital probes associated with inappropriate extubation during prehospital rapid sequence intubation in head injury patients: Case examples. *J Emerg Med* 2012;42:424–428.

Benumof JL, Dagg R, Benumof R. Critical hemoglobin desaturation will occur before return to an unparalyzed state following 1 mg/kg intravenous succinylcholine. *Anesthesiology* 1997;87:979–982.

Levitan RM, Everett WW, Ochroch EA. Limitations of difficult airway prediction in patients intubated in the emergency department. *Ann Emerg Med* 2004;44:307–313.

Weingart SD. Preoxygenation, reoxygenation, and delayed sequence intubation in the emergency department. *J Emerg Med* 2011;40:661–667.

Weingart SD, Levitan RM. Preoxygenation and prevention of desaturation during emergency airway management. *Ann Emerg Med* 2012;59:165–175.

3

Mechanical Ventilation

JAKE HOYNE AND JOSHUA KOLIKOF

Introduction

- Mechanical ventilation is the utilization of positive pressure to ventilate a patient via an endotracheal tube or tracheostomy tube.
- Mechanical ventilation drastically alters normal respiratory physiology. We normally breathe by generating negative pressure in the thoracic cavity, while mechanical ventilation uses positive pressure to drive the flow of gas into the lungs.
- If mechanical ventilation is done inappropriately, morbidity and mortality can dramatically increase because of the development of certain complications:
  - **Ventilator-induced lung injury (VILI):**
    - Lung disease does not take place uniformly throughout the lungs.
    - Tidal volumes preferentially inflate healthy lung tissue. Therefore, high tidal volumes can cause stress to the alveolar–capillary interface of the normal lungs.
    - This injury can cause and worsen outcomes in patients with acute respiratory distress syndrome (ARDS)
    - **Barotrauma** occurs as a result of excessive airway pressures and can result in pneumothorax, pneumomediastinum, or alveolar rupture.

- **Volutrauma** occurs as a result of high tidal volumes.
- **Atelectrauma** occurs with the continuous closing and reopening of alveoli.
  - **Ventilator-associated pneumonia (VAP):**
    - VAP is defined as a pneumonia that develops more than 48 hours following the initiation of mechanical ventilation.
    - The endotracheal tube bypasses many of the body's defenses against pathogens and acts as a direct conduit for bacteria into the lungs.

Definitions

- **Inspiration:** Gas flows into the lungs.
- **Expiration:** Ventilator flow is stopped to allow gas to escape from the lungs.
- **Triggering:** Initiation of a breath.
  - Can be machine-initiated after a set amount of time has elapsed since the last breath.
  - Can be patient-initiated in response to a reduction of airway pressure below a preset threshold, or in response to the detection of inspiratory flow.
- **Limit:** A parameter that is used to control inspiration. Ventilation can be either volume- or pressure-limited.
- **Cycling:** Switching from inspiration to expiration.
  - Can occur because a certain amount of time has passed, a preset volume has been delivered, or a preset decrease in flow rate has occurred.
- **Minute ventilation (V_E)** = Tidal volume (V_t) × Respiratory rate (RR).

Common Ventilator Settings

- **Fraction of inspired oxygen (FiO_2):** The percentage of oxygen being delivered to the patient. It ranges between 21% and 100%.
- **Positive end-expiratory pressure (PEEP):** Positive airway pressure applied by the ventilator at the end of expiration. PEEP prevents alveolar collapse at the end of expiration and "recruits" alveoli to participate in respiration, thereby improving gas exchange.
- **Respiratory rate (RR):** Number of breaths delivered per minute.
- **Tidal volume (V_t):** Volume in mL delivered in a single breath.
- **Inspiratory flow rate (IFR):** The rate of air entry in L/minute during inspiration.

- **Inspiratory pressure**: Set pressure used to inflate the lungs during inspiration.
- **Inspiratory time (T_i)**: The time over which the V_t is delivered.
- **I:E ratio**: The ratio of inspiratory time to expiratory time. A normal I:E ratio is 1:2 to 1:3. Increasing the I:E ratio can improve oxygenation by increasing the mean airway pressure. A longer inspiration will result in a longer period of high pressure, thus increasing the mean airway pressure over the entire respiratory cycle.

Airway Pressures

- **Peak Inspiratory Pressure (PIP):** Sum of all inspiratory pressures generated in the alveoli, bronchi, endotracheal tube, and ventilator tubing; reflects *resistance* in the airways; automatically measured by ventilator.
- **Plateau Pressure (P_{plat}):** Pressure affecting small airways & alveoli, reflects *compliance* (change in volume divided by change in pressure) of lung and chest wall; measured manually by performing end-inspiratory hold. **This is the primary determinant of VILI.**

Common Modes of Ventilation

See Table 3.1.

- **Assist volume control**: Commonly referred to just as Assist Control **(AC)**. This is a volume-cycled mode of ventilation that delivers the same V_t during every breath. Breaths can be triggered by the patient or the machine. There is a set RR, FiO_2, PEEP and V_t but the patient can breathe over the set RR. If the patient does not initiate a breath after a set time, the ventilator will initiate the breath. All patient-triggered breaths are assisted by the ventilator to produce the set V_t. This is commonly used and the **mode of choice in the ED**. Pitfalls include the inability to control for pressure which can lead to barotrauma.
- **Controlled mandatory ventilation (CMV)**: The ventilator controls all aspects of ventilation. A set RR and V_t are delivered by the ventilator. This mode is usually a volume-controlled mode but can also be a pressure-controlled mode. **The patient has no ability to initiate breaths**, breathe over the set RR, or influence the characteristics of the breath. This mode is mostly **used in heavily sedated and paralyzed patients** in the operating room.

Table 3.1 Common ventilator modes

Mode	Trigger	Breaths	Limit	Cycle	Variables set
CMV	Ventilator (time)	Mandatory	Volume	Ventilator (volume)	V_t, RR, IFR, FiO_2, PEEP
AC	Ventilator (time) and/or patient (flow or pressure)	Mandatory or assisted	Volume	Ventilator (volume)	V_t, RR, IFR, FiO_2, PEEP
SIMV	Ventilator (time) and/or patient (flow or pressure)	Mandatory or assisted; breaths above set RR are spontaneous and unassisted (unless PS used)	Volume, pressure	Ventilator (volume), breaths above set RR are patient cycled (flow)	V_t, RR, FiO_2, PEEP, PS (can be used for breaths above set RR)
PC	Ventilator (time) and/or patient (flow or pressure)	Mandatory or assisted	Pressure	Ventilator (time)	Inspiratory pressure, RR, T_i, FiO_2, PEEP
PS	Patient (flow or pressure)	Assisted by pressure support	Pressure	Patient (flow)	PS, PEEP

- **Pressure control (PC)**: PC is an assist control mode of ventilation in which the desired inspiratory pressure is set. This mode is similar to assist volume control but instead of a set V_t being delivered, a set pressure is delivered. Breaths can be triggered by the machine or the patient. In this mode, the RR and T_i are set which will determine the I:E ratio. Each breath is assisted by the machine and the set pressure is delivered. An advantage of this mode is the pressure limit can be set to **limit barotrauma** and this may improve patient ventilator synchrony. A disadvantage of this mode is that V_t **will vary with each breath** based on the patient's thoracic compliance, airway resistance, and patient effort. Therefore, a set minute ventilation will not be guaranteed.
- **Pressure support (PS)**: This mode of ventilation provides partial support. The patient is spontaneously breathing and the ventilator will augment each breath with a set inspiratory pressure. The patient sets his or her own respiratory rate and V_t. This mode necessitates an intact ventilatory drive and is **commonly used as patients improve**.
- **Synchronized intermittent mandatory ventilation (SIMV)**: SIMV represents a **combination of breathing types**. It is a mix of ventilator triggered and controlled breaths and the patient's spontaneously triggered and controlled breaths. If the patient is breathing **below the set RR**, then the **breaths are machine assisted**. If the patient is breathing **above the set RR**, then the **patient's breaths are spontaneous and unassisted**. Unlike AC, there is no guarantee of a set V_t for every breath because the V_t for the unassisted breaths depends on the patient's respiratory effort and lung mechanics. Therefore, this is **not a good initial mode when respiratory muscles are fatigued**.

Strategies of Ventilation

Outlined below are two ventilation strategies that can be used in critically ill patients in the emergency department. Both strategies utilize the assist control (AC) volume cycled mode of ventilation.

Lung Protective Strategy

See Figure 3.1.

- This strategy is designed for patients with or at risk for ARDS. The majority of patients fit into this category. Therefore, this strategy should be employed on **most critically ill patients** who are on a ventilator.
- This ventilation strategy is derived from the ARDSNet study and has been shown to **decrease mortality** in patients with ALI/ARDS by avoiding over-distension of the alveoli and preventing atelectrauma and other forms of VILI.
- *ARDSNet Protocol:*
  - ○ "Low" physiological tidal volumes (6 mL/kg of ideal body weight).
  - ○ Maintain a plateau pressure (P_{plat}) <30 cm H_2O.
  - ○ Oxygenation is maintained with protocol driven PEEP and FiO_2 values.

LUNG PROTECTIVE STRATEGY

- **Calculate** the predicted body weight (**PBW**):
  - ○ Males = 50 + 2.3 [height(in) − 60]
  - ○ Females = 45.5 + 2.3 [height(in) − 60]
- Select **Assist Control** Mode
- Set initial **Vt to 6 mL/kg** PBW
- Set initial **RR to 18** and **adjust** to target **pH > 7.30** (keep RR < 35)
- Adjust Vt and RR to achieve pH and plateau pressure goals
- Set inspiratory flow rate above patient demand (usually 60–80 L/min)
- **PLATEAU PRESSURE GOAL: ≤30 cm H_2O**
  - ○ Check Pplat (0.5–1 second inspiratory pause), SpO2, RR, Vt, and pH (if available) at least every 4 hours and after any change in PEEP and Vt.
  - ○ If P_{plat} > 30: Decrease Vt by 1 mL/kg steps (minimum = 4 mL/kg).
  - ○ If P_{plat} < 25 and Vt < 6 mL/kg: Increase Vt by 1 mL/kg until Pplat > 25 or Vt = 6 mL/kg.
  - ○ If P_{plat} < 30 and **breath stacking** or **dyssynchrony** occurs: may increase Vt in 1 mL/kg increments (maximum = 8 mL/kg) if Pplat remains < 30

- **OXYGENATION GOAL: SpO2 92–96%**
  - ○ Use incremental FiO_2/PEEP combinations such as shown below to achieve goal.

FiO₂	0.3	0.4	0.4	0.5	0.5	0.6	0.7	0.7	0.7	0.8	0.9	0.9	0.9	1.0	1.0	1.0
PEEP	5	5	8	8	10	10	10	12	14	14	14	16	18	20	22	24

Figure 3.1 Ventilator settings for lung protective strategy.

(Courtesy of Scott D. Weingart, MD.)

Obstructive Strategy

See Figure 3.2.

- This strategy is designed for patients with obstructive lung disease (i.e., **asthma or COPD**) whose airways are constricted and therefore require a longer time to fully exhale.
- They also require respiratory support during inspiration due to fatigued respiratory muscles.
- The basis of this strategy is to **decrease the RR** and adjust the IFR to achieve a **prolonged I:E ratio** (1:4 to 1:5). This will allow the patient sufficient time to fully exhale and **avoid auto-PEEP** or breath stacking.
- Breath stacking is the phenomenon of delivering another breath before the lungs have completely exhaled. This results in an increased intrathoracic pressure and can cause a pneumothorax or hemodynamic instability due to decreased venous return.
- Decreasing the respiratory rate results in retention of CO_2 which may lead to a respiratory acidosis; this is tolerated to a certain extent ($PaCO_2$ < 85, pH > 7.2) — known as **permissive hypercapnia**.

OBSTRUCTIVE STRATEGY

- Select **Assist Control** Mode
- Set initial **Vt to 6–8 mL/kg** PBW
- Set initial **RR to 10** and adjust to achieve **I:E ratio of 1:5**
- Set inspiratory flow rate to 80 L/min
- Set **PEEP to 5**
- Titrate FiO_2 to maintain SpO_2 > 88–90%

PLATEAU PRESSURE GOAL: ≤ 30 cm H_2O
 CHECK EXPIRATORY FLOW CURVE:

- Make sure the expiratory flow reaches zero before the next breath is initiated to avoid breath stacking.

Figure 3.2 Ventilator settings for obstructive strategy.

(Courtesy of Scott D. Weingart, MD.)

Sudden Deterioration

- **Use the mnemonic DOPES on patients that are deteriorating while on the ventilator:**

- **D**islodgement of tubes:
  - ○ Check the ET tube position by direct visualization or by connecting it to quantitative EtCO$_2$ capnography and looking for a loss of waveform.
- **O**bstruction:
  - ○ Usually from kinking of the ET tube or from a mucous plug.
  - ○ Confirm with fiberoptic bronchoscopy if available.
    - ▪ Insert a suction catheter through the ET tube to remove the plug.
    - ▪ In some cases, the tube will have to be replaced.
- **P**neumothorax:
  - ○ Place a chest tube on the affected side. Might need emergent chest decompression.
  - ○ If the patient is hypotensive and the side of the pneumothorax is not clear, bilateral chest tubes should be placed.
- **E**quipment failure:
  - ○ Disconnect the patient from the ventilator and ventilate with a bag valve apparatus until another ventilator is available.
- **S**tacking of breaths:
  - ○ Remove the patient from the ventilator and allow for a full expiration.
  - ○ Gentle pressure can be applied to the chest to accelerate the exhalation process.
- The relationship between PIP & P_{plat} may provide diagnostic clues:
  - ○ If **PIP is high and P_{plat} is normal**, airway resistance is likely high.
    - ▪ DDX: obstruction of the ETT, proximal airway, or ventilator circuit.
  - ○ If **PIP is high and P_{plat} is high**, lung compliance is likely low.
    - ▪ DDX: pneumothorax, ARDS, pulmonary edema, abdominal distension, or pleural effusion.
  - ○ If **PIP is low and P_{plat} is low**, suspect an air leak or tube dislodgement.
    - ▪ DDX: displaced tube or cuff leak.

BIBLIOGRAPHY

Acute Respiratory Distress Syndrome Network. Ventilation with lower tidal volumes as compared with traditional tidal volumes for acute lung injury and the acute respiratory distress syndrome. *N Engl J Med* 2000;342:1301–1308.

Weingart S. Dominating the vent: Part I. *EMCrit Blog* 2010 [updated May 24, 2010; cited August 1, 2012]. Available from: http://emcrit.org/lectures/vent-part-1/ [last accessed February 14, 2023].

4

· · · · · · · ·

The Boarding ICU Patient in the Emergency Department

ROBERT L. SHERWIN

Introduction

- Critical illness should be viewed as a continuum from prehospital development of disease, through emergency department (ED) presentation to ICU admission to post-ICU care and ultimately to hospital discharge.
- Over two million patients are admitted to intensive care units (ICUs) from EDs each year in the United States (US).
- Critical care visits increased by 80% between 2006 and 2014.
- More than 50% of ICU admissions remain in the ED in excess of 6 hours.
- ICU patients who board in the ED have been shown to have worse outcomes.
- There is no current consensus definition of an ED boarder, though mortality increases at **6 hours**.
- This chapter is meant to represent best practice, evidence-based guidelines for common ICU patients boarding in the ED. It is not intended to be a comprehensive review of any specific topic or disease process.

Ongoing Assessment of the ICU Boarder

- For ICU patients boarding in the ED, it is reasonable to completely reassess the patient every 2–4 hours (or sooner if unstable).
- Assessments should focus on fundamentals of critical care and disease-specific goals.
- Recommended general management:
  - Avoid blood transfusion for non-bleeding patients with hemoglobin > 7 mg/dL.
  - Place central venous lines using maximum barrier and aseptic techniques and avoid femoral site if possible.
- When a patient requires an indwelling urinary catheter, ensure that all CDC guidelines are adhered to in order to avoid a catheter-associated UTI (CAUTI).
- For ongoing reassessments, use the mnemonic: **BOARDER**

Bloodwork: reconcile new critical labs and/or labs requiring trending (e.g., troponin, lactate).

Orders: reconcile medications for any essential home meds or new meds requiring re-dosing (e.g., stress dose steroids, antibiotics).

Advanced directives & goals of care: engage patient, family +/− palliative care services early regarding goals of care and critical decisions.

Resuscitation endpoints: ensure "ins and outs" are accurate; review resuscitation endpoints (below).

Documentation: ensure history, events, and interventions are well-documented for ICU team that will eventually admit the patient.

Evolving data & diagnosis: consider changing or expanding differential diagnosis as new information comes in to avoid premature closure and anchoring.

Rounds: it is essential to round or huddle frequently with ancillary staff (nursing, RT).

Resuscitation Endpoints

- Monitoring **resuscitation endpoints** is vital to avoid under- or over-resuscitation (knowing that only 50% of critically ill patients are volume responsive).
- Target multiple endpoints and use overall clinical judgement as no single endpoint is ideal.

- **Static endpoints:** These include **vital signs** (e.g., heart rate, blood pressure), **urine output** (> 0.5 mL/kg/hr), or **labs** (e.g., lactate, hemoglobin, base deficit, etc.) and may be helpful but should not be used exclusively as they have limited reliability for predicting volume responsiveness.
- **Dynamic endpoints:** these are metrics that assess volume responsiveness in real-time and are thus more reliable than static markers.
  - **Fluid challenge:** Ideally volume responsiveness should increase stroke volume (SV) by ≥ 10% following a fluid challenge (usually 500 cc); the downside of this is the risk for volume overload with repeated challenges.
  - Passive leg raise (PLR) maneuver is a quick, noninvasive predictor of volume responsiveness that does not risk volume overload.
- Other available endpoints:
  - Central venous pressure – not a reliable indicator of volume responsiveness.
  - Ultrasound and echocardiography (e.g., filling pressures, IVC diameter, and EF).
  - Cardiac output monitoring (cardiac index, stroke volume, stroke volume variation).
  - There are several non-invasive methods/devices that offer the ability to facilitate the measurement of more advanced hemodynamic and dynamic endpoints including transpulmonary thermodilution, pulse contour analysis, bioreactance or bioimpedance.

Septic Patients Boarding in the ED

- Globally, sepsis has a 25% case fatality rate.
- Current sepsis and septic shock definitions include both SIRS- (used by CMS) and SOFA- (consensus and literature standard) based identification strategies.
- Recommended management:
  - *Antibiotics:* Prompt, **broad spectrum antibiotics** as early as possible (within the first 1–3 hours). The sickest patients benefit most; do not forget to re-dose these in ICU boarders.
  - *Fluid resuscitation:* 30 cc/kg of crystalloid bolus for septic patients with any SBP < 90 mmHg a serum lactate of > 4.0 mmol/dL (within the first 3 hours).

- The caveat is that fluid overload is harmful and leads to poorer clinical outcomes.
- Patients at highrisk for overload or with current evidence of fluid overload should be managed judiciously: e.g., renal failure, congestive heart failure (HFpEF or HFrEF), and known pulmonary hypertension.
- Balanced fluids appear to be more beneficial than isotonic solutions.
- Avoid anchoring on sepsis as the cause of shock, which risks excessively volume resuscitating patients.
- *Vasopressors:* **Norepinephrine** is the consensus recommendation as a first line vasopressor to maintain MAP $\geq$ 65 mmHg if not achieved after initial fluid bolus. **Vasopressin** or **epinephrine** should be considered for second line, particularly if norepinephrine requirements are rapidly escalating.
- *Blood cultures:* Obtain appropriate routine microbiologic cultures prior to antibiotic administration.
- *Lactate measurement:* Measure lactate at initial workup as a marker of tissue perfusion. Best practice to trend lactate until normalization.
- *Source control:* Identify source of infection promptly within 6 hours.
- *Steroids:* Hydrocortisone (50 mg every 6 hours) should be considered as steroids appear to reduce vasopressor requirements in **refractory septic shock;** do not forget to re-dose these in ICU boarders
- Deep vein thrombosis (DVT) and gastrointestinal stress ulcer prophylaxis.

Intubated Patients Boarding in the ED

- Intubated patients should be managed with the following parameters:
  - Determine an accurate height and predicted body weight for each patient.
  - Tidal volume of 6 mL/kg.
  - Minimize FiO_2 delivery; target normoxia (SPO$_2$ 92–96%).
  - Continuous end tidal CO_2 monitoring.
  - Keep head of bed > 30 degrees.
  - Implement oral hygiene within 1 hour of intubation, then Q4H.
  - Maintain the endotracheal tube cuff pressure between 25 and 30 cm H_2O.

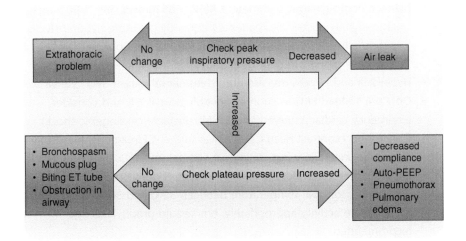

Figure 4.1 Suggested algorithm to assess PAP in troubleshooting intubated patients.

- Pain and agitation should be routinely assessed using validated scoring tools.
  - In general, target light sedation such that the patient still responds to significant stimuli but is not agitated or at risk for self-extubation.
  - However, if the patient is at risk for ARDS and dyssynchronous with ventilator, deeper sedation may be required.
  - Non-benzodiazepine sedation is suggested (e.g., propofol).
- Deep vein thrombosis (DVT) and gastrointestinal stress ulcer prophylaxis.
- Proximal airway pressures (PAP) should be regarded as a vital sign in intubated patients and monitored regularly to keep < 30 cmH$_2$O (Figure 4.1).
- Ensure Plateau Pressure (P$_{plat}$) remains < 30 cmH$_2$O
- Watch for auto-PEEP (also known as intrinsic PEEP or dynamic hyperinflation) due to obstructive physiology.

Adult Post-Cardiac Arrest Care

- Early placement of an endotracheal tube, if not already established, and follow recommended ventilation parameters.

- Manage hemodynamic parameters: MAP > 65 mmHg, SBP > 90 mmHg.
  - Immediately post-ROSC, patients frequently get more hypotensive or potentially re-arrest; have norepinephrine or epinephrine drips ready and cycle blood pressure frequently.
- Hyperoxia and hypoxemia are both detrimental (target SPO_2 92–98%).
- Obtain a 12-lead EKG as soon as possible post ROSC and consider emergency cardiac intervention (STEMI, unstable cardiogenic shock).
- Obtain a non-contrast Head CT as well as further CT imaging if there is any diagnostic uncertainty (e.g., pulmonary embolism, aortic dissection, etc.)
- Initiate targeted temperature management (if does not follow commands) for goal temperature between 32°C and 36°C.
- Treat seizure activity appropriately, but seizure prophylaxis not recommended.
- Prophylactic antibiotics are not recommended.
- Evaluate and treat for rapidly reversible causes.
- Neuro-prognostication involving a multimodal approach; unreliable before 72 hours.

Specific Strategies to Manage ICU Boarders in the ED

- **ED-centric model:** The ED is completely responsible for care with minimal input from the ICU. The ICU team takes over care when the patient arrives in the ICU.
- **ICU-centric model:** The ICU is completely responsible for patient care, orders, and management. The emergency physician is still available for emergent interventions and acute deterioration while the patient is located in the ED.
- **Hybrid-model:** Shared responsibility of care is often dictated by a consensus interdepartmental policy or may include an ED–CC consultant service.
  - **ED-based Critical Care Rotations:** Several emergency medicine programs have ED-based critical care rotations during which the resident's duties focus solely on the care of critically ill patients, including ICU boarders.

BIBLIOGRAPHY

Bednarczyk JM, Fridfinnson JA, Kumar A, et al. Incorporating dynamic assessment of fluid responsiveness into goal-directed therapy: A systematic review and meta-analysis. *Crit Care Med* 2017;45:1538–1545.

Jayaprakash N, Pflaum-Carlson J, Gardner-Gray J, et al. Critical care delivery solutions in the emergency department: Evolving models in caring for ICU boarders. *Ann Emerg Med* 2020;76:709–716.

Mathews KS, Durst MS, Vargas-Torres C, et al. Effect of emergency department and ICU occupancy on admission decisions and outcomes for critically ill patients. *Crit Care Med* 2018;46:720–727.

Mohr NM, Wessman BT, Bassin B, et al. Boarding of critically ill patients in the emergency department. *Crit Care Med* 2020;48:1180–1187.

Rhodes A, Evans LE, Alhazzani W, et al. Surviving sepsis campaign: International guidelines for management of sepsis and septic shock: 2016. *Crit Care Med* 2017;45:486–552.

Rose L, Scales DC, Atzema C, et al. Emergency department length of stay for critical care admissions: A population-based study. *Ann Am Thorac Soc* 2016;13:1324–1332.

SECTION 2

Infectious Disease Emergencies

MARK ANDREAE

5

· · · · · · · ·

Covid-19

JOHN ROZEHNAL AND MELISSA VILLARS

Introduction

- Severe acute respiratory syndrome coronavirus 2 (SARS-CoV-2) caused the pandemic declared in March 2020. While many of the manifestations (i.e., ARDS) are similar to other severe respiratory viruses, there are an increasing number of specific therapeutics found to be effective in combating Coronavirus Disease 2019 (COVID-19).
- As data emerge on the optimal treatment of COVID-19, the recommendations that follow are based upon the current consensus from large global health and infectious disease authorities but are subject to evolution of the evidence.

Epidemiology

Transmission

- Evidence of aerosolized transmission supports in-hospital use of N95 or higher respiratory protection as well as eye protection, in addition to contact precautions.
- Outdoor transmission risk is decreased by ten- to twenty-fold.

- Variants emerging may have increased or decreased transmissibility or virulence, but timing of symptoms and manner of transmission appear unchanged.

Natural History

- Symptoms tend to occur from two to 14 days after exposure.
- Clinical risk factors for severe morbidity and mortality include obesity, hypertension, diabetes, smoking, age > 65, kidney disease, lung disease, cardiovascular disease, pregnancy, immunocompromised states, neurological conditions, cancer.
- mRNA and vector vaccines provide high levels of protection from illness, serious illness and some degree of reduction of asymptomatic spread.

Presentation

Classic Presentation

Patient presentations of COVID-19 are currently described in two phases: the initial stage is marked by mild respiratory symptoms; after the first week, approximately 20% will progress to bilateral pneumonia with supplemental oxygen requirements.

- The predominant symptomatic presentation includes fever, dry cough, myalgia, malaise, and headache.
- Depending on source, 80–99% of symptomatic presentations have at least one of these symptoms.
- Patients may present with symptoms outside the respiratory system.
  - Anosmia (loss of smell) and ageusia (loss of taste) is present in up to 40% of cases, and may be the only presenting symptom.
  - Diarrhea and vomiting may also be present (or may be the only symptom). When in conjunction with classic symptoms, GI symptoms are associated with a more severe clinical course.
  - Neurologic symptoms, distinct from anosmia and ageusia, are also common, including dizziness, altered mental status, ataxia, acute cerebrovascular disease, and seizure.

Critical Presentation

Severe pneumonia/respiratory failure manifests as ARDS.

Diagnosis and Evaluation

Basic workup for patients with COVID-19 should include labs, EKG, and imaging.

- Basic Labs: CBC, CMP, inflammatory markers.
  - CBC: Neutropenia or lymphopenia may limit the ability to use some therapies in the medications section below.
  - CMP: Elevated Creatinine, AST, ALT have been associated with increased risk of disease progression.
  - Inflammatory markers provide insight on the risk of developing severe disease and are used in determining eligibility for therapeutic medications. (Confer with local infectious disease specialists for institutional protocols.)
    - Elevated CRP, D-dimer, Ferritin and LDH are all associated with increased risk of disease progression.
- Imaging
  - CXR findings from more frequent to least include normal CXR, consolidation opacities, peripheral ground glass opacities, reticular interstitial thickening, pulmonary nodules, and pleural effusions.
  - CT scans are not routinely used. Findings are similar to that of CXRs including ground glass opacities, mixed ground glass opacities and consolidations, vascular enlargement, and traction bronchiectasis.
  - CTA scans can be used if clinical suspicion for PE is present; however, there are no current data to help risk stratify for PE in COVID-19 infection.
- COVID-19 testing
  - PCR tests have higher sensitivity and specificity than rapid antigen tests.
  - In areas with no rapid PCR testing available, the risks and benefits of a rapid result compared to a more accurate result need to be considered.

Disposition

Admission Criteria

- Patients with resting $SpO_2 < 94\%$, desaturation with ambulation, or decreased capability or resources to care for themselves should be admitted.
- The level of care for admission (general floor, step down unit, or ICU) is based on institutional practices.
- Discharged patients should be sent home with strict return precautions for shortness of breath and, if available, a pulse oximeter.
- Nirmatrelvir-ritonavir twice daily for 5 days substantially decreases the risk of progression to severe disease, and should be offered to discharged patients within 5 days of symptom onset.
- Drug-drug interactions are common, and patients' home medications should be screened for dangerous interactions with one of several readily available tools

Critical Management

Brief Summary Checklist

- ☑ **Oxygenation**
- ☑ **Proning**
- ☑ **Fluid Balance**
- ☑ **Anticoagulation**
- ☑ **Medications**

Oxygenation

- Oxygen therapy is an aerosolizing procedure with varying distances of particle spread based on modality.
  - Safety measures such as viral filters for all NIPPV and invasive ventilation and proper PPE should be utilized.

Non-Invasive Ventilation

- Oxygen support should be titrated to $SpO_2 \geq 95\%$ with progressive escalation of oxygen support modalities as needed and with observation of clinical work of breathing as a proxy for lung injury.
  - Nasal cannula versus high-flow nasal cannula versus BIPAP should be administered as needed to maintain $SpO_2 \geq 95\%$.

Invasive Ventilation

- Optimal timing of intubation is controversial and may represent a trade-off between ventilator-induced lung injury in early intubation versus patient self-induced lung injury and evolving critical illness in late intubation.
- Management of mechanical ventilation in the COVID-19 patient does not differ much from the standard of care approach for severe ARDS.
  - Ventilation strategies should be managed according to Low-TV ARDS table.
  - For more details, please refer to Chapter 22.

Proning

- Self-proning in non-intubated patients has been shown to be feasible with potential to avoid intubation.
- Proning intubated COVID-19 patients for 12–16 hours daily is recommended with similar guidelines as severe ARDS prone position protocols.

Fluid Balance

Please refer to Chapter 22.

Anticoagulation

- While thromboembolic disease is present at higher rates, we have not found clear evidence that therapeutic dosing of anticoagulation in admitted patients improves outcomes over prophylactic dosing. Management of anticoagulation varies by institution and may vary on a patient-by-patient basis

Medications

- Steroids
  - All patients requiring supplemental oxygen should receive corticosteroids. Robust evidence supports 6 mg dexamethasone daily for up to 10 days, or 50 mg hydrocortisone q6h, but equivalent doses of other corticosteroids are reasonable choices. Steroids may be harmful in patients who do not require oxygen.
- IL-6 inhibitor (e.g., tocilizumab or sarilumab)
  - In adults requiring supplemental oxygen and CRP > 75 mg/L, a dose of 8 mg/kg of tocilizumab is recommended in combination with steroids.
    - This appears most helpful when given early in the course of rapidly progressive disease.
- JAK inhibitor (e.g., baricitinib or tofacitinib)
  - With remdesivir, JAK inhibitor can be considered in patients with progressive disease and in those on organ support
  - Baricitinib, given either with or without remdesivir, is an appropriate alternative to tocilizumab in patients with rapidly progressing disease. Best given within 24-48 hours of initiation of ICU-level care and within 96h of hospitalization. Avoid in severe renal injury or leukopenia
- Several trials show remdesivir is associated with improved outcomes in patients requiring supplemental oxygen but not mechanical ventilation, however these benefits are usually slight and statistically not significant. IDSA recommends a 5-day course of remdesivir
- Avoid in patients with renal disease
- Patients who are otherwise eligible for discharge should not have their hospitalization extended to complete the course of treatment.
- Routine convalescent plasma does not improve mortality, length of stay or ventilator-free days, but may be indicated in certain populations.
- Antibody therapy
  - At the time of writing, the efficacy of monoclonal antibodies appears to have been evaded by circulating viral lineages, therefore monoclonal antibody therapy is no longer recommended

- Other novel or experimental therapies and management strategies should only be followed in the context of clinical trials.

VV-ECMO

- Young healthy patients, including pregnant patients, with a short duration of mechanical ventilation should be considered for transfer to a facility with capability to perform ECMO.
- In general, the criteria established by the EOLIA trial are followed in determining eligibility for ECMO.

Sudden Deterioration

- Worsening hypoxia is the most likely underlying issue. Escalate oxygenation from non-invasive to invasive if required.
- Consider interval development of pneumothorax or pulmonary embolus.
- Myocarditis and cardiogenic shock are also possible. Stat echocardiogram and possible need for ECMO should be considered.
- The long ventilator courses of critically ill COVID-19 patients expose them to common risks often seen in severe ARDS; consider ventilator-associated pneumonia, pneumothorax or mucus plugging in the acutely deteriorating patient.

Pediatric Considerations

General

- Likelihood of severe infection is lower than in adults; however, there is a risk of post-viral multisystem inflammatory syndrome (MIS-C) linked to SARS-Cov2.
- MIS-C is often present in children after asymptomatic infections.
- Increasing male predominance, especially in older children. Increased incidence of MIS-C in patients of African, Afro-Caribbean, and Hispanic descent, but lower in those of East Asian descent.

- MIS-C is defined as hyperinflammatory state involving at least two organ systems, but 90% of cases involved at least four systems.
- MIS-C most commonly includes abdominal pain, vomiting, diarrhea, rash, conjunctival hyperemia, cough, shortness of breath, or chest pain.
- Most likely clinical findings include hypotension, shock, cardiac dysfunction, myocarditis, coronary aneurysm, pericardial effusion, pneumonia, ARDS, pleural effusion.

Workup

- Assessment for MIS-C should be done alongside assessment for other causes of the child's symptoms.
- A well-appearing child can be screened with CBC, CMP, ESR, CRP and both PCR and antibody testing for SARS-Cov2 infection.
- A positive screen is (1) an elevation in ESR or CRP and one of the following: ALC > 1000/uL, platelet count < 150K/uL, Na < 135, neutrophilia, hypoalbuminemia.
- A patient with a positive screen and/or a patient with concerning history and signs of shock should have a broader workup including EKG, echocardiogram, cardiac markers, procalcitonin, d-dimer, fibrinogen, pt/ptt, LDH, urinalysis, cytokine panel, triglycerides, blood smear.

Management

- The child should be admitted for monitoring and treatment. Infectious Disease specialists should be consulted.
- Treatment: IVIG 2 g/kg in addition to supportive care. Methylprednisolone 1–2 mg/kg/day is recommended for refractory or severe cases, with escalating doses of steroids (methylprednisone 10–30 mg/kg/day and/or high-dose Anakinra) for refractory shock.

BIBLIOGRAPHY

Avari H, Hiebert RJ, Ryzynski AA, et al. Quantitative assessment of viral dispersion associated with respiratory support devices in a simulated critical care environment. *Am J Respir Crit Care Med* 2021;203(9):1112–1118. https://doi.org/10.1164/rccm .202008-3070OC

Brower RG, Matthay MA, Morris A, et al. Ventilation with lower tidal volumes as compared with traditional tidal volumes for acute lung injury and the acute respiratory distress syndrome. *New Engl J Med* 2000;342(18):1301–1308.

Gottlieb RL, Nirula A, Chen P, et al. Effect of bamlanivimab as monotherapy or in combination with etesevimab on viral load in patients with mild to moderate COVID-19: A randomized clinical trial. *JAMA* 2021;325(7):632–644. https://doi.org/10.1001/jama.2021.0202

Janiaud P, Axfors C, Schmitt AM, et al. Association of convalescent plasma treatment with clinical outcomes in patients with COVID-19: A systematic review and meta-analysis. *JAMA* 2021;325(12):1185–1195. https://doi.org/10.1001/jama.2021.2747

Korley FK, Durkalski-Mauldin V, Yeatts SD, et al. Early convalescent plasma for high-risk outpatients with COVID-19. *N Engl J Med* 2021;385(21):1951–1960. https://doi.org/10.1056/NEJMoa2103784

Libster R, Pérez MG, Wappner D, et al. Early high-titer plasma therapy to prevent severe COVID-19 in older adults. *N Engl J Med* 2021;384(7):610–618. https://doi.org/10.1056/NEJMoa2033700

Saniasiaya J, Islam MA, Abdullah B. Prevalence of olfactory dysfunction in coronavirus disease 2019 (COVID-19): A meta-analysis of 27,492 patients. *Laryngoscope* 2021;131(4):865–878. https://doi.org/10.1002/lary.29286

Silva FAFD, Brito BB, Santos MLC, et al. COVID-19 gastrointestinal manifestations: A systematic review. *Rev Soc Bras Med Trop* 2020;53:e20200714. https://doi.org/10.1590/0037-8682-0714-2020

Solomon IH, Normandin E, Bhattacharyya S, et al. Neuropathological features of Covid-19. *N Engl J Med* 2020;383(10):989–992. https://doi.org/10.1056/NEJMc2019373

Wong HYF, Lam HYS, Fong AHT, et al. Frequency and distribution of chest radiographic findings in patients positive for COVID-19. *Radiology* 2020;296(2):E72–E78.

Zhao W, Zhong Z, Xie X, et al. Relation between chest CT findings and clinical conditions of coronavirus disease (COVID-19) pneumonia: A multicenter study. *Am J Roentgenol* 2020;214(5):1072–1077.

6

. . . .

Sepsis and Septic Shock

ERICA CHIMELSKI

Introduction

- **Definitions**
  - ○ Sepsis is currently defined as life-threatening organ dysfunction caused by dysregulated host response to infection.
  - ○ Septic shock is sepsis with persistent hypotension requiring vasopressor to maintain MAP $\geq$ 65 mmHG and having a serum lactate > 2 mmol/dL despite adequate fluid resuscitation.
  - ○ There is wide variation in test characteristics for screening scores like systemic inflammatory response syndrome (SIRS), quick Sequential Organ Failure Assessment (qSOFA), National Early Warning Score (NEWS), and Modified Early Warning Score (MEWS). A qSOFA score of $\geq$ 2, or a change in SOFA score of $\geq$ 2 can promptly identify these patients; however, qSOFA is not recommended as a single screening tool over comparable scores like SIRS, NEWS, or MEWS.
- Usual care was found in a series of trials (ProCESS, ProMISe, ARISE) to be noninferior to the previous algorithmic approach of Early Goal Directed Therapy. Effective sepsis management still includes early initiation of fluid resuscitation, antibiotic therapy, and source control but does not require invasive measures such as CVP or SvO_2.

Presentation

Classic Presentation

qSOFA Score (≥ 2 of the following are required)	
Altered Mental Status	GCS ≤ 13
Tachypnea	RR > 22
Hypotension	SBP ≤ 100

Critical Presentation

- Hypotension: systolic blood pressure <90 mmHg or mean arterial pressure <65 mmHg.
  - Beware of relative hypotension in patients with chronic hypertension.
- Encephalopathy and altered mental status.
- Acute kidney injury presenting as oliguria or anuria.
- Myocardial dysfunction/cardiogenic shock: decreased left ventricular ejection fraction on echocardiogram, troponin leak.
- Lung injury or acute respiratory distress syndrome (ARDS).
- Disseminated intravascular coagulation (DIC).

Diagnosis and Evaluation

Step 1 : Confirm the diagnosis of sepsis (qSOFA score of ≥ 2, or a change in SOFA score of ≥ 2), and determine the severity of illness.
  - Basic metabolic panel: ↑creatinine (acute kidney injury), ↑glucose (increased insulin resistance).
  - CBC with differential: WBC, ↓platelets (DIC).
  - Coagulation profile: ↑PT/INR/PTT (DIC).
  - Lactate: ≥2 mmol/L after adequate fluid resuscitation (evidence of cellular anaerobic respiration).
  - Arterial blood gas: ↓pH (metabolic acidosis), PaO_2 (ARDS)
  - Liver function tests: ↑AST, ↑ALT, ↑bilirubin (shock liver).
  - Cardiac markers: ↑troponin (cardiac injury).

Step 2: Identify source of infection
- ○ Chest radiograph to evaluate for pulmonary processes.
- ○ Urine analysis if symptoms of dysuria (burning, urgency, flank, or pelvic pain).
- ○ Lumbar puncture if symptoms are concerning for meningitis (sepsis with altered mental status without alternate explanation).
- Cultures
  - ○ Blood (minimum two sets from two different sites).
  - ○ Urine (if there is clinical suspicion for a urinary source).
  - ○ Sputum if there is a suspicion for pneumonia.
  - ○ Cerebrospinal fluid if clinically indicated.
- Imaging as indicated by symptoms (computed tomography [CT] of the abdomen and pelvis, ultrasound, etc.).

Critical Management

Step 1: Early Antimicrobial Therapy
- ☐ Broad initial empiric therapy to cover relevant gram negative and gram-positive organisms (empiric methicillin-resistant Staphylococcus aureus [MRSA] coverage for those at high risk).
- ☐ Review patient's prior microbiology data and risk factors for multidrug resistant (MDR) organisms with low threshold for empiric coverage.
- ☐ Consider empiric antifungal coverage in high-risk populations (e.g., immunocompromised state, transplant history, or long-term critical illness).
- ☐ Consider empiric antiviral therapy in the appropriate clinical context.

Step 2: Fluid resuscitation
- ☐ 30 mL/kg of lactated ringers or other balanced crystalloid is appropriate initial resuscitation in most patients within the first 3 hours.
- ☐ There is no evidence to recommend colloid over crystalloid resuscitation outside of specific clinical scenarios (hepatorenal syndrome or spontaneous bacterial peritonitis).
- ☐ Additional fluid resuscitation should be guided by dynamic reassessments (i.e., effect of passive leg raise on pulse pressure variation or other invasive or noninvasive measure of change in stroke volume) over static measures such as CVP.

☐ Initiate vasopressors promptly in patients who do not respond to additional fluid resuscitation.

Step 3: Source control

☐ Consult interventionalist (surgery, urology, interventional radiology, gastroenterology, etc.) early to control sources of infection identified on imaging or physical exam (abscess, cholangitis, cholecystitis, necrotizing soft tissue infection, etc.)

☐ Remove indwelling catheters with concern for catheter-associated bloodstream infection.

☐ Place foley catheters in patients with urinary source of sepsis in the setting of urinary retention.

Monitoring Criteria

Criterion	Goal	Necessary lines
Mean arterial pressure (MAP)	≥ 65 mmHg	Arterial line
Urine output (UOP)	≥ 0.5 mL/kg/hour	Foley or non-indwelling
Lactate clearance	Normalization < 2	None
Glucose	140–180 mg/dL	None

Sudden Deterioration

Patients with persistent hypotension (MAP < 65 mmHg) despite adequate fluid administration will require additional interventions.

- Vasopressors
  - First line: norepinephrine
  - Second line: vasopressin (0.03 units/minute) or epinephrine (0.01–0.5 micrograms/kg/minute).
  - Other as appropriate: Angiotensin II, phenylephrine, dopamine, methylene blue.
- If hypotension persists despite adequate vasopressor dose, consider administering steroids (hydrocortisone 200 mg/day + fludrocortisone 50 μg/day).
- Mixed cardiogenic/vasodilatory shock: consider inotropes (epinephrine versus dobutamine+norepinephrine).

- Respiratory failure: If intubation and mechanical ventilation are required:
  - ○ Volume-controlled ventilation at 6 mL/kg *ideal* body weight (i.e., based upon patient height) targeting plateau pressure $\leq$ 30 cmH$_2$O if at-risk for ARDS
  - ○ Minimize FiO$_2$ and increase PEEP to achieve an O$_2$ saturation goal of 88–95% while avoiding oxygen toxicity.
- Renal failure: Timing of renal replacement therapy (RRT) in septic shock is controversial. Consult nephrology early in oliguric or anuric patients with refractory metabolic acidosis despite initial resuscitation or other emergent indications for RRT.

BIBLIOGRAPHY

ARISE Investigators, ANZICS Clinical Trials Group, Peake SL, et al. Goal-directed resuscitation for patients with early septic shock. *N Engl J Med* 2014; 371:1496–1506.

Evans L, Rhodes A, Alhazzani W, et al. Surviving sepsis campaign: International guidelines for management of sepsis and septic shock 2021. *Intensive Care Med* 2021;47(11):1181–1247. https://doi.org/10.1007/s00134-021-06506-y

ProCESS Investigators, Yealy DM, Kellum JA, et al. A randomized trial of protocol-based care for early septic shock. *N Engl J Med* 2014;370:1683–1693.

ProMISe Investigators, Mouncey PR, Osborn TM, et al. Trial of early, goal-directed resuscitation for septic shock. *N Engl J Med* 2015;372:1301–1311.

Rhodes A, Evans LE, Alhazzani W, et al. Surviving sepsis campaign: international guidelines for management of sepsis and septic shock: 2016. *Crit Care Med* 2017;45:486–552.

Rivers E, Nguyen B, Havstad S, et al. Early goal-directed therapy in the treatment of severe sepsis and septic shock. *N Engl J Med* 2001;345:1368–1377.

Singer M, Deutschman CS, Seymour CW, et al. The third international consensus definitions for sepsis and septic shock (Sepsis-3). *JAMA* 2016;315:801–810.

7

Pneumonia

NAVDEEP SEKHON AND CALVIN LEE

Introduction

- **Classification of Pneumonia**
  - **Community-acquired pneumonia (CAP)** is a pneumonia that is not acquired in a hospital. Usual pathogens include *Streptococcus pneumoniae, Haemophilus influenzae, Mycoplasma pneumoniae, Staphylococcus Aureus, Chlamydophila pneumoniae, Legionella pneumophila and Moraxella catarrhalis.*
  - Healthcare-associated pneumonia (HCAP) is no longer recognized as a clinical entity by the 2019 ATS/IDSA Guidelines on the Management of Community Acquired Pneumonia. HCAP designation did not uniformly predict drug-resistant organisms, so management is driven on an individual basis.
  - **Hospital-acquired pneumonia (HAP)** is defined as a pneumonia not incubating at the time of hospital admission and occurring more than 48 hours after admission.
  - **Ventilator-associated pneumonia (VAP)** is defined as a pneumonia occurring more than 48 hours after intubation.

Presentation

Classic Presentations of Community-Acquired Pneumonia

- "Typical" pneumonia presents with a sudden onset of fever and chills accompanied by productive cough with purulent sputum. Traditionally, it is caused by *Streptococcus pneumoniae* and *Haemophilus influenzae*.
- "Atypical" pneumonia presents subacutely with a nonproductive cough, fever, headache, myalgias, and malaise. It is traditionally caused by *Mycoplasma pneumoniae, Chlamydophila pneumoniae, Legionella pneumophila,* and *Coxiella burnetii.*

Critical Presentation

- Patients can present with hypoxia, tachycardia, and hypotension.
- Hypoxia is frequently related to shunt through consolidated lung, and may not be responsive to supplemental oxygen alone.

Diagnosis and Evaluation

- **History**
  - Duration and progression of symptoms.
  - Risk factors for severe disease, e.g., diabetes, immunocompromised state.
  - Relevant environmental and nosocomial exposures.
  - Risk factors for multidrug-resistant organisms, atypical infections, and fungal infection.
- Lab Testing
  - **Blood cultures and sputum gram stain with cultures should not be performed routinely** in the patient with community-acquired pneumonia except for the following situations according to ATS/IDSA 2019 guidelines:
    - Patients with severe community-acquired pneumonia.
    - Patients receiving empiric treatment for MRSA or pseudomonas.
    - Patients with prior history of MRSA or pseudomonas infection, especially if in the respiratory tract.

Table 7.1 Chest radiographic findings and their associated etiology

Chest radiographic finding	Suggested organism
Lobar consolidation	S. pneumoniae, Klebsiella pneumoniae
Patchy infiltrates	Atypical and fungal organisms
Interstitial pattern	Mycoplasma or viral organisms
Miliary pattern	Tuberculosis or fungal organisms
Apical infiltrate	Tuberculosis
Infiltrate in superior part of lower lobes or posterior part of the upper lobes	Aspiration pneumonia, anaerobic organisms
Cavitary lesion	Tuberculosis, S. aureus, anaerobic organisms, Gram-negative bacilli
Pneumothorax or pneumatocele	Pneumocystis jirovecii

- Patients who have been hospitalized and received intravenous antibiotics in the past 90 days.
  - Pneumococcal urine antigen testing should be performed in severe cases of community-acquired pneumonia.
  - Legionella urine antigen should be collected in patients who have epidemiological risk factors for Legionella (local outbreak or recent travel).
  - Influenza and COVID-19 testing can be performed to aid in diagnosis based on their prevalence in the community.
- **Chest X-Ray**
  - The pattern of the infiltrate on a chest radiograph can suggest an etiology (Table 7.1).
- Diagnostic thoracentesis should be performed if the pleural effusion is greater than 5 cm on chest radiograph. Appropriate studies on the pleural fluid include: cell count with differential, pH, Gram stain and culture.

Critical Management

Critical Management Checklist
☑ Airway management as needed.
☑ Administer oxygen for a goal oxygen saturation greater than 88%.

☑ Timely administration of antibiotics.

☑ Fluid resuscitation and initiation of vasopressors as needed.

☑ Obtain sputum and blood cultures as needed.

☑ Place patients with concern for droplet and airborne communicable diseases (tuberculosis, influenza, COVID-19) in appropriate isolation.

☑ Provide supplemental oxygen to maintain an oxygen saturation higher than 88% (or $PaO_2 > 60$).

- High flow nasal cannula (HFNC) reduces 90-day mortality in patients with hypoxemic respiratory failure without hypercapnea when compared to noninvasive positive pressure ventilation (NIPPV) or conventional supplemental oxygen therapy.
- The evidence for the use of NIPPV is mixed in patients with hypoxemic respiratory failure secondary to pneumonia.
- Intubation may be required for patients with refractory hypoxemia, hypercapnia, mental status changes, or concerns for impending respiratory failure related to unsustainable respiratory effort.
- NIPPV or HFNC should be considered for preoxygenation of hypoxic patients prior to endotracheal intubation.
- Patients with associated distributive shock should be resuscitated with crystalloids and vasopressors.
- Two clinical decision rules can assist the physician in deciding whether a patient needs to be admitted for inpatient management, or can be discharged home with outpatient follow-up:
  - The Pneumonia Severity Index.
  - The CURB-65 rule (Table 7.2). Two or more points warrant hospital admission. Three or more points suggests the need for an ICU admission.

Table 7.2 CURB-65 criteria for patients with a diagnosis of pneumonia

CURB-65 criterion	Points
Confusion	1
Uremia (> 20 mg/dL)	1
Respiratory rate > 30/minute	1
Blood pressure (systolic < 90 mmHg, diastolic < 60)	1
Age > 65 years	1

- **Initiate appropriate antibiotic therapy promptly**, as decreased time to administration has been shown to improve outcomes. Below are appropriate regimens:
  - *Community-acquired pneumonia; outpatient therapy:*
    - If the patient has no comorbidities and no antibiotic use in the past 3 months, one of the following classes can be used as monotherapy:
      - Beta-lactam
      - Tetracycline
      - Macrolide
    - If the patient has comorbidities such as diabetes mellitus; asplenism; chronic heart, liver, lung or kidney disease; immunosuppression; alcoholism; malignancy; and patients who have received antibiotics in the last 3 months:
      - Beta-lactam and a macrolide/doxycycline
      - Respiratory fluoroquinolone
  - *Community-acquired pneumonia; inpatient therapy, non-severe:*
    - Appropriate regimens
      - Beta-lactam plus a macrolide
      - Respiratory quinolone
  - *Community-acquired pneumonia; severe:*
    - Beta-lactam *and* a macrolide (for dosing see above); should also include cover for pseudomonas and MRSA.
    - Beta-lactam *and a* respiratory fluoroquinolone (for dosing see above); should also include coverage for pseudomonas and MRSA.
- *Indications for adding MRSA and Pseudomonas coverage for patients with CAP*
  - Prior respiratory isolation of MRSA and/or Pseudomonas (only add coverage for what has been isolated previously).
  - Hospitalization in the past 90 days with the administration of intravenous antibiotics.
  - Locally validated risk factors for MRSA and Pseudomonas.
- *Hospital-acquired pneumonia/ventilator-associated pneumonia*
  - The antibiotics given should treat *Staphylococcus Aureus* and Pseudomonas.
- Based on local susceptibilities, the antibiotics should cover MRSA as needed
- The patient should be double covered for pseudomonas if the patient has a high risk for mortality, has received intravenous antibiotics in the past 90 days, or has other risk factors for multidrug-resistant organisms.

It is preferred that the anti-Pseudomonal antibiotics be one beta-lactam and one non-beta-lactam, like an aminoglycoside or a fluoroquinolone.

Sudden Deterioration

- Patients' ability to oxygenate and ventilate can decompensate rapidly. If this occurs, intubation and mechanical ventilation will be required.
- Aggressive resuscitation for hypotension from septic shock should be initiated with aggressive fluid resuscitation and vasopressor and/or inotrope support as needed.
- Patients presenting with pneumonia whose blood pressure is deteriorating should be treated as septic shock. Norepinephrine is the first-line vasopressor for this condition.

Special Considerations

- Steroids – Consider steroids for CAP patients with high markers of inflammation (e.g., C-reactive protein [CRP] > 15 mg/dL).
- *Aspiration pneumonia* – More prevalent in patients who have difficulty protecting their airway. Infiltrates can be found in the dependent lung segments. Standard antimicrobial coverage is appropriate for most patients. Anaerobic coverage should be added to patients with specific risk factors or findings consistent with anaerobic infection (witnessed aspiration, lung abscess, necrotizing infection, periodontal disease).
- *Influenza pneumonia* – Consider antiviral medication such as oseltamivir in patients with severe disease or at risk for complications.
- *Parapneumonic effusion and empyema* – Large, complicated parapneumonic effusions or empyema should be drained by thoracentesis or tube thoracostomy.
  - Do not delay antibiotics prior to fluid sampling.
  - Patients in whom drainage fails may require intrapleural tPA/DNase or video-assisted thoracic surgery for decortication.
- *Pneumonia in the immunocompromised patient (e.g., AIDS, active chemotherapy, solid organ and hematopoietic stem cell transplant)*
  - In general, we advocate a multidisciplinary approach involving infectious disease specialists.

- Community-acquired organisms remain the most common pathogens.
- Tuberculosis and bacterial pneumonia can be challenging to distinguish on chest X-ray. Hence, it is prudent to place immunocompromised patients with infiltrates on X-ray on respiratory isolation.
- Consider empiric treatment for fungal pneumonia in patients with risk factors and classic radiographic findings (nodular findings or cavitary lesions). Invasive aspergillosis is a particular concern in the transplant population. Specific therapies depend on relevant exposures, radiographic findings, and disease severity.
- *Pneumocystis jirovecii pneumonia (PJP)*
  - All patients with HIV who have CD4 count < 200 cells/μL with pneumonia should be treated for PJP pneumonia.
  - Typically, LDH levels are typically elevated in PJP pneumonia.
  - Classic X-ray findings of PJP pneumonia include bilateral reticular interstitial infiltrates and hilar lymphadenopathy.
  - Treatment with trimethoprim-sulfamethoxazole is first line. For patients who are allergic to sulfa, clindamycin-primaquine or pentamidine can be used.
  - Steroids are indicated if the PaO_2 is < 70 mmHg or the A-a gradient is > 35 mmHg on arterial blood gas analysis. A common dosing regimen is prednisone 40mg BID for five days with subsequent taper.

BIBLIOGRAPHY

Kalil AC, Metersky ML, Klompas M, et al. Management of adults with hospital-acquired and ventilator-associated pneumonia: 2016 Clinical Practice Guidelines by the Infectious Diseases Society of America and the American Thoracic Society [published correction appears in *Clin Infect Dis* 2017;64(9):1298] [published correction appears in *Clin Infect Dis* 2017;65(8):1435] [published correction appears in *Clin Infect Dis* 2017;65(12):2161]. *Clin Infect Dis* 2016;63(5):e61–e111. https://doi.org/10.1093/cid/ciw353

Metlay J P, Waterer GW, Long AC, et al. Diagnosis and treatment of adults with community-acquired pneumonia. An official clinical practice guideline of the American Thoracic Society and Infectious Diseases Society of America. *Am J Resp Crit Care Med* 2019;200(7):e45–e67. https://doi.org/10.1164/rccm.201908-1581ST

Walls RM, Hockberger RS, & Gausche-Hill M. *Rosen's Emergency Medicine: Concepts and Clinical Practice*, 9th ed. Philadelphia, PA: Elsevier, 2018.

8

Meningitis and Encephalitis

CHRISTOPHER ALLISON

Chapter 8:
Meningitis and Encephalitis

 ## Presentation

Classic Presentation:
Fever, headache, nuchal
rigidity, with possible
prodromal illness or
petechiae/purpura.

Critical Presentation:
Seizures, sepsis, altered
mental status, focal
neurological deficits.

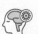

Encephalitis may
present with
non-convulsive
seizures.

 ## Diagnosis and Evaluation

Place patient on
droplet precautions if
bacterial meningitis is
suspected.

LP with CSF analysis.
⚙ *Cell count and differential,*
glucose, protein,
Gram stain and culture,
HSV PCR, other PCRs
for suspected pathogens.

Perform head CT
before LP in patients at
risk for CNS mass
lesions or with signs of
increased ICP.

 ## Management

Airway management and
hemodynamic monitoring.

Prompt initiation of
CNS penetrating antibiotics.
🌀 *Consider adjunctive dexamethasone.*

Optimize for CPP > 60 mmHg;
consider CSF drainage to decrease
ICP.

Sudden deterioration may be due
to seizure or herniation.

Vasopressor of choice:
norepinephrine.

Introduction

- Meningitis is inflammation of the meningeal membranes of the brain and spinal cord.
- Encephalitis is inflammation of the brain parenchyma with or without inflammation of the meninges.
- Cerebral perfusion is a function of arterial pressure and intracranial pressure (i.e., cerebral perfusion pressure = mean arterial pressure – intracranial pressure).
- Hypoperfusion results from cerebral edema and increased intracranial pressure (ICP).
- Meningitis is a life-threatening condition with up to 30% mortality and high risk of long-term neurological complications.
- The differential diagnosis for meningitis and encephalitis includes subarachnoid hemorrhage, cerebral venous thrombosis, metabolic/toxic encephalopathy, and other infections not involving the central nervous system (CNS).

Presentation

Classic Presentation

- Fever, headache, and nuchal rigidity.
- Prodromal upper respiratory tract infection with nausea, vomiting, and photophobia can also occur.
- Petechial or purpuric rash may be present.

Critical Presentation

- Altered mental status
- Seizures
- Sepsis
- Rapid onset over hours in meningococcal meningitis.
- Focal neurological deficits including palsy of cranial nerves III, VI, VII, and VIII.

Diagnosis and Evaluation

- If bacterial meningitis is suspected, place the patient on droplet precautions.
- Absence of leukocytosis does not exclude the diagnosis.
- Physical exam is neither sensitive nor specific for meningitis and encephalitis. Consider lumbar puncture (LP) in patients with fever and altered mental status without an identified source of infection, or with risk for contiguous spread.
- **Obtain a computed tomography (CT) scan of the head prior to LP in patients at risk for central nervous system (CNS) mass lesions or with signs of increased ICP (further indications for head CT prior to LP below in "Critical Management" section).** In case of a CNS mass lesion, defer LP prior to neurosurgical consultation.
- Encephalitis may present with nonconvulsive seizures.
- **LP with evaluation of the cerebrospinal fluid (CSF) is the diagnostic test of choice** (Table 8.1).
  - CSF tests to perform: gram stain and culture, cell count and differential, as well as glucose and protein levels. HSV PCR is routinely sent. Specific antigen or PCR tests can be considered for special pathogens (VZV, *Cryptococcus*, etc.).
- CSF WBC count: Elevation of the WBC count is expected in meningitis. There is neutrophil predominance in ~90% of cases bacterial meningitis, although lymphocytes can sometimes predominate.

Table 8.1 Interpretation of lumbar puncture results

Infection	Glucose (mg/dL)[a]	Protein (mg/dL)	CSF glucose to blood glucose ratio	WBC count (cells/microliter)
No infection	45–80	15–45	> 0.6	< 5
Bacterial meningitis	Decreased	Elevated	< 0.4	Elevated (500–5000)
Viral meningitis	Normal	Elevated	> 0.6 (normal)	Elevated (10–500)

[a] Glucose: 1mg/dL = 0.0555 mmol/L

- CSF glucose concentration is typically decreased in bacterial meningitis, but may be falsely normal if serum hyperglycemia is present (in which case use the CSF:blood glucose ratio).
- HSV encephalitis may have elevated CSF red blood cells due to hemorrhage.
- Brain MRI may have findings supportive of meningitis or encephalitis, but should not guide empiric treatment, given time delay to results.

Critical Management

Critical Management Checklist

- ☑ CT
- ☑ Antibiotics
- ☑ Intracranial pressure control

- **CT prior to lumbar puncture should be obtained for the following:**
  - ○ Age older than 60 years
  - ○ Immunocompromised patients
  - ○ History of CNS lesion(s)
  - ○ Recent seizure
  - ○ Papilledema on retinal examination
  - ○ Altered mental status
  - ○ Focal neurological deficit on examination
- **Antibiotic treatment should not be delayed** for CT scan or lumbar puncture results. If CSF is obtained promptly (ideally within 1 hour of presentation), give antibiotics immediately after LP. If CSF cannot be safely obtained promptly, give antibiotics prior to LP.
- Empiric antibiotics are based on common organisms by age:
  - ○ 2–50 years old: *N. meningitides, S. pneumoniae.*
  - ○ > 50 years old: *S. pneumoniae, N. meningitides, L. monocytogenes.*
- A standard empiric regimen for meningitis in adults is
  - ○ **Ceftriaxone** 2 g IV every 12 hours and **vancomycin** 30 mg/kg loading and dosing every 12 hours for trough concentration of 15–20 micrograms/mL.
  - ○ **AND ampicillin** 2 g IV every 4 hours for patients older than 50 years.
  - ○ **AND acyclovir** 10 mg/kg IV every 8 hours for suspected HSV encephalitis (one of the most common causes of encephalitis).

- Antibiotics must have good CNS penetration. For example, ceftriaxone or cefepime is chosen over piperacillin-tazobactam.
- Adjunctive dexamethasone is also recommended at 10 mg IV every 6 hours initiated prior to or concurrent with antibiotic therapy for bacterial meningitis.
- Cerebral perfusion pressure (CPP = MAP – ICP) should be optimized. Intracranial pressure should be decreased via consideration of CSF drainage or lumbar drain.

Special Circumstances

- Patients with shunt, recent neurosurgery or trauma should be managed with multidisciplinary input. These patients should be covered for Pseudomonas and skin flora. Consider carbapenems over cefepime in patients prone to seizure as cefepime decreases seizure threshold.
- CSF WBC count is less sensitive and specific in the setting of external ventricular drains.
- Infected shunts should be removed and replaced with external drains if needed.
- Clinical findings and lumbar puncture results can be much more subtle in immunocompromised patients.
- Consider testing for pathogens depending on exposure history such as tuberculosis, Lyme disease, arboviruses, and endemic mycoses.

Sudden Deterioration

- Patients at risk of aspiration should be endotracheally intubated.
- A sudden decline in mental status may be from seizure, or less commonly, herniation. Seizure should be emergently managed with benzodiazepines and subsequently loaded with first-line antiepileptic drug (levetiracetam, fosphenytoin, valproic acid).
- Cerebral perfusion pressure = mean arterial pressure – intracranial pressure. Targets vary by age but generally, goal is CPP > 60 mmHg.
- Intracranial pressure measured by lumbar puncture is in cm of H_2O. ICP in mmHg = (0.7 mmHg/1 cm H_2O) (LP pressure in cm H_2O).

- Herniation is temporized by preservation of CPP via vasopressors, hyperosmolar therapy and CSF drainage pending neurosurgical intervention.

Vasopressor of choice: Hypotensive patients are likely septic and should be managed with norepinephrine as a first-line agent. POCUS of heart can show if inotrope is needed.

BIBLIOGRAPHY

Attia J, Hatala R, Cook DJ, et al. Does this adult patient have acute meningitis? *JAMA* 1999;282:175–181.

McIntyre PB, Berkey CS, King SM, et al. Dexamethasone as adjunctive therapy in bacterial meningitis: A meta-analysis of randomized clinical trials since 1988. *JAMA* 1997;278:925–931.

Straus SE, Thorpe KE, Holroyd-Leduc J, et al. How do I perform a lumbar puncture and analyze the results to diagnose bacterial meningitis? *JAMA* 2006;296:2012–2022.

Tunkel AR, Glaser CA, Bloch KC, et al. The management of encephalitis: Clinical practice guidelines by the Infectious Diseases Society of America. *Clin Infect Dis* 2008;47:303–327.

Tunkel AR, Hartman BJ, Kaplan SL, et al. Practice guidelines for the management of bacterial meningitis. *Clin Infect Dis* 2004;39:1267–1284.

van de Beek D, de Gans J, Tunkel AR, et al. Community-acquired bacterial meningitis in adults. *N Engl J Med* 2006;354:44–53.

van de Beek D, Drake JM, Tunkel AR. Nosocomial bacterial meningitis. *N Engl J Med* 2010;362:146–154.

9

Infective Endocarditis

JASON M. BLOCK

Introduction

- Infective endocarditis (IE) is a microbial infection of the endothelial layer of the heart, the valves, or both.
- The mitral valve is most commonly affected, except in patients with intravenous drug use (IVDU), where the tricuspid valve is more commonly affected.
- Risk factors include age, chronic hemodialysis, poor dentition, valvulopathy, immunocompromised status, diabetes, IVDU, prosthetic valve, and implanted cardiac devices.
- More than 50% of cases of IE occur in patients older than 60 years.
- The majority of cases are due to Gram-positive cocci such as Staphylococcus and Streptococcus species (Table 9.1).
- In patients with negative blood cultures and no recent antibiotic use, the organisms are often the HACEK group (*Haemophilus, Actinobacillus, Cardiobacterium, Eikenella, Kingella*).
- Approximately 50% of patients require surgical management.

Presentation

Classic Presentation

- The presentation of IE is highly variable, but the most common symptoms are fever and malaise.
- The classic triad of fever, new murmur, and anemia is rare.
- The spectrum of clinical findings range from non-specific infectious symptoms or embolic phenomena to heart failure or cardiogenic shock.
- Extracardiac physical examination findings are due to embolic vegetations and immune complexes (Table 9.1).

Critical Presentation

- Shock (septic, cardiogenic, or mixed) may be present, especially with acute valvular insufficiency.
- Heart block and dysrhythmia are also possible as the infection may infiltrate the conduction system.
- Embolization of valve vegetations is common. These emboli may affect any organ system:

Table 9.1 Physical findings in infective endocarditis

Finding	Location	Description	Frequency
Petechiae	Buccal mucosa, conjunctiva, extremities	Nonblanching erythematous pinpoint macules	20–40%
Osler's nodes	Pads of fingers and toes	Tender, small subcutaneous nodules	10–25%
Splinter hemorrhages	Under fingernails or toenails	Linear dark streaks	15%
Roth spots	Retina	Oval retinal hemorrhages with pale lefts near optic disc	< 10%
Janeway lesions	Palms and soles	Nontender, small hemorrhagic plaques	< 10%

- Central nervous system: mycotic cerebral aneurysm, ischemic stroke, intracranial hemorrhage, monocular blindness, toxic encephalopathy
- Pulmonary: pneumonia, abscess, infarction, edema
- Renal: acute renal failure, glomerulonephritis
- Gastrointestinal: splenic infarction, mesenteric ischemia

Diagnosis and Evaluation

- The Duke Criteria are used to diagnose IE and have a sensitivity of about 90% (Table 9.2). A positive diagnosis consists of:
  - Two major criteria, *or*
  - One major criterion and three minor criteria, *or*
  - All five minor criteria.
- Transthoracic echocardiography (TTE) should be performed as early as possible.
- A transesophageal echocardiogram is more sensitive and should be performed in patients where there is intermediate to high clinical suspicion and a normal TTE. It may also identify complications of endocarditis such as perivalvular abscess or valve perforation.

Table 9.2 Duke Criteria for the diagnosis of infective endocarditis

Major criteria	Minor criteria
Two separate positive blood cultures with typical IE organisms: • *Staphylococcus aureus* • *Streptococcus viridans* • *Staphylococcus epidermidis* • HACEK group	Risk factor: IVDU or predisposing heart condition Fever > 38°C Immunological phenomena: glomerulonephritis, Osler nodes, Roth spots
Echocardiographic evidence: • Vegetation • Abscess • New dehiscence of prosthetic valve • New valvular regurgitation	Embolic phenomena: pulmonary infarct, arterial emboli, Janeway lesion, conjunctival hemorrhage Positive blood culture that does not meet major criteria above

- Laboratory findings are non-specific and include leukocytosis, normocytic anemia, elevated C-reactive protein (CRP), elevated erythrocyte sedimentation rate (ESR), and hematuria.
- Patients may have conduction abnormalities on ECG. They may also have embolic infiltrates or pulmonary edema on chest radiography, but these findings are neither sensitive nor specific.

Critical Management

Critical Management Checklist

☑ Antibiotics and cultures
☑ Shock assessment
☑ Echocardiography and electrocardiogram
☑ Vasopressors

- Intravenous (IV) antibiotics should be initiated early. Empiric regimens are listed in Table 9.3 but microbiological cultures are integral in guiding therapy.
- Patients may present with mixed septic and cardiogenic shock and require resuscitation with judicious IV fluid and inopressors.
- Echocardiography will reveal valvulopathy (i.e., regurgitation) and cardiac function to guide inotropes and/or vasopressors.
- Intubation should be considered if there is evidence of encephalopathy or respiratory compromise.

Sudden Deterioration

- Perform repeat point-of-care ultrasound (POCUS) to assess for acute valvulopathy. Surgical evaluation for valve replacement should be considered.

Table 9.3 Empiric therapy for suspected infective endocarditis*

Native valve	Vancomycin 15 mg/kg IV *and* cefepime 1g IV *or* gentamicin 1–3 mg/kg IV
Prosthetic valve	Vancomycin 15 mg/kg IV *and* gentamicin 1–3 mg/kg IV *and* rifampin 300 mg PO

* There are slight variations in recommended empiric therapy in the literature; always follow institutional guidelines.

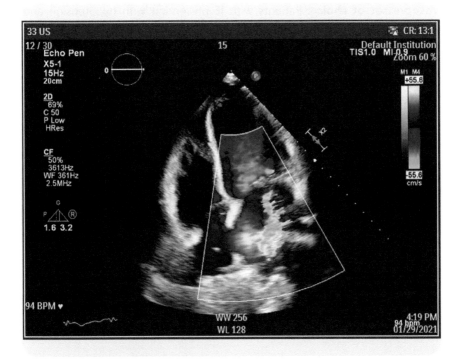

Figure 9.1 Echocardiogram demonstrating acute mitral regurgitation with mitral leaflet vegetation.

(Credit to Jason Block, MD)

- Consider expanding antibiotic coverage for unusually resistant staphylococcal infection. Unusually resistant staphylococcal infections may have success with vancomycin plus beta-lactam, daptomycin plus beta-lactam, ceftaroline, linezolid, or telavancin.
  - The most likely cause for sudden deterioration in the patient with suspected IE is acute insufficiency of the aortic or mitral valve (Figure 9.1) resulting in cardiogenic shock and pulmonary edema.
  - An intra-aortic balloon pump may temporize the patient with acute mitral regurgitation, but is contraindicated in aortic regurgitation.
  - Early conduction abnormalities include PR prolongation due to perivalvular extension of infection to the conduction system. Complete heart block may ensue and require temporary transcutaneous or transvenous pacing.
- If there is sudden neurologic deterioration, consider embolic stroke, ruptured mycotic cerebral aneurysm, or intracranial abscess.

Vasopressor of choice: Patients with IE presenting with hypotension and evidence of hypoperfusion will usually be in septic shock. Norepinephrine is generally the vasopressor of choice in this scenario. However, in patients with aortic or mitral valve insufficiency, inotropic agents should be considered (e.g., epinephrine).

BIBLIOGRAPHY

Marx JA, Hockberger RS, Walls RM, et al., eds. *Rosen's Emergency Medicine: Concepts and Clinical Practice*, 9th ed. Philadelphia, PA: Mosby Elsevier, 2018.

Tintinalli JE, Stapczynski JS, Cline DM, et al., eds. *Emergency Medicine: A Comprehensive Study Guide*, 9th ed. New York, NY: McGraw-Hill Medical, 2016.

Habib G, Lancellotti P, Antunes MJ, et al. 2015 ESC Guidelines for the Management of Infective Endocarditis: The Task Force for the Management of Infective Endocarditis of the European Society of Cardiology. *Eur Heart J* 2015;36(44):3075–3128.

Wang A, Gaca JG, Chu VH. Management considerations in infective endocarditis: A review. *JAMA* 2018;320(1):72–83. https://doi.org/10.1001/jama.2018.7596

10

Necrotizing Soft Tissue Infections

JENNIFER CARNELL

Introduction

- For the clinical applications of this chapter, necrotizing soft tissue infections (NSTIs) will refer to infection of deep subcutaneous tissues and adjacent fascia.
- Mortality is estimated to be around 20–50% in observational literature with variation by infection site and specific organism.
- **Paucity of early physical examination findings can lead to a delay in diagnosis as classic superficial findings do not manifest until later in the disease course**.
  - ○ Infection leads to toxin production, cytokine activation, and microthrombosis which all contribute to ischemia, impaired antibiotic delivery, and rapid progression.
- **Early surgical intervention decreases morbidity and mortality.**
- NSTIs can be classified based on microbial etiology, with polymicrobial etiology being the most common (Table 10.1). Type I necrotizing fasciitis is polymicrobial in origin. Type II is monomicrobial, often caused by group A Streptococcus (typically, *S. pyogenes*). Staphylococcal NSTIs are increasing in prevalence due to community-associated methicillin-resistant *S. aureus*.

Table 10.1 Classification of necrotizing soft tissue infections

Type of microbial etiology
Type I Polymicrobial (most common)
Type II Monomicrobial (streptococci, staphylococci, clostridia)
Type III Vibrio vulnificus (associated with seawater exposure)

- Exotoxin release by clostridia, staphylococci, and streptococci can enhance cytokine release and promote an inflammatory cascade which can lead to death if untreated.
- NSTIs are more common in patients with comorbidities including diabetes mellitus, chronic alcoholism, chronic renal failure, HIV, liver failure (which is classically associated with Vibrio vulnificus), and other immunosuppressed states.

Presentation

Classic Presentation

- **NSTIs are notoriously difficult to diagnose early in the disease course.** Initial pain, swelling, and erythema are often indistinguishable from typical cellulitis.
- Frequently there is either minor trauma or no identified bacterial portal of entry.
- Classically the pain is out of proportion to physical examination findings. As infection rapidly spreads along the fascial planes, pain and swelling may extend beyond the areas of overlying erythema.

Critical Presentation

- **As an NSTI progresses, patients may present with ecchymoses, bullae, and crepitus** as a result of subcutaneous emphysema. **However, these occur later in the disease process** (Figure 10.1).
- **It is more common to see signs of systemic toxicity with NSTIs versus soft tissue infections without necrotizing component**. This is

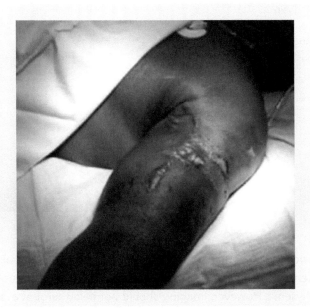

Figure 10.1 Ecchymosis and bullae of the upper extremity of a patient with an NSTI.

due to the systemic inflammatory response from cytokine release, which can manifest as abnormal vital signs or abnormal laboratory markers.

Diagnosis and Evaluation

- **No test, whether radiologic or laboratory, should delay surgical intervention when there is a strong clinical suspicion for NSTI.** However, it should be noted that CT with IV contrast is often obtained when there is uncertainty with the diagnosis.
- **No scoring system has adequate sensitivity to rule out NSTI.**
- The Laboratory Risk Indicator for Necrotizing Fasciitis (LRINEC) score includes six variables (C-reactive protein, total white cell count, hemoglobin, serum sodium, creatinine, glucose) associated with NSTIs that are used to calculate a score, ranging from 0 to 13, that correlates with the magnitude of the risk. Recent studies indicate variable sensitivity for NSTI, especially in an emergency department setting.
- Plain radiographs can demonstrate subcutaneous emphysema, but this is a late finding and should not be used to rule out NSTI (Figure 10.2).

Figure 10.2 Plain radiograph of the foot demonstrating subcutaneous emphysema.

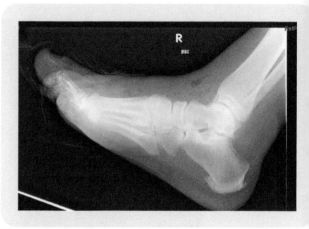

- Advanced imaging modalities such as CT and MRI can reveal fascial thickening, edema, fluid along the fascial planes, and subcutaneous emphysema. However, imaging should not delay surgical evaluation/ intervention.
- Point-of-care ultrasound (POCUS) revealing fluid collections along the deep fascia can aid in the diagnosis of NSTI but cobblestone appearance of cellulitis of the subcutaneous tissue can look similar. (Figure 10.3).
- **The gold standard for diagnosis remains surgical exploration** for direct visualization of the deep subcutaneous tissues with histological confirmation. If the diagnosis is equivocal, local exploration of the area/ fascia at the bedside under local anesthetic may reveal the diagnosis.
- The classic intraoperative finding is friable fascia, dishwater gray fluid (notably absent of pus), and tissue necrosis.

Critical Management

Critical Management Checklist
- ☑ **Adequate IV access**
- ☑ **IVF**
- ☑ **Blood cultures (should not delay antibiotic therapy)**
- ☑ **Surgical consultation and operative intervention**
- ☑ **Broad spectrum antibiotics including a protein synthesis inhibitor (clindamycin or linezolid)**
- ☑ **Vasopressors**

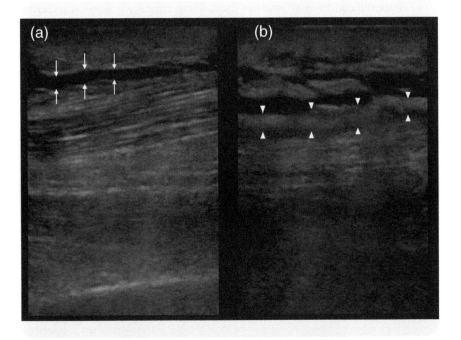

Figure 10.3 (a) Arrows indicate anechoic (black) fluid tracking along the echogenic (bright white) deep fascial plane. (b) Arrowheads delineate the thickened irregular fascia. In addition, anechoic fluid can be seen tracking along the deep fascial plane.

Glycemic control (insulin)

- Aggressive resuscitative measures should be initiated by placing two large-bore catheters and administering resuscitative intravenous fluids. Early aggressive therapy for sepsis caused by NSTI should be implemented when indicated per sepsis guidelines.
- **Antibiotic therapy should be initiated early with broad-spectrum coverage** of Gram-positive, Gram-negative, and anaerobic organisms. Clindamycin or linezolid inhibit protein synthesis, and should be added to decrease exotoxin production/release. Empiric regimens include: Vancomycin, piperacillin-tazobactam, and clindamycin; or linezolid and piperacillin-tazobactam.
- Vasopressor support can be started as necessary for hypotension refractory to fluid resuscitation. Exotoxins and toxins can have a direct myocardial depressant effect; some patients may require inotropic support.

- Glycemic control may improve mortality in critically ill surgical patients. It is reasonable to consider initiation of insulin early in management.
- Less well-studied are use of intravenous immunoglobulin (IVIG) and/or hyperbaric oxygen (HBO) for necrotizing fasciitis. IVIG has been investigated as adjunctive therapy for the extracellular toxins from group A Streptococcus. HBO has been studied with the mechanism thought to be enhanced oxygen delivery to infected, hypoxic tissues.

Sudden Deterioration

- POCUS may help in differentiating the etiology of shock, especially as a distributive picture may evolve to have a cardiogenic component.
  - Early and aggressive surgical debridement remains the key intervention.
  - Given the paucity of high-quality data, possibly consider cost/benefit tradeoff of adjunctive therapies as listed above (IVIG or HBO).

BIBLIOGRAPHY

Stevens DL, Bryant AE, Goldstein EJ. Necrotizing soft tissue infections. *Infect Dis Clin North Am* 2021;35(1):135–155. https://doi.org/10.1016/j.idc.2020.10.004

11

Complications of Human Immunodeficiency Virus (HIV) and Acquired Immunodeficiency Syndrome (AIDS)

ABEER ALMASARY AND ZUBAID RAFIQUE

Introduction

- Human immunodeficiency virus (HIV) pathophysiology is driven by the degree to which the patient is immunocompromised, reflected by the $CD4^+$ count roughly stratifying into three groups: > 500 cells/μL, 200–500 cells/μL, and < 200 cells/μL.
- Stages:
  - Viral transmission
  - Acute HIV infection (primary infection or acute seroconversion syndrome)

- ○ Chronic HIV infection, subdivided into:
  - ▪ Chronic without acquired immunodeficiency syndrome (AIDS): relative stability of the viral level and progressive decline in CD4 count. May manifest in nonspecific symptoms such as fatigue, sweats, or weight loss and persistent generalized lymphadenopathy.
  - ▪ AIDS: CD4 < 200 cells/ μL or the presence of any AIDS defining condition
  - ▪ Advanced HIV infection: CD4 < 50 cells/μL
- AIDS is defined as evidence of HIV infection with either a CD4 count < 200 cells/μL or at least one AIDS-defining illness (Table 11.1).
- AIDS is a reportable disease in all 50 states of the United States.

Table 11.1 AIDS-defining illnesses

Infections:

- ○ Pneumocystis jirovecii pneumonia (PCP)
- ○ Candidiasis: Esophageal, bronchial or tracheal,
- ○ Tuberculosis
- ○ Cytomegalovirus (CMV) disease (other than liver, spleen, or nodes), onset at age > 1 month, CMV retinitis (with loss of vision)
- ○ Recurrent bacterial pneumonia
- ○ Toxoplasmosis of brain
- ○ Chronic cryptosporidiosis intestinal
- ○ Disseminated histoplasmosis or extrapulmonary
- ○ Chronic herpes simplex: chronic ulcers or bronchitis, pneumonitis, or esophagitis
- ○ Coccidioidomycosis, disseminated or extrapulmonary
- ○ Cryptococcosis, extrapulmonary
- ○ Isosporiasis, chronic intestinal
- ○ Mycobacterium avium complex (MAC) or Mycobacterium kansasii, (or other species) disseminated or extrapulmonary
- ○ Salmonella septicemia, recurrent

- **Cancers**

Table 11.1 (*cont.*)

Infections:

o Kaposi sarcoma

o High-grade Non-Hodgkin's Lymphoma (NHL)

o Cervical cancer: Invasive cervical cancer

o Immunoblastic lymphoma

o Burkitt lymphoma (or equivalent term)

o Lymphoma, primary, of brain

● **Other:**

o Progressive multifocal leukoencephalopathy

o HIV-associated encephalopathy

o HIV-associated dementia

o Wasting syndrome

Presentation

- Primary HIV infection:
  - ○ **Acute seroconversion occurs 2–6 weeks** after initial exposure.
  - ○ Symptoms may include: fever, fatigue, lymphadenopathy, pharyngitis, diarrhea, weight loss, and rash.
- A number of complications can result from HIV and its progression to AIDS. The presentation of some of these complications is summarized in Table 11.2.

Diagnosis, Evaluation, and Critical Management

- **Enzyme-linked immunoassay (ELISA) or rapid HIV test followed by Western blot analysis for confirmation is the current gold standard for diagnosis of the condition**. If there is a discrepancy between ELISA and Western blot, further testing is warranted.

Table 11.2 Opportunistic infections in patients with HIV

Opportunistic infection	CD4 count (cells/μL)	Presentation	Diagnosis	Treatment
Cryptococcal infection	< 50	Fever, malaise, headache, meningoencephalitis	CSF analysis for cryptococcal antigen, elevated CSF pressure (> 20 mmH$_2$O), pleocytosis	Liposomal amphotericin B and Flucytosine Therapeutic LP to relieve intracranial pressure is effective
Cytomegalovirus retinitis	< 50	Decreased visual acuity, floaters, scotomata	Dilated fundus examination. CMV antigen level in serum and PCR can be positive before developing clinical features	Intravitreal Ganciclovir or Foscarnet and Valganciclovir
Mycobacterium avium complex	< 50	Cough, weight loss, fever, night sweats	AFB smear of blood, tissue or stool culture	Clarithromycin or azithromycin and ethambutol (may add rifabutin)
Toxoplasmosis	< 100	Headache, confusion, weakness, fever	Ring-enhancing lesions on CT or MRI, serum anti-toxo IgG, brain biopsy. CSF analysis and PCR	Pyrimethamine and Sulfadiazine or TMP-SMX
Aspergillosis	< 100	Fever, cough, dyspnea, chest pain, hemoptysis, hypoxemia	Isolation from respiratory secretions, CXR or CT with suggestive findings. Beta-D-glucan (sensitive) galactomannan (specific) are promising assays	Voriconazole, isavuconazonium sulfate or Posaconazole
Candida esophagitis	< 100	Odynophagia, retrosternal burning pain, white plaques	Plaques visualized with upper endoscopy, cultures	Fluconazole
Cryptococcal diarrhea	< 100	Nausea, vomiting, watery diarrhea, crampy abdominal pain	Stool studies for oocysts	Initiate ART. Consider Nitazoxanide

	CD4 count	Clinical features	Diagnosis	Treatment
Microsporidia diarrhea	< 100	Diarrhea, cholangitis, hepatitis	Light microscopy or small-bowel biopsy	Albendazole or Itraconazole
Bartonella	< 100	Cutaneous lesions, osteomyelitis, fever, night sweats, weight loss, peliosis hepatis	Tissue biopsy. Blood cultures may be unreliable	Doxycycline and Gentamicin or Rifampin
Histoplasma (disseminated)	< 200	Fever, fatigue, weight loss, hepatosplenomegaly, lymphadenopathy. Muco-cutaneous manifestations, abdominal pain, and diarrhea	Histoplasma antigens in blood or urine or BAL. Gold standard: staining and culture of all tissues or body fluids	Liposomal amphotericin B or Posaconazole
Candida albicans (thrush)	< 200	Painless white plaques	Clinical (plaques easily scrape off), light microscopy with KOH preparation	Fluconazole
Pneumocystis Jirovecii (PCP) pneumonia	< 200	Dyspnea, hypoxia, fever, nonproductive cough	CXR (diffuse interstitial infiltrates), BAL culture, sputum PCR	TMP-SMX. Consider steroids when hypoxia is present
Varicella zoster virus	Any but more commonly < 200	Typical rash (may have atypical pattern in immunocompromised patients)	Clinical diagnosis; swab open lesions for culture or PCR	Acyclovir or Valcyclovir (outpatient); Acyclovir IV (inpatient)
Salmonella, Shigella, Campylobacter	Any	Watery diarrhea, crampy abdominal pain, anorexia, malaise, fever	Stool studies	Ciprofloxacin or Levofloxacin or Azithromycin
Coccidiodomycosis	< 250	Diffuse pneumonia or meningitis	IgG study, specimen culture	Fluconazole, Itraconazole or amphotericin B
EB virus (oral hairy leukoplakia)	Any	Painless plaques along lateral tongue borders	Unable to scrape off; biopsy	Initiate ART. Consider steroids

Table 11.2 (cont.)

Opportunistic infection	CD4 count (cells/µL)	Presentation	Diagnosis	Treatment
Mycobacterium tuberculosis	Any	Cough, hemoptysis, weight loss, fever, night sweats	CXR, AFB smear	Isoniazid and Rifampin and Pyrazinamide and Ethambutol Consider dexamethasone for CNS infection. Consider consulting Infectious Disease prior to treatment initiation.
Streptococcal pneumonia	Any	Fever, chills, rigors, productive cough with purulent sputum, dyspnea	CXR	Antibiotic choice same as non-HIV patients; Beta-lactam and macrolide (always dual therapy)
JC virus (PML)	Any	Altered mental status, speech disturbances, visual deficits, discoordination	MRI shows hypodense white matter lesions, CSF analysis for JC virus by PCR	ART and cidofovir
Talaromycosis (formerly known as Penicilliosis; not common in the US)	< 100	Disseminated disease with fever, weight loss, hepatosplenomegaly lymphadenopathy, abdominal pain, and diarrhea. Skin and genital lesions	Culture, histopathology, ELISA and PCR	Liposomal amphotericin B or Itraconazole (mild disease)

AFB: acid-fast bacillus; ART: antiretroviral therapy; BAL: bronchoalveolar lavage; CSF: cerebrospinal fluid; CT: computed tomography; CXR: chest radiograph; EBV: Epstein–Barr virus; IgG: immunoglobulin G; JC: John Cunningham; KOH: potassium hydroxide; MRI: magnetic resonance imaging; PCR: polymerase chain reaction; PML: progressive multifocal leukoencephalopathy; TMP: trimethoprim; SMX: sulfamethoxazole; IV: intravenous.

- If patient is not already taking antiretroviral therapy (ART), this should be initiated in consultation with an HIV specialist.
- Opportunistic infections should be evaluated according to Table 11.2.

Sudden Deterioration

- In the deteriorating patient with HIV/AIDS, the usual considerations of *a*irway, *b*reathing, and *c*irculation (ABC) should be assessed and supported.
- Broad-spectrum antimicrobials should be initiated with additional coverage for suspected opportunistic infections (Table 11.2).
- Medication side effects and drug interactions can cause organ dysfunction, cardiac arrhythmias, or electrolyte abnormalities, and offending agents should be stopped.
- **Immune reconstitution inflammatory syndrome (IRIS)** should be considered.
  - IRIS is a constellation of symptoms characterized by fever and worsening of the clinical manifestations of the underlying opportunistic infection after starting ART.
  - In this condition, the immune system begins to recover after the initiation of ART and starts responding to the opportunistic infection with an excessive inflammatory response that is worse than the initial symptoms.
  - It is **typically seen within the first 4–8 weeks after initiation of ART**, and most commonly with mycobacterial infections.
  - It is a clinically challenging diagnosis since the differentiation from progression of the initial opportunistic infection, the development of a new opportunistic infection, an unrelated organ dysfunction, or drug toxicity cannot be easily made.
  - Patients should receive supportive care. **Systemic corticosteroids should be considered** after consultation with an infectious disease specialist.
- **Special considerations for the pregnant patient**
  - **Immediate initiation of ART** should be considered when opportunistic infections are diagnosed in pregnant patients. **This can minimize transmission of disease to the fetus**.
- **System-specific complications and special considerations**
  - *Central nervous system:*
    - Reported complications: encephalitis, seizure, lymphoma, meningitis, myelopathy, myopathy, space-occupying lesions and infections.

- Altered mental status should be worked up. Appropriate brain imaging to evaluate for mass-occupying lesions, and lumbar puncture to evaluate for opportunistic infections.
- Broad-spectrum antibiotics, antivirals, and antifungals should be started if there is suspicion for meningitis in the setting of a low CD4 count.
  - *Pulmonary:*
    - Reported complications: pneumonia, tuberculosis, PJP-related pneumothorax, fungal infections, and HIV-associated pulmonary arterial hypertension.
    - A chest radiograph (CXR) may be nonspecific. A chest computer tomography (CT) should be considered in the setting of hypoxia or dyspnea with non-diagnostic CXR.
- *Cardiovascular:*
  - Reported complications: pericardial effusion, dilated cardiomyopathy, myocarditis, coronary artery disease, endocarditis.
  - An electrocardiogram and troponin analysis should be performed if the patient presents with chest pain.
  - Consider bedside ultrasonography to evaluate for pericardial effusion left ventricular contractility in the patient presenting with heart failure symptoms.
- *Gastrointestinal:*
  - Reported complications: infectious colitis and gastroenteritis esophagitis, pancreatitis, pancreatic exocrine insufficiency, AIDS cholangiopathy, infiltrative hepatobiliary and pancreatic infection, and liver failure.
  - Check for hepatitis B and C co-infections.
- *Renal:*
  - Reported complications: HIV nephropathy, acute kidney injury, and chronic kidney disease.
  - Stop all nephrotoxic medications and hydrate the patient.
  - Certain antiretroviral drugs are associated with nephrolithiasis and should be avoided.
  - Decreased renal function and proteinuria are associated with increased mortality.
- *Metabolic and endocrine:*
  - Reported complications: disorders of hypothalamic-pituitary-adrenal and gonadal axes.

- *Genital tract*:
  - ○ Elevated rates of human papillomavirus infection, increasing the risk of anogenital tract dysplasia. Outpatient screening for cervical cancer for women is recommended within 1 year of the onset of sexual activity and before the age of 21.

BIBLIOGRAPHY

AIDSinfo. Guidelines for the use of antiretroviral agents in HIV-1-infected adults and adolescents [Internet]. 2011 [updated March 27, 2012]. Available from: https://clinicalinfo.hiv.gov/en/guidelines [last accessed February 15, 2023).

Ayoade F, Chandranesan JAS. HIV-1 associated toxoplasmosis. In: StatPearls [Internet]. Treasure Island, FL: StatPearls Publishing; 2021. Available from: www.ncbi.nlm.nih.gov/books/NBK441877/ [last accessed February 15, 2023].

Centers for Disease Control and Prevention. 1993 Revised classification system for HIV infection and expanded surveillance case definition for AIDS among adolescents and adults. *JAMA* 1993;269:729–730.

Chu C, Pollock LC, Selwyn PA. HIV-associated complications: A systems-based approach. *Am Fam Physician* 2017;96(3):161–169. https://pubmed.ncbi.nlm.nih.gov/28762691/

Kaplan JE, Benson C, Holmes KK, et al. Guidelines for prevention and treatment of opportunistic infections in HIV-infected adults and adolescents: Recommendations from CDC, the National Institutes of Health, and the HIV Medicine Association of the Infectious Diseases Society of America. *MMWR Recomm Rep* 2009;58(RR-4):1–207.

Limper AH, Adenis A, Le T, et al. Fungal infections in HIV/AIDS. *Lancet Infect Dis* 2017;17 (11):e334–e343. https://doi.org/10.1016/s1473-3099(17)30303-1

Marco CA, Rothman RE. HIV infection and complications in emergency medicine. *Emerg Med Clin North Am* 2008;26:367–387.

Marochi-Telles JP, Muniz R Jr, Sztajnbok J, et al. Disseminated mycobacterium avium on HIV/AIDS: Historical and current literature review. *Aids Revs* 2020;22(1). https://doi.org/10.24875/aidsrev.20000104

Munro M, Yadavalli T, Fonteh C, et al. Cytomegalovirus retinitis in HIV and non-HIV individuals. *Microorganisms* 2019;8(1). https://doi.org/10.3390/microorganisms8010055

Sarwar M, Gardezi SAH, Zaman G, et al. Evaluation of galactomannan and beta-d-glucan assays for the diagnosis of invasive aspergillosis in clinically suspected cases. *J Pak Med Assoc* 2020;70(3):442–446. https://doi.org/10.5455/JPMA.1476

Shiels MS, Engels EA. Evolving epidemiology of HIV-associated malignancies. *Curr Opin HIV AIDS* 2017;12(1):6–11. https://doi.org/10.1097/COH.0000000000000327

Venkat A, Piontkowsky DM, Cooney RR, et al. Care of the HIV-positive patient in the emergency department in the era of highly active antiretroviral therapy. *Ann Emerg Med* 2008;52:274–285.

Wood B, Sax, & Mitty J. The natural history and clinical features of HIV infection in adults and adolescents. Published March 8, 2021. Available from: www.uptodate.com/contents/the-natural-history-and-clinical-features-of-hiv-infection-in-adults-and-adolescents/print [last accessed February 15, 2023].

1993 revised classification system for HIV infection and expanded surveillance case definition for AIDS among adolescents and adults. *MMWR Recomm Rep* 1992;41(RR-17):1–19.

SECTION 3

Neurological Emergencies

MICHAEL COCCHI

12

Ischemic Strokes

JOSHUA W. JOSEPH

Chapter 12:

Ischemic Stroke

Presentation

Classic Presentation: Constellation of neurological symptoms including but not limited to: ataxia, aphasia, visual deficits, facial weakness, sensory and motor deficits, apraxia, vestibular symptoms, incontinence, and cranial nerve palsies.

Critical Presentation: AMS and subsequent airway compromise.

Diagnosis and Evaluation

Thorough history to determine eligibility for thrombolysis.

Physical exam guided by National Institutes of Health Stroke Scale.

ECG.

Non-contrast head CT to exclude intracranial hemhorrhage.

⚙ *MRI most sensitive if available, but should not delay tPA administration in eligible patients.*

Labwork: Glucose, CBC, BMP, coagulation studies, and serial cardiac enzymes.

Management

Airway managment and hemodynamic monitoring.

Maintain oxygen saturation ≤ 94%, with supplemental oxygen as necessary.

Consult neurology.

 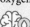

Careful consideration of eligibility for throm-bolysis; if appropriate, administer tPA.

Sudden deterioration may indicate intracranial hemorrhage.

⚠ *Stop tPA infusion, check pupillary reflex, repeat non-contrast head CT.*

Goal blood glucose: 140–180 mg/dL.

Blood pressure managment *(i.e. labetalol, nicardipine).*

⚠ *tPA candidates: Begin antihypertensives when systolic BP ≥ 185 mmHg and/or diastolic BP ≥ 110.*

⚠ *non-tPA candidates: Begin antihypertensives when systolic BP ≥ 220 mmHg and/or diastolic BP ≥ 120.*

Introduction

- Cerebrovascular accident (CVA) or stroke is an interruption of blood supply due to **thrombosis** or **embolization.**
- Thrombosis is caused by an in-situ clot at a site of atherosclerotic plaque.
- Embolization is caused by an intravascular embolus. Sources include atrial fibrillation, ventricular aneurysm, hypokinetic ventricle, myocardial infarction, prosthetic valve, infective endocarditis, and proximal friable atherosclerotic plaques.

Presentation

Classic Presentation

- Middle cerebral artery syndrome
  - The **most common** stroke syndrome
  - Contralateral hemiplegia of the upper extremity > the lower extremity
  - Facial hemiplegia
  - Dominant hemisphere: aphasia
  - Nondominant hemisphere: inattention, neglect, apraxia
  - Contralateral homonymous hemianopia: eyes point toward side of lesion
- Anterior cerebral artery syndrome (less common, accounting for approximately 0.6–3% of acute ischemic strokes)
  - Contralateral hemiplegia and sensory neglect of the lower extremity > the upper extremity
  - Apraxia
  - Mutism and/or aphasia
- Posterior cerebral artery syndrome
  - Homonymous hemianopia
  - Patient unaware of defect (visual agnosia)
  - Third nerve palsy
  - Sensation deficits (pinprick, light touch)
- Vertebrobasilar artery syndrome
  - Ipsilateral cranial nerve palsy and contralateral hemiplegia
  - Ipsilateral facial paresthesia, vertigo, Horner syndrome, dysphagia, and dysphonia

- ○ Contralateral sensory deficits (pain and temperature)
- ○ Abnormal gait and cerebellar coordination testing
- Basilar artery occlusion
  - ○ Quadriplegia
  - ○ Coma
  - ○ Locked-in syndrome
- Cerebellar infarction
  - ○ Ataxia
  - ○ Can have headache, central vertigo, nausea, and vomiting
  - ○ Herniation from edema may manifest as decreased level of consciousness, abnormal respiratory pattern, and pupillary dilation
- Lacunar syndromes
  - ○ Pure motor stroke (most common)
  - ○ Pure sensory stroke
  - ○ Clumsy hand-dysarthria syndrome

Critical Presentation

- Patients may present with altered mental status or airway compromise requiring immediate treatment.

Diagnosis and Evaluation

- **History** is important in identifying:
  - ○ Time last *witnessed* "normal," establishing time of onset of CVA
    - ▪ Patients waking from sleep with stroke symptoms are considered "normal" when last witnessed at their baseline while awake.
- Exclusion criteria for thrombolytics (Table 12.1).
- **Physical examination**
  - ○ National Institutes of Health Stroke Scale (NIHSS) (Table 12.2).
- **Ancillary testing**
  - ○ Bedside glucose
  - ○ Complete blood count, electrolyte panel and coagulation profile
  - ○ ECG, as cardiac abnormalities are prevalent in stroke patients
  - ○ Serial cardiac enzymes (i.e., troponin)
- **Imaging**
  - ○ Noncontrast head CT: can be normal in the first 24 hours, especially in the first 3 hours from presentation

Table 12.1 Indications for thrombolytics (tPA)

These statements must be true in order to consider systemic tPA administration:

1. Ischemic stroke onset within 3 hours, or in certain cases within 4.5 hours

2. Measurable deficit on NIH Stroke Scale examination

3. CT does not show hemorrhage or non-stroke cause of deficit

4. Patient's age is > 18 years

Contraindications to thrombolytics (tPA)

Do NOT administer tPA if any of these statements are true:

1. Patient's symptoms are minor (NIHSS < 5) and nondisabling

2. Patient has had another stroke or serious head trauma within the past 3 months

3. Patient has known history of intracranial hemorrhage

4. Patient has known intracranial neoplasm, AVM, or aneurysm

5. Recent intracranial or intraspinal surgery

6. Patient has sustained systolic blood pressure > 185 mmHg

7. Patient has sustained diastolic blood pressure > 110 mmHg

8. Imaging shows evidence of subarachnoid hemorrhage

9. Active internal bleeding

10. Blood glucose concentration < 50 mg/dL (2.7 mmol/L) – if corrected and otherwise, eligible, may be reasonable

11. CT demonstrates large infarction (hypodensity > 1/3 cerebral hemisphere)

12. Active bleeding diathesis, including:

   - Patient has received heparin within the last 48 hours and has elevated PTT
   - Patient's prothrombin time (PT) is > 15 seconds or INR > 1.7
   - Patient's platelet count is < 100, 000
   - Direct thrombin inhibitor or direct factor Xa inhibitor use

Relative contraindications to thrombolytics (tPA)

1. Patient has a large stroke with NIH Stroke Scale score > 22

2. Seizure at onset with postictal residual neurological impairments

Table 12.1 (*cont.*)

These statements must be true in order to consider systemic tPA administration:
3. Major surgery or serious trauma within previous 14 days
4. Recent gastrointestinal or urinary tract hemorrhage (within previous 21 days)
5. Recent acute myocardial infarction (within previous 3 months)
6. Pregnancy
7. Patient has had arterial puncture at noncompressible site within the last 7 days

Additional warnings to consider

1. Age > 80 years

2. History of prior stroke *and* diabetes

3. Any anticoagulant use prior to admission (even if INR < 1.7)

4. NIHSS > 25

- o MRI: more sensitive than CT during the immediate period, but is more time consuming to obtain and less available emergently at most institutions.
- o CTA/MRA: used to identify large-vessel occlusions in patients presenting between 6 and 24 hours from symptom onset to identify candidates for endovascular therapy and a potential extended window (4.5–9.0 hours) for thrombolysis as guidelines evolve

Critical Management

Critical Management Checklist

☑ Airway management as needed

☑ Oxygen

☑ IV access

☑ Cardiac monitors

☑ Fingerstick blood glucose test

☑ Noncontrast head CT

☑ Neurology consultation

☑ Thrombolytics (if meet all criteria)

☑ Blood pressure control

☑ Glucose control

☑ Temperature control

Table 12.2 NIH Stroke Scale

1a. Level of consciousness:
Alertness and response to stimuli

1. **Alert**; keenly responsive.

2. **Not alert**, but arousable by minor stimulation to obey, answer, or respond.

3. **Not alert**; requires repeated stimulation to attend, or is obtunded and requires strong or painful stimulation to make movements (not stereotyped).

4. Responds only with reflex motor or autonomic effects or is totally unresponsive, flaccid, and areflexic

1b. LOC questions:
The month and patient's age

1. **Answers** both questions correctly.

2. **Answers** one question correctly.

3. **Answers** neither question correctly.

1c. LOC commands:
Opening and closing eyes, opening and closing non-paretic hand

1. **Performs** both tasks correctly.

2. **Performs** one task correctly.

3. **Performs** neither task correctly.

2. Best gaze:
Horizontal eye movements

1. Normal.

2. **Partial gaze palsy**; gaze is abnormal in one or both eyes, but forced deviation or total gaze paresis is not present.

3. **Forced deviation**, or total gaze paresis not overcome by the oculocephalic maneuver.

3. Visual:
Test visual fields to confrontation

1. **No visual loss.**

2. **Partial hemianopia.**

3. **Complete hemianopia.**

4. Bilateral hemianopia (blind including cortical blindness).

Table 12.2 (cont.)

4. Facial Palsy: Ask patient to show teeth, open/close eyes	1. **Normal** symmetrical movements.
	2. **Minor paralysis** (flattened nasolabial fold, asymmetry on smiling).
	3. **Partial paralysis** (total or near-total paralysis of lower face).
	4. **Complete paralysis** of one or both sides (absence of facial movement in the upper and lower face).
5. Motor Arm: Extend arm, test for drift	1. **No drift**; limb holds 90 (or 45) degrees for full 10 seconds.
5a. Left Arm	2. **Drift**; limb holds 90 (or 45) degrees, but drifts down before full 10 seconds; does not hit bed or other support.
5b. Right Arm	3. **Some effort against gravity**; limb cannot get to or maintain (if cued) 90 (or 45) degrees, drifts down to bed, but has some effort against gravity.
	4. **No effort against gravity**; limb falls.
	5. **No movement.** UN = Amputation or joint fusion
6. Motor Leg: Extend leg, test for drift	1. **No drift**; leg holds 30-degree position for full 5 seconds.
6a. Left Leg	2. **Drift**; leg falls by the end of the 5-second period but does not hit bed.
6b. Right Leg	3. **Some effort against gravity**; leg falls to bed by 5 seconds, but has some effort against gravity.
	4. **No effort against gravity**; leg falls to bed immediately.
	5. **No movement.** UN = Amputation or joint fusion

Table 12.2 (*cont.*)

7. **Limb Ataxia**: Finger–nose and heel–shin tests	1. Absent. 2. Present in one limb. 3. Present in two limbs. UN = Amputation or joint fusion
8. **Sensory**: Sensation to pinprick, withdrawal to noxious stimuli	1. **Normal**; no sensory loss. 2. **Mild-to-moderate sensory loss**; patient feels pinprick is less sharp or is dull on the affected side; or there is a loss of superficial pain with pinprick, but patient is aware of being touched. 3. **Severe to total sensory loss**; patient is not aware of being touched in the face, arm, and leg.
9. **Best Language**: Patient is asked to describe a standard picture, name objects, read sentences	1. **No aphasia**; normal. 2. **Mild-to-moderate aphasia**; some obvious loss of fluency or facility of comprehension, without significant limitation on ideas expressed or form of expression. Examiner can identify picture or naming card content from patient's response. 3. **Severe aphasia**; all communication is through fragmentary expression; great need for inference, questioning, and guessing by the listener. Examiner cannot identify materials provided from patient response. 4. **Mute, global aphasia**; no usable speech or auditory comprehension.

Table 12.2 (*cont.*)

10. **Dysarthria:** Patient reads/repeats words	1. Normal.
	2. **Mild-to-moderate dysarthria**; patient slurs at least some words and, at worst, can be understood with some difficulty.
	3. **Severe dysarthria;** patient's speech is so slurred as to be unintelligible in the absence of or out of proportion to any dysphasia, or is mute/anarthric. UN = Intubated or other physical barrier
11. **Extinction and inattention:** Extinction to bilateral visual/sensory stimuli	1. **No abnormality.**
	2. **Visual, tactile, auditory, spatial, or personal inattention** or extinction to bilateral simultaneous stimulation in one of the sensory modalities.
	3. **Profound hemi-inattention or extinction** to more than one modality; does not recognize own hand or orients to only one side of space.

Sentences for Best Language Task:	**Words for Dysarthria Task:**
You know how.	MAMA
Down to earth.	TIP-TOP
I got home from work.	FIFTY-FIFTY
Near the table in the dining room.	THANKS
They heard him speak on the radio last night.	HUCKLEBERRY
	BASEBALL PLAYER

- If the patient is not protecting his/her airway due to neurological deficits or level of consciousness, **intubation** will be required. If possible, try to assess the neurological examination prior to intubation.
- Supplemental **oxygen** is only necessary in patients with oxygen saturation ≤94%.
- Patient should be placed on a **cardiac monitor** for evaluation of atrial fibrillation or other cardiac arrhythmias.
- After **fingerstick blood glucose** (to assess for hypoglycemia), obtain a STAT **noncontrast head CT**. Head CT will exclude intracranial hemorrhage as the etiology of the patient's presentation and is essential before consideration of intravenous thrombolytic therapy.
- Additional diagnostic testing **should not delay tPA administration in eligible patients** without suspected coagulopathy.
- **Neurology consultation** should be obtained early in the patient's presentation.
- Consider **systemic thrombolysis** for those patients meeting criteria for tissue plasminogen activator (tPA) and presenting within 3–4.5 hours of symptom onset (Table 12.1).
  - Dose 0.9 mg/kg, maximum 90 mg:
    - 10% of the dose is given as an initial bolus over 1 minute.
    - Remainder of the dose is infused over 60 minutes.

  Placement of arterial catheters, indwelling urinary catheters, and nasogastric tubes should be avoided for at least 24 hours if the patient can be safely managed without.

  Admit the patient to an intensive care unit setting.
- **Blood pressure monitoring** is essential for maintaining brain perfusion and decreasing the risk of conversion to hemorrhagic stroke.
  - *For tPA candidates*
    - Begin treatment at systolic BP ≥ 185 mmHg and/or diastolic BP ≥ 110 mmHg. Consider labetalol IV push or nicardipine infusion.
    - If blood pressure does not decline and remains ≥ 185/110 mmHg, do not administer tPA.
    - During infusion, monitor blood pressure every 15 minutes, more frequently if the blood pressure is ≥ 185/110.

- ○ *For those excluded from tPA administration*, permissive hypertension is allowed.
  - ▪ Begin hypertensive treatment at systolic BP $\geq$ 220 mmHg and/or diastolic BP $\geq$ 120 mmHg.
  - ▪ Consider nicardipine, labetalol, esmolol, or enalaprilat for BP control.
  - ▪ The goal is BP reduction of ~15% during the first 24 hours after onset.
- • **Blood glucose control** should be maintained with a goal of **140–180 mg/dL.**
- • Normothermia should be targeted; patients with **fever** should be given antipyretics.

Sudden Deterioration

- • The most likely cause of sudden decompensation is **intracranial hemorrhage** during tPA administration or increased **intracranial pressure** due to cerebral edema.
- • Signs and symptoms include new/worsening neurological deficits, nausea/vomiting, severe headache, acute hypertension, or decreased level of consciousness.
- • If any of these develop during infusion, immediately stop the infusion. Check pupillary response and obtain a repeat noncontrast head CT. Recommendations vary, but consider TXA, cryoprecipitate and fresh frozen plasma.
- • If there is concern for increased intracranial pressure:
  - ○ Begin medical management with hyperosmolar therapy, elevating the head of the bed to 30°, keeping the jugular neck veins straight, treating fever, pain, and agitation.
  - ○ Hyperventilation is not recommended except as a bridge to decompressive therapy, as it reduces ICP by reducing cerebral blood flow, which can worsen infarction.
  - ○ The goal should be to maintain normocarbia while minimizing excessive positive end-expiratory pressure (PEEP). Increased PEEP can lower venous return to the heart, leading to reduced cardiac output and worsening cerebral perfusion.
  - ○ Consult **neurosurgery** for consideration of cerebral fluid drainage or decompressive surgery. This can be pivotal during cerebellar infarcts or massive hemispheric infarcts.

BIBLIOGRAPHY

Demaerschalk BM, Kleindorfer DO, Adeoye OM, et al. Scientific rationale for the inclusion and exclusion criteria for intravenous alteplase in acute ischemic stroke: A statement for healthcare professionals from the American Heart Association/American Stroke Association. *Stroke* 2016;47(2):581–641.

Ma H, Campbell BC, Parsons MW, et al. Thrombolysis guided by perfusion imaging up to 9 hours after onset of stroke. *New Engl J Med* 2019;380(19):1795–1803.

National Institutes of Health. NIH Stroke Scale. Bethesda, MD: National Institutes of Health, National Institute of Neurological Disorders and Stroke; 2013. Available from: http://stroke.nih.gov/documents/NIH_Stroke_Scale.pdf [last accessed February 15, 2023].

Phipps MS, Cronin CA. Management of acute ischemic stroke. *BMJ* 2020;368.

Powers WJ. Acute ischemic stroke. *New Engl J Med* 2020;383(3):252–260.

Powers WJ, Rabinstein AA, Ackerson T, et al. Guidelines for the early management of patients with acute ischemic stroke: 2019 update to the 2018 guidelines for the early management of acute ischemic stroke: A guideline for healthcare professionals from the American Heart Association/American Stroke Association. *Stroke* 2019;50(12):e344–e418.

13

Intracranial Hemorrhage

MATTHEW L. WONG AND JOSHUA W. JOSEPH

Chapter 13:
Intracranial Hemorrhage

Includes:

- subarachnoid hemorrhage
- epidural hematoma
- subdural hematoma
- intracerebral hemorrhage

 Presentation

Varies widely according to location and severity.

Aneurysmal subarachnoid hemorrhage may present as thunderclap headache.

Patients with epidural hemorrhage may have a lucid interval.

Patient may have history of trauma or use of anticoagulants.

 Diagnosis and Evaluation

Imaging: CT.

✿ *Negative head CT not sufficient to rule out aneurysmal SAH after 6 hours from symptom onset, LP is indicated.*

Labwork: CBC, coagulation studies, serum glucose, type and screen, urine pregnancy, consider cardiac enzymes/ECG and toxicology.

Chapter 13:
Intracranial Hemorrhage

 Management

Airway management.

- *Beware! Laryngeal manipulation may transiently increase ICP.*
- *Goal PaCO2 35–40 mmHg.*

ICP Control

- *Consider use of osmotic diuretics (i.e. mannitol, hypertonic saline) as a temporizing measure prior to surigical intervention/invasive ICP monitoring.*

Blood Pressure Control.

- *Consider nicardipine, clevidipine, or labetalol.*
- *aSAH.*
  + *Goal SBP: < 160 mmHg, goal MAP: < 110 mmHg.*
  + *Administer nimodipine.*
- *Spontaneous intracerebral hemhorrage with presenting SBP 150–220 mmHg.*
  + *Goal SBP: < 140 mmHg.*
- *Spontaneous intracerebral. hemhorrage with presenting SBP > 220mmHg.*
  + *Goal SBP: 140–160 mmHg.*

Anticoagulation reversal.

Invasive ICP monitoring.

Sudden deterioration likely due to acutely increased ICP.

Goal CPP **> 60 mmHg**

$$CPP = MAP - ICP$$

Introduction

- Intracranial hemorrhage (ICH) occurs when blood occupies space within the calvarium.
- ICH irritates brain parenchyma and impairs outflow of cerebral spinal fluid (CSF) from the dural sinus venous network, which raises intracranial pressure (ICP) with a resultant decrease in cerebral perfusion.
- ICH types are defined by the location of the bleeding: intracerebral (within the parenchyma), epidural (between the skull and the dura), subdural (between the dura and arachnoid membrane) and subarachnoid (between arachnoid membrane and pia mater).
- The skull is inelastic so blood accumulation increases intracranial pressure.
- Cerebral blood flow is modulated by vascular resistance. Cerebral perfusion pressure (CPP) is the difference between mean arterial pressure (MAP) and ICP.

$$CPP = MAP - ICP (normal\ CPP = 50 - 70mmHg)$$

- Blood has several effects on surrounding tissues: inflammation, edema, and irritation (vasospasm, thrombosis, and seizures). Intraventricular hemorrhage may block CSF flow and cause an acute noncommunicating hydrocephalus.
- There are several types of intracranial hemorrhage, and diagnostic and therapeutic approaches differ (Table 13.1).
- *Subarachnoid hemorrhage (SAH)*
  - SAH that results from trauma is considered a form of traumatic brain injury (TBI) and is covered in a separate chapter.
  - Non-traumatic SAH is considered a form of stroke, and has a mortality rate approaching 45%.
  - The most common and feared cause of non-traumatic SAH is a ruptured cerebral aneurysm, but it may also result from venous bleeding.
- *Subdural hemorrhage (SDH)*
  - SDH is classically from shearing of the bridging veins that extravasate into the space between the arachnoid and dura.
  - The majority of SDHs are acute and managed as a TBI.
  - SDH is a common injury of the elderly with even minor mechanisms of head injury.

Table 13.1 Types of intracranial hemorrhage categorized by location

Type	Location
Subarachnoid hemorrhage	The potential space between the arachnoid and pia mater
Subdural hematoma	The potential space between the dura and arachnoid membrane
Epidural hematoma	The space between skull and the dura
Intracerebral hemorrhage	Brain parenchyma

- ○ SDH can also be caused by low CSF pressure, such as in those with significant brain atrophy or iatrogenically after a procedure.
- *Epidural hemorrhage (EDH)*
  - ○ Epidural hematomas most often form secondary traumatic injury to the meningeal arteries.
  - ○ If the condition is recognized and treated early, the prognosis is excellent.
  - ○ About 50% of patients have a "lucid interval," which is a window of consciousness that occurs between an initial transient loss of consciousness and eventual coma.
- *Intracerebral hemorrhage (ICH)*
  - ○ ICH as the result of trauma is also known as a contusion, and is better classified and managed as a form of traumatic brain injury.
  - ○ Non-traumatic, or spontaneous, intracerebral hemorrhage is considered a form of stroke, and has very high morbidity and mortality.
  - ○ The most common causes of spontaneous ICH are hypertensive arteriopathy, cerebral amyloid angiopathy, hemorrhagic conversion of ischemic stroke, cerebral venous sinus thrombosis, tumors, arteriovenous malformation, cavernous angiomas, posterior reversible encephalopathy syndrome, and vasculitis.

Presentation

Classic and Critical Presentation

- Patient presentation varies widely depending on location and extent of the hemorrhage.

- The classic presentation of aneurysmal SAH (aSAH) is the sudden onset of "the worst headache of one's life." SAH is the most common life-threatening cause of such "thunderclap headaches."

Diagnosis and Evaluation

- **Radiology**
  - CT is the cornerstone imaging modality for all forms of intracranial hemorrhage. Though it may eventually be used, MRI is not a practical initial test of choice.
  - For aSAH, a noncontrast head CT is highly sensitive if performed within 6 hours of symptom onset. Lumbar puncture (LP) following an early negative CT is often not performed, though some pursue an LP to evaluate for presence of RBCs and xanthochromia.
  - A negative head CT is not sensitive enough to rule out aSAH after 6 hours from symptom onset and LP is still indicated.
- **Laboratory tests**
  - Serum glucose as hypoglycemia can mimic the signs and symptoms of intracranial hemorrhage
  - Coagulation studies, and complete blood count to identify coagulopathy and thrombocytopenia.
  - Troponin and an EKG if there is concern about cardiac complications.
  - Type and screen/cross-matched blood products
  - Consider toxicology screens.
  - Pregnancy test as needed.

Critical Management

Critical Management Checklist

☑ Airway
☑ Blood pressure/cerebral perfusion pressure
☑ Anticoagulation reversal
☑ Intracranial pressure management

- **Securing the airway**
  - Laryngeal manipulation transiently increases ICP. Consider an awake technique with topical anesthesia.

- Utilize hemodynamically neutral induction agent dosing (often lower than cited dose recommendations are appropriate in the critically ill).
- Nondepolarizing neuromuscular blockers do not cause muscle contraction but have longer durations of action. ICH patients need frequent neurological exams, so if rocuronium is used, sugammadex should be available for reversal.
- Adequate sedation prevents agitation and subsequent elevations in ICP.
- Mechanical ventilation settings should be adjusted to a goal $PaCO_2$ of 35–40 mmHg to prevent cerebral vasodilation and elevations in ICP.
- Avoid hyperoxemia and target normal SpO_2 or PaO_2.

- **Blood pressure control**
  - Hypertension in ICH may be associated with hematoma expansion (as in epidural, subdural, or spontaneous intracerebral hematoma) or rebleeding of an unsecured aneurysm (as in aneurysmal SAH).
  - In cases of **spontaneous intracerebral hemorrhage**, the recommended target blood pressure depends on their presenting blood pressure. For patients whose presenting systolic blood pressure is 150–220 mmHg, medications should be used to decrease the blood pressure to less than 140 mmHg. For patients whose presenting systolic blood pressure is greater than 220 mmHg, their blood pressure should be reduced to a range of 140–160 mmHg.
  - In cases of **aneurysmal SAH**, until the aneurysm is surgically controlled, a systolic blood pressure of less than 160 mmHg, a MAP less than 110 mmHg, or both, should be targeted.
  - Consider nicardipine, clevidipine, or labetalol for blood pressure control agents. Nitroprusside is generally avoided given potential to increase ICP. Hydralazine may cause reflex tachycardia.
  - Nimodipine should be administered to all patients with aSAH to prevent vasospasm (oral or NGT).
  - Pain relief and control of nausea should also be addressed.
  - Patients with traumatic brain injury, which includes EDH, SDH, non-traumatic ICH, and non-traumatic SAH, depend on the balance between MAP and ICP to maintain CPP goals typically > 60 mmHg.
  - Consider arterial line insertion to help monitor all patients requiring anti-hypertensive drips or pressors for MAP management.

- **Anticoagulation reversal** (Table 13.2)
  - Reversal of anticoagulation can prevent hematoma expansion and improve clinical outcomes (see Table 13.2).

Table 13.2 Reversal of anticoagulation

Medication	Reversal agent
Warfarin	Vitamin K
	Fresh frozen plasma
	Prothrombin complex concentrates
Aspirin/Clopidogrel	Platelets
	DDAVP
Heparin/Enoxaparin	Protamine
Direct Acting Oral Anticoagulants	Prothromin complex concentrates
	Andexanet alfa
	Idarucizumab

- **ICP management**
  - ○ Elevate the head of the bed to 30° to promote venous drainage from the head to reduce ICP.
  - ○ Maintain the head in a midline position to ensure drainage of the neck veins.
  - ○ Empiric treatment for presumed herniation includes use of osmotic agents to reduce cerebral edema. These are purely temporizing measures until invasive ICP monitoring is established to guide therapy, or until surgical interventions become available.
    - ▪ *Mannitol* is an osmotic diuretic to draw hypotonic fluid (edema) into the hypertonic intravascular space. Use with caution in patients with low MAP, as well as in patients with renal failure.
    - ▪ *Hypertonic saline* is generally not associated with hypotension unless infused rapidly. There are various concentrations of hypertonic saline with dosing regimens that may be chosen based on the clinical scenario. Ultimately, close monitoring of serum sodium levels and serum osmolarity dictates infusion volume.
- **Invasive ICP monitoring** is crucial for aggressive management of patients with presumed ICP elevations.
  - ○ Extraventricular drains (EVDs) allow real-time ICP monitoring while allowing drainage of CSF to help lower ICP.
  - ○ Other devices including Camino bolts and intraparenchymal pressure catheters can also be used for ICP monitoring but do not offer the option of draining CSF to lower ICP.

- **General neurointensive care**
  - ○ Patients should be evaluated for other active underlying medical issues, such as myocardial infarction, renal failure, rhabdomyolysis, or DKA.
  - ○ Blood sugars should be managed to avoid hypoglycemia and hyperglycemia.
  - ○ Patients should be maintained at normothermia; avoid fever.
  - ○ Seizure prophylaxis depends on the underlying cause of the hemorrhage and local practices.

Sudden Deterioration

- Sudden deterioration may represent acutely increased ICP.
- Temporize ICP changes, avoid secondary insults (e.g., hypoxia and hypotension), and protect CPP (vasopressors as needed) while expediting neurosurgical evaluation for possible life-saving surgical intervention.
- Secure the airway and use osmotic agents like mannitol or hypertonic saline (e.g., administer 30 mL of 23.4% hypertonic saline) to empirically temporize impending herniation.
- Other quick measures to reduce ICP include adequate sedation, neuromuscular blockade, elevation of the head of bed to 30°, and adjustment of the respiratory rate for goal $PaCO_2$ of 35 mmHg. Hyperventilation is a temporizing strategy pending more definitive treatment.
- Reverse coagulopathy in concert with neurosurgical consultants (as some reversal is controversial [i.e., platelets per PATCH trial]).

Vasopressor of choice: norepinephrine is generally safe; however, increased ICP could cause myocardial dysfunction necessitating inotrope (use POCUS).

BIBLIOGRAPHY

Carney N, Totten AM, O'Reilly C, et al. Guidelines for the management of severe traumatic brain injury. *Neurosurgery* 2017;80(1):6–15.

Gross BA, Jankowitz BT, Friedlander RM. Cerebral intraparenchymal hemorrhage: a review. *JAMA* 2019;321(13):1295–1303.

Hemphill JC 3rd, Greenberg SM, Anderson CS, et al. Guidelines for the management of spontaneous intracerebral hemorrhage: a guideline for healthcare professionals from the American Heart Association/American Stroke Association. *Stroke* 2015;46:2032–2060.

Marcolini E, Stretz C, DeWitt KM. Intracranial hemorrhage and intracranial hypertension. *Emerg Med Clin* 2019;37(3):529–544.

Qureshi AI, Huang W, Lobanova I, et al. Outcomes of intensive systolic blood pressure reduction in patients with intracerebral hemorrhage and excessively high initial systolic blood pressure: post hoc analysis of a randomized clinical trial. *JAMA Neurology* 2020;77(11):1355–1365.

14

Status Epilepticus

MATTHEW L. WONG

Chapter 14:
Status Epilepticus

Presentation

Seizure lasting more than 5 minutes, or multiple seizures within 5 minutes without return to baseline.

Critical Presentation: Seizures associated with CNS infections. *(Administer antimicrobials without delay.)*

Diagnosis and Evaluation

Immediate bedside glucose and ECG.

Consider head CT to rule out structural cause.

Consider LP if infectious etiology suspected.

Labwork: CMP, CK, toxicology, anti-epileptic drug levels, urine pregnancy.

Consider STAT EEG in intubated patients or suspected nonconvulsive SE.

Management

Airway management and hemodynamic monitoring.
- *In RSI, consider propofol for induction and continued sedation.*

Benzodiazepine administration.

Second line antiepileptics.
- *Levetiracetam, valproic acid, fosphenytoin, or phenytoin.*

Address underlying cause *(i.e. infectious agent, hyponatremia, eclampsia).*

Monitor for hyperthermia, hyperkalemia, rhabdomyolysis, and AKI.

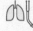

In sudden deterioration, consider airway compromise, sepsis, or recurrent seizure activity.

Introduction

- Generalized convulsive status epilepticus (GCSE) is when a seizure lasts longer than 5 minutes or when two seizures occur without an interval return to baseline.
- The most common error in managing status epilepticus is not administering enough benzodiazepine.
- If the patient is refractory to benzodiazepines, there are multiple appropriate agents for second-line treatment (e.g., leviteracetam, valproate, fosphenytoin).
- A timely and early intubation may be the safest option and provide the best outcome for the patient.
- Nonconvulsive status epilepticus (NCSE) presents without muscle involvement, and may be suspected clinically, but needs electroencephalography (EEG) to make the diagnosis.

Presentation

Classic Presentation

- Unresponsive with rhythmic movement of one or more body parts, or tonic eye deviation; of note, myotonic movements and incontinence may be seen in syncope as well as seizure.
- Less commonly, patients with altered mental status may actually be in NCSE.
- Seizures are followed by a postictal state – an altered mental status of variable duration.
- A postictal state may include a Todd's paralysis in which focal neurological deficits may mimic a stroke.

Critical Presentation

- Seizures associated with CNS infection require early and empiric antimicrobials (targeted at bacterial and viral pathogens) and possibly steroids, ideally before lumbar puncture is performed. Do not delay administration of these medications while awaiting lumbar puncture.

- It is not uncommon that seizures will require additional treatment and can be refractory to first-line agents (i.e., benzodiazepines) and second-line agents (e.g., levetiracetam, phenytoin, valproate, and phenobarbital).
- Be aware that patients could be seizing with little or no muscle twitching because of fatigue, or concomitant administration of neuromuscular blockade medications.

Diagnosis and Evaluation

- **Immediate bedside tests**
  - Bedside glucose level to rapidly evaluate for hypoglycemia.
  - Electrocardiogram to screen for hyperkalemia or toxidrome.
- **Laboratory tests**
  - Obtain basic serum electrolytes, calcium, magnesium, phosphorus, and glucose.
  - Lactate will be elevated if blood is drawn during or immediately after seizure activity. Recheck the lactate level after seizures have successfully been aborted.
  - Get total creatine phosphokinase (CK/CPK) to assess for associated rhabdomyolysis.
  - Consider drug levels such as antiepileptic drug levels, ethanol, salicylate, acetaminophen, and tricyclic level.
  - Urine toxicology test to screen for cocaine or other ingestions.
  - Urine/serum pregnancy test to screen for pregnancy.
- **Imaging studies**
  - Consider noncontrast head CT to evaluate for structural cause for the seizure such as hemorrhage or mass, particularly for first-time seizures.
- **Further testing**
  - Consider lumbar puncture and empiric administration of antibiotics/antiviral medications if an infectious etiology is suspected.
  - Consider STAT EEG in the emergency department if the patient is intubated or there is concern about NCSE.

Critical Management

- Assess **airway** security. Patients unable to protect the airway may require rapid sequence intubation (RSI). Start with a nasopharyngeal airway if indicated.
- Rapidly identify and correct hypoglycemia and hypoxia with dextrose and high-flow oxygen.
- Administer **benzodiazepines** as first-line therapy:
  - ○ Typically lorazepam IV (2-4 mg every 3 to 5 minutes), diazepam IV (5 to 10 mg every 3 to 5 minutes), or midazolam IV/IM (0.2 mg/kg every 5 minutes).
  - ○ Inadequate benzodiazepine dosing is a common error.
  - ○ Midazolam is the preferred intramuscular benzodiazepine if no IV access.
- Administer **second-line agents** if necessary:
  - ○ Levetiracetam 60 mg/kg (max of 4.5 g) over 10 minutes.
  - ○ Valproic acid 40 mg/kg (max of 3 g) over 10 minutes.
  - ○ Fosphenytoin 20 mg/kg at 150 mg/minute or phenytoin 20 mg/kg at 50 mg/minute.
- While administering the second-line agent, prepare to intubate and do so if the seizure is not terminated. Use propofol for induction and continue for sedation.

Treat the Underlying Cause

- *Infectious:* Early administration of antimicrobials and steroid before lumbar puncture if infectious etiology is suspected.

- *Hyponatremia:* If seizures are due to hyponatremia, administer **hypertonic saline** (3% NS) as a 100 mL bolus over 10 minutes, followed by up to two additional 100 mL doses, as needed. Then recheck sodium level hourly; the goal of therapy is to rapidly increase the serum sodium by 4 to 6 mEq/L over a period of a few hours, while avoiding too rapid correction and **osmotic demyelination syndrome**.
  - *Eclampsia:* If seizures are from **eclampsia**, administer magnesium (4–6 g over 15–20 minutes then 2 g/hour).
  - *Toxic ingestion:* Consider antidotes and extracorporeal removal as appropriate, and contact the local poison control center and toxicology service.
- Monitor and treat expectantly for hyperthermia, rhabdomyolysis, hyperkalemia, and acute kidney injury.
- Patients with status epilepticus should be admitted to an intensive care unit (ICU) setting.

Sudden Deterioration

Assess for recurrent seizures

Secure airway

Assess for other reasons for clinical decline (i.e., sepsis)
- The most likely causes for sudden decompensation are airway compromise/ respiratory failure, sepsis/septic shock, and recurrent seizure activity.
- Patients requiring multiple boluses of medications or continuous infusions should be considered for intubation for airway protection.
- Patients with an infectious etiology may rapidly progress to sepsis and require additional hemodynamic support.
- Prolonged seizure activity with or without overt muscle twitching is associated with increased mortality.

Vasopressor of choice: norepinephrine, but may depend on underlying etiology and hemodynamic status.

BIBLIOGRAPHY

Kapur J, Elm J, Chamberlain J, et al. Randomized trial of three anticonvulsant medications for status epilepticus. *N Engl J Med* 2019;381(22):2103–2113. https://doi .org/10.1056/NEJMoa1905795

Silbergleit R, Durkalski V, Lowenstein D, et al. Intramuscular versus intravenous therapy for prehospital status epilepticus. *N Engl J Med* 2012;366:591–600.

Treiman DM, Meyers PD, Walton NY, et al. A comparison of four treatments for generalized convulsive status epilepticus. Veterans Affairs Status Epilepticus Cooperative Study Group. *N Engl J Med* 1998;339:792–798.

15

Acute Spinal Cord Compression

CRISTAL CRISTIA[1]

[1] Thank you to Timothy C. Peck for his contribution to the original "Acute Spinal Cord Compression" chapter in the first edition of this book.

Chapter 15:
Acute Spinal Cord Compression

 ## Presentation

 Neck or back pain.

 Neurological signs/symptoms.
i.e. gait abnormality, neurogenic bladder, autonomic dysfunction, weakness, or paresthesias.

 Most commonly due to metastatic lesion, but may be traumatic, infectious, vascular, **structural, or inflammatory** in origin.

 ## Diagnosis and Evaluation

 Emergent MRI can best evaluate soft tissue structures.
Consider CT myelogram if unable to obtain MRI.

 ## Management

 Airway management and hemodynamic monitoring.

 Obtain serial FVC measurements to monitor progression of respiratory fatigue.

 Maintain strict spinal precautions.

 Analgesia, antibiotics if indicated.

 Consider dexamethasone administration.

 Surgical consultation.

 Sudden deterioration often due to neurogenic shock or high thoracic/cervical lesion causing respiratory/hemodynamic compromise.

Introduction

- Acute spinal cord compression results from impingement on the spinal cord due to a variety of etiologies, including neoplasm, hemorrhage, infection, or other structural abnormality at any vertebral level (Table 15.1).
- Any patient who presents with a history of trauma, intravenous drug use (IVDU), or immunocompromised state with associated neurological deficit and/or back pain should be evaluated for acute cord compression.
- Neoplastic disease is rarely confined to a single location; therefore, **the entire spine should be evaluated when metastatic disease is suspected**.
- Cervical spine injury accounts for 50% of traumatic spinal cord injury, while thoracolumbar injuries comprise the remaining 50%.

Table 15.1 Etiologies of acute spinal cord compression

Neoplastic disease

- Most common presentation is metastatic lesion (lung/prostate/breast > renal/gastrointestinal/lymphoma)

Infectious causes

- Extradural spinal abscess (IVDU, HIV, tuberculosis, immunosuppression)
- Diskitis/osteomyelitis

Vascular causes

- Ischemic
- Hemorrhagic (anticoagulation)

Mechanical/structural abnormalities

- Traumatic/bony injury
- Osteoporosis/pathological fracture
- Degenerative joint disease
- Postsurgical complication

Inflammatory disease

- Rheumatoid arthritis (C1/2 dislocation)

Presentation

Classic Presentation

- **Neck or back pain**
  - ○ May be acute, subacute, or chronic
  - ○ May be associated with symptoms of the underlying disease process (e.g., fever)
- **Neurological signs and symptoms**
  - ○ Associated limb weakness/paresthesias in more advanced cases
  - ○ Neurogenic bladder and/or bowel
  - ○ Autonomic dysfunction is expected with cervical/high thoracic lesions
  - ○ Gait abnormality

Critical Presentation

- Spinal shock differs from neurogenic shock
- **Spinal shock is loss of cord function caudal to specific injury level manifesting as flaccidity, loss of sensation, areflexia and bowel/bladder dysfunction lasting for weeks.**
- **Neurogenic shock is the hemodynamic manifestation of typically cervical or thoracic [typically T1–T5] spinal cord injury resulting in loss of sympathetic outflow (hypotension, bradycardia and vasodilation).**
- Priapism may also be present, due to loss of sympathetic innervation below the level of the lesion.
- Cervical and thoracic lesions may be associated with respiratory compromise.

Diagnosis and Evaluation

- Spinal imaging:
  - ○ **Emergent MRI is the preferred imaging modality.**
  - ○ Plain radiographic films may show bony destruction in infectious, metastatic disease, or traumatic fracture. However, **plain films may be falsely negative in up to 20% of cases.**

- CT scan of the spine provides improved evaluation of bony structures.
- **MRI preferred over CT** because it can better evaluate soft tissue structures such as spinal cord and ligamentous pathology.
- CT myelography is useful for identifying spinal canal compromise in patients unable to undergo MRI. However, it does not provide distinction between various soft tissue lesions such as hematoma, epidural abscess, etc.

Critical Management

Critical Management Checklist

☑ Airway management as needed

☑ Maintain spinal precautions, especially in the setting of trauma

☑ Vasopressors

☑ ± Antibiotics

☑ Neurosurgery consultation and admission

- **Manage airway**
  - **Patients with a cervical lesion may require intubation** for definitive airway control and to assist with ventilation and oxygenation.
  - If the patient is breathing spontaneously, obtain an FVC (forced vital capacity) to assess for impending airway compromise. **Serial FVC measurements should be obtained to monitor for progression of respiratory fatigue.**
  - Respiratory muscle weakness and paralysis as evidenced by poor FVC or concerning clinical signs such as shallow rapid breathing should be managed immediately with endotracheal intubation.
  - **Manual cervical in-line spinal stabilization should be maintained during intubation** if a direct laryngoscopy approach is used, particularly in the setting of trauma. Fiberoptic intubation using a bronchoscope may be necessary.
- **Strict spinal precautions** (e.g., cervical collar, backboard) to prevent further neurological injury should be continued until imaging has been obtained.

- **IV narcotic analgesia** will likely be necessary. In patients with subacute onset, such as with neoplastic disease, pain may have been present for days to weeks prior to presentation.
- Maintain **NPO** status; patients with spinal cord compromise may require emergent operative intervention.
- If an infectious process is suspected, draw blood cultures and administer broad-spectrum **IV antibiotic coverage**. Prompt recognition of infection based on history and physical examination, or other indicators such as the presence of SIRS or elevated ESR/CRP, is important to minimize delays in antibiotics.
- **Check a post-void residual** via bladder ultrasound or catheterization, as **urinary retention is very sensitive** for spinal cord injury and cauda equina syndrome.
- Steroid treatment for spinal cord injury is controversial, especially in the setting of trauma, and is beyond the scope of this discussion. In contrast, administration of corticosteroids (most commonly **dexamethasone**) is an important component in the **treatment of spinal cord compression secondary to metastatic disease**. In this population, steroids have been shown to improve clinical outcomes and may also alleviate pain related to bony metastases and compression of neural structures.
- **Surgical consultation** should be obtained for all patients with acute cord compression. Radiation therapy may have a role in relieving cord compression caused by malignancy. Continued management should occur in an intensive care setting.

Sudden Deterioration

- The mostly likely causes for sudden decompensation includes expansion of the offending lesion causing worsening neurological compromise, or a high cervical/thoracic lesion resulting in respiratory or hemodynamic compromise. Both scenarios require urgent surgical consultation $\pm$ surgical decompression. Endotracheal intubation may also be required.
- Risk factors for sudden deterioration include weakened diaphragmatic function (poor FVC), advanced age, history of cardiopulmonary disease, and tachypnea at presentation.

- **Respiratory compromise** occurs with spinal cord lesions above the high thoracic level. Monitor closely for diaphragmatic or respiratory muscle weakness with FVC (forced vital capacity) and intubate as needed.
- **Cardiopulmonary collapse** may occur. Hypotension and bradycardia are hallmarks. Remember that neurogenic shock does not always present with bradycardia and depends on the level of the lesion.
  - Provide IV fluids and vasopressor therapy as needed to maintain adequate perfusion.
  - Symptomatic or unstable bradycardia may require administration of atropine or cardiac pacing.
  - Vasopressors with chronotropic properties, such as epinephrine and norepinephrine, may be of particular advantage in patients with persistent bradycardia.
  - Adequate perfusion may be assessed by standard resuscitation parameters, such as appropriate urine output and resolution of systemic acidosis.

Special Circumstances

- **Cauda equina syndrome** is not a compression of the spinal cord, but rather a syndrome whereby compression occurs at the spinal nerve roots below the level of the spinal cord.
  - A clinical diagnosis that classically presents with bilateral lumbosacral back pain with radiation to the legs, subjective urinary retention or overflow incontinence, bowel incontinence, and saddle anesthesia.
  - **Presentation may be subtle: a high index of suspicion is required to prevent delay in diagnosis.**
  - Examination should include a rectal examination and evaluation of sensory function in the perineal area.
  - Urinary retention (at least 500 mL) is a concerning late finding.
- Emergent MRI and surgical consultation should be obtained in all patients in whom the diagnosis is being considered.

Vasopressor of choice: If heart rate is normal, phenylephrine may be appropriate to treat low peripheral vascular resistance. If bradycardia is prominent, use epinephrine or norepinephrine.

BIBLIOGRAPHY

Fehlings MG, Cadotte DW, Fehlings LN. A series of systematic reviews on the treatment of acute spinal cord injury: A foundation for best medical practice. *J Neurotrauma* 2011;28:1329–1333.

George R, Jeba J, Ramkumar G, et al. Interventions for the treatment of metastatic extradural spinal cord compression in adults. *Cochrane Database Syst Rev* 2008;4: CD006716.

Markandaya M, Stein DM, Menaker J. Acute treatment options for spinal cord injury. *Curr Treat Options Neurol* 2011;14:175–187.

SECTION 4

Cardiovascular Emergencies

TODD SIEGEL

16

Post-Cardiac Arrest Care

DI PAN

Introduction

- Major advances in post-cardiac arrest care research – particularly targeted temperature management (TTM) – have been made in recent years.
- The general approach to post-arrest care focuses on treating the etiology of the arrest while optimizing hemodynamics and neurologic protection.
- General considerations for post-arrest care are listed in Table 16.1.

Diagnosis and Evaluation

- An immediate assessment of a patient after the return of spontaneous circulation (ROSC) should include a focused history (usually from families, bystanders, or emergency medical services personnel in case of out-of-hospital cardiac arrest [OHCA]), physical examination, diagnostic testing, and imaging studies to determine a cause for the cardiac arrest.
- The physical examination should parallel an ATLS approach:
  - (1) Evaluate and establish airway.
  - (2) Address breathing issues.

Table 16.1 General considerations for post-cardiac arrest care

Neurologic
CT head
EEG between 24–48 hours
Targeted temperature management/fever avoidance/shivering control
Sedation and analgesia (avoid drugs with long half-time [i.e., fentanyl])
Neuromuscular blockade if severe shivering
Neuroprognostication labs, imaging and exam after 72 hours
Cardiovascular
Delayed versus immediate coronary revascularization
Antiarrhythmic drugs
Echocardiography
ECG
Pulmonary
CXR
CT angiography for pulmonary embolism
Lung protective ventilation
Avoidance of hyperoxia
Renal and acid/base
Titrate acid/base in setting of eucapnia and avoidance of hyperoxia
ID
Consideration of septic shock in differential
Endocrine
Intermediate glucose control

- (3) Assess circulatory status and blood pressure.
- (4) Identify disability with neurological response (Glasgow Coma Scale).
- (5) Exposure to fully perform the examination.

- **Electrocardiogram (ECG)**
  - ECG should be performed as soon as possible to look for evidence of myocardial infarction and other reversible abnormalities such as arrhythmias, conduction abnormalities, or prolonged QTc.
  - If acute myocardial infarction is suspected, interventional cardiology should be immediately involved.
- **Imaging studies**
  - Chest radiography (CXR): it can help determine both pulmonary and cardiac causes of cardiac arrest. Examples include pulmonary edema and cardiogenic shock, cardiac tamponade, aortic dissection, pneumothorax, and parenchymal lung diseases such as pneumonia and acute respiratory distress syndrome (ARDS).
  - Echocardiography: it may help detect wall motion abnormalities, assess left ventricular (LV) and right ventricular (RV) function, and rule out cardiac tamponade.
  - CT scan: it can be performed to exclude a primary intracranial process, or to evaluate the chest, abdomen, and pelvis.
- **Laboratory studies**
  - Basic serum electrolytes, complete blood count, arterial blood gas, serum troponin, serum lactate, and specific toxicological studies should be drawn as part of the patient workup.

Critical Management

Critical Management Checklist

- ☑ End-organ perfusion
- ☑ Target eucapnia and avoid hyperoxia
- ☑ Targeted temperature management (avoid fever)
- ☑ Neuroprognostication after 72 hours

- **Hemodynamic optimization**
  - End-organ perfusion should be optimized early and aggressively.
  - The mean arterial pressure (MAP) should be at least above 65 mmHg and ideally within the 80–100 mmHg range to optimize cerebral perfusion; vasopressors may be required to achieve this goal.

- If ventricular fibrillation (VF) or ventricular tachycardia (VT) preceded the cardiac arrest, an antiarrhythmic agent such as amiodarone may be started.
- Patients should be placed on continuous telemetry with serial 12-lead ECGs performed.

- **Cardiac catheterization**
  - High probability of acute coronary occlusion should prompt consultation with cardiac catheterization lab
  - However, no difference in 90-day mortality between delayed and immediate coronary angiography strategies was found for VT/VF OHCA without ST-elevation.

- **Pulmonary optimization**
  - An endotracheal tube should be placed in unconscious patients to protect the airway. If cardiopulmonary resuscitation is ongoing, care should be taken to avoid interruption of quality chest compressions for the purpose of endotracheal tube placement. A temporary device such as an extraglottic airway may be temporarily placed until ROSC is achieved.
  - Titrate the minute ventilation on the ventilator to keep partial pressure of carbon dioxide ($PaCO_2$) at 40–45 mmHg.
  - Hypocarbia can potentially cause cerebral vasoconstriction, leading to decreased cerebral perfusion and neurological injury.
  - FiO_2 should also be titrated down to keep the oxygen saturation (SpO_2) at 94% or above in order to reduce the potential for oxygen toxicity.

- **Neurological protection**
  - Avoidance of fever has been shown to associate with meaningful neurological outcomes for patients who remain unresponsive after cardiac arrest from shockable rhythms (VF and VT), though it has also been utilized in patients who suffered PEA or for whom the etiology of arrest is unclear.
  - Patients who remain unresponsive after ROSC should receive targeted temperature management with the goal of normothermia (< 37.8C).
  - Hyperpyrexia should be avoided in these patients as it has been shown to exacerbate the extent of brain damage, especially within the first 48 hours.

- **Neuroprognostication after 72 hours**
  - ○ Multimodal prognostication strategies are recommended in comatose patients after 72 hours following ROSC.
  - ○ Poor outcome is likely if two or more of the following are present:
    - Absent pupillary or corneal reflexes $\geq$ 72 hours
    - Absent bilateral N20 SSEP wave $\geq$ 24 hours
    - Malignant EEG (suppressed background or burst suppression) $\geq$ 24 hours
    - Neuron specific enolase > 60 µg/L at 48 hours and/or 72 hours
    - Status myoclonus $\leq$ 72 hours
    - Diffuse anoxic brain injury on CTH or MRI

Targeted Temperature Management (TTM) after Cardiac Arrest

- **Contraindications to cooling**
  - ○ The only absolute contraindications for TTM in comatose patients are a do not resuscitate (DNR) order or arrest secondary to traumatic injury.
  - ○ Relative contraindications include active bleeding, pregnancy, and septic shock as a cause of the arrest. Follow institutional guidelines.
  - ○ Induction of TTM can begin before cardiac catheterization and can safely be continued throughout the procedure.
- **Shockable and non-shockable rhythms**
  - ○ TTM is recommended for both initial shockable and non-shockable rhythms for patients with either in-hospital or out-of-hospital cardiac arrests who survive but remain comatose.
- **Cooling methods and monitoring**
  - ○ There are multiple methods of cooling and none have been proven to be superior.
  - ○ Internal systems using intravascular catheters and surface cooling devices are common.
  - ○ Cooling blankets and ice bags can be used but patients should be monitored closely as the rate of cooling and the goal temperature cannot be programmed.
  - ○ Intravascular cooling with cool IVF is an easy way to initiate cooling in the prehospital setting or in the emergency department: 30 mL/kg of 4°C (39°F) isotonic saline is administered through peripheral access.

- A patient's core temperature should always be monitored through an esophageal thermometer, pulmonary artery catheter, or bladder catheter.
- The goal temperature should ideally be reached within 6 hours and maintained for 24 hours.

- **Sedation and paralytics**
  - Sedation decreases agitation, pain, and anxiety, during therapeutic hypothermia. Agents of choice are propofol, fentanyl, and midazolam.
  - Midazolam may cause less hypotension than propofol but its effects are longer lasting, which can affect neurological examinations.
  - Paralytics can be used to prevent shivering, which can increase temperature and delay reaching the hypothermia goal; unless shivering occurs, paralytics are not required for TTM.

Sudden Deterioration

- **Seizures**
  - Continuous electroencephalogram (EEG) monitoring should be used on all patients requiring neuromuscular blockade in order to monitor for seizures.
  - If seizures occur, propofol, midazolam, phenytoin, and phenobarbital can be used and are similarly effective. Multiple medications may be required.
- **Coagulopathy**
  - Hypothermia impairs coagulation and therefore any active bleeding should be controlled before the initiation of cooling.
  - In the event of significant bleeding, therapeutic hypothermia should be stopped and the patient rewarmed to at least 35°C.
- **Infection**
  - Hypothermia longer than 24 hours has been shown to increase the risk of infection due to decreased leukocyte function.
  - Hence sepsis and septic shock as the cause of arrest is a relative contra-indication to the initiation of hypothermia.
- **Arrhythmias**
  - Hypothermia can lead to bradyarrhythmia and QT interval prolongation.
  - If the blood pressure remains adequate then the bradycardia does not need to be addressed.

- **Hyperglycemia**
  - ○ Hyperglycemia due to insulin resistance has been shown to result in worse neurological outcomes and increased mortality in post-cardiac arrest patients. However, intense glucose control can also lead to episodes of hypoglycemia and adverse outcomes.
  - ○ Glucose control should therefore aim to maintain glucose between 140 and 180 mg/dL (7.77–9.99 mmol/L).
- **Electrolyte abnormalities**
  - ○ Hypothermia can lead to increased urine output, a condition known as "cold diuresis," which in turn can lead to hypovolemia and electrolyte abnormalities.
  - ○ Fluid balance should be continuously monitored in all patients and electrolytes measured every 3–4 hours and replaced as needed.
- **Reversible causes of cardiac arrest**
  - ○ POCUS is useful to workup undifferentiated shock including tamponade, pneumothorax or severe decrease in cardiac output (i.e., systolic dysfunction in the post-arrest period).
  - ○ The clinical scenario can prompt administration of blood products or intravenous fluids.
  - ○ Repeat CXR and/or ECG for cardiorespiratory instability.

Special Circumstances

- In post-cardiac arrest patients where arrest is secondary to known or suspected pulmonary embolism, fibrinolytics should be considered.
- If adequate hemodynamic stability cannot be achieved through IVF and inotropic support, placement of an intra-aortic balloon pump may be necessary.
- If these therapies fail, a left ventricular assist device, or extracorporeal membrane oxygenation (ECMO), may be considered.

Vasopressor of choice: Patients who are hypotensive post cardiac arrest from a shockable rhythm (VT or VF) are likely suffering from a degree of cardiogenic shock. In such cases, norepinephrine, epinephrine, or dobutamine can be used for circulatory support but will increase myocardial oxygen demand and risk for arrhythmia. Phenylephrine should be avoided.

BIBLIOGRAPHY

Arrich J, Holzer M, Havel C, et al. Hypothermia for neuroprotection in adults after cardiopulmonary resuscitation. *Cochrane Database Syst Rev* 2012;9:CD004128.

Cronberg T, Lilja G, Horn J, et al. Neurologic function and health-related quality of life in patients following targeted temperature management at 33°c vs 36°c after out-of-hospital cardiac arrest: A randomized clinical trial. *JAMA Neurol* 2015;72(6):634–641.

Lemkes JS, Janssens GN, van der Hoeven NW, et al. Coronary angiography after cardiac arrest without st-segment elevation. *New Engl J Med* 2019;380(15):1397–1407. https://doi.org/10.1056/NEJMoa1816897

Nolan JP, Neumar RW, Adrie C, et al. Post-cardiac arrest syndrome: Epidemiology, pathophysiology, treatment, and prognostication. A Scientific Statement from the International Liaison Committee on Resuscitation; the American Heart Association Emergency Cardiovascular Care Committee; the Council on Cardiovascular Surgery and Anesthesia; the Council on Cardiopulmonary, Perioperative, and Critical Care; the Council on Clinical Cardiology; the Council on Stroke. *Resuscitation* 2008;79:350–379.

Nolan JP, Sandroni C, Böttiger BW, et al. European Resuscitation Council and European Society of Intensive Care Medicine guidelines 2021: Post-resuscitation care. *Intensive Care Med* 2021;47:369–421. https://doi.org/10.1007/s00134-021-06368-4

Peberdy MA, Callaway CW, Neumar RW, et al. Part 9: Post-cardiac arrest care: 2010 American Heart Association Guidelines for Cardiopulmonary Resuscitation and Emergency Cardiovascular Care. *Circulation* 2010;122(18 Suppl 3):S768–786.

Reynolds JC, Lawner BJ. Management of the post-cardiac arrest syndrome. *J Emerg Med* 2012;42:440–449.

Schenone AL, Cohen A, Patarroyo G, et al. Therapeutic hypothermia after cardiac arrest: A systematic review/meta-analysis exploring the impact of expanded criteria and targeted temperature. *Resuscitation* 2016;108:102–110.

Stub D, Bernard S, Duffy SJ, et al. Post cardiac arrest syndrome: A review of therapeutic strategies. *Circulation.*2011;123:1428–1435.

17

Acute Coronary Syndrome

STEVEN C. ROUGAS

Chapter 17:
Acute Coronary Syndrome

 ## Presentation

 General: Chest pain, diaphoresis, dyspnea, nausea, vomiting, radiation to arm/jaw/neck, may present atypically in women and diabetics.

 AMI: ECG changes and cardiac biomarker elevation.

 Stable Angina: Transient, usually resolving with rest or nitroglycerin.

 Unstable Angina: Episodes lasting longer than 20 minutes, not relieved by rest or nitroglycerin, no elevated cardiac biomarkers or ST Elevation.

 Critical Presentation: cardiogenic shock, arrhythmia, new murmur, pulmonary edema, cardiac arrest.

 ## Diagnosis and Evaluation

 Serial ECGs.
- *ST elevation indicates infarction; depression indicates ischemia.*

 Cardiac Biomarkers: Troponin I, CK-MB.

 ## Management

 STEMI: Immediate reperfusion indicated, ideally with percutaneous coronary intervention.
- *If no PCI available within 2 hrs of arrival, use fibrinolytics.*
  - *Review absolute contraindications before administration.*
- *Adjunctive pharmacological therapies (i.e. analgesia, nitrates, aspirin, consider beta blockers).*

 NSTEMI/UA: No immediate reperfusion indicated.
- *Monitor with serial ECGs and cardiac enzymes.*
- *Adjunctive pharmacological therapies (i.e. analgesia, nitrates, aspirin, consider beta blockers).*

Introduction

- Ischemic heart disease is the leading non-infectious cause of death in adults in the United States.
- Acute coronary syndrome (ACS) refers to symptoms attributable to atherosclerotic disease of the epicardial coronary arteries, usually caused by a fixed atherosclerotic lesion of varying severity.
- ACS is a spectrum of disease and can present as acute myocardial infarction (AMI) or unstable angina (UA).
  - AMI: myocardial ischemia *with* necrosis; can occur with or without ST segment elevation. The latter is referred to as non-ST-segment elevation myocardial infarction (NSTEMI).
  - UA: reversible myocardial ischemia *without* necrosis.
- The etiologies for ACS can be divided into primary and secondary (see Table 17.1).

Presentation

Classic Presentation

- **General signs and symptoms:**
  - Substernal or left-sided chest discomfort (heaviness, pressure, tightness, or squeezing).
  - Pain radiation to the arms, jaw, or neck.
  - Nausea, vomiting.
  - Diaphoresis.
  - Dyspnea.
  - Atypical presentations are common, particularly in women.

Table 17.1 Etiologies of acute coronary syndrome

Primary etiologies	Secondary etiologies
Coronary artery spasm	Increased myocardial oxygen demand
Disruption or erosion of atherosclerotic plaques	Reduced myocardial blood flow
Platelet aggregation or thrombus formation at	Reduced myocardial oxygen delivery

- **Stable angina** (chest pain syndrome brought on by exertion or supply–demand mismatch)
  - Transient, episodic chest pain.
  - Exercise or stress may induce symptoms.
  - Episodes usually last < 10 minutes.
  - Usually resolves with rest or nitroglycerin.
- **Unstable angina** (clinical diagnosis of chest pain without elevated cardiac biomarkers or ST elevation on ECG)
  - Occurs more suddenly with minimal exertion or at rest.
  - Episodes usually last > 20 minutes despite nitroglycerin or cessation of activity.
- **Acute myocardial infarction** (cardiac ischemia with biomarker elevation and a variety of ECG changes depending on nature of ischemic injury)
  - Prolonged, continuous, severe chest discomfort at rest.
  - May not respond to immediate symptomatic management.

Critical Presentation

- Patients may present with cardiogenic shock:
  - Hypotension
  - Pallor
  - Diaphoresis
  - Cardiac arrhythmias (ventricular fibrillation [VF] or ventricular tachycardia [VT])
  - Variations in systolic blood pressure
  - Bradycardia or heart block
  - New murmur secondary to papillary muscle rupture
  - Pulmonary edema manifested by shortness of breath and rales on auscultation
- Patients in extremis may also present in cardiac arrest.

Diagnosis and Evaluation

- There are four main elements in the diagnosis of ACS:
  - Clinical history

Table 17.2 ECG findings in acute coronary syndrome

	Male < age 40	Male > age 40	Female (all ages)
V2 or V3	≥ 2.5 mm	≥ 2 mm	≥ 1.5 mm
All other leads	≥ 1 mm	≥ 1 mm	≥ 1 mm

- ○ Physical examination
- ○ Electrocardiogram (ECG) findings:
- ○ Serial ECG are important to assess evolution of ischemia or myocardial injury.
- ○ Myocardial distress manifests in the ST segments of the ECG; ST segment depression indicates myocardial ischemia, whereas ST segment elevation (STE) indicates acute myocardial infarction.
- ○ ECG changes occur in patterns on the ECG and may be suggestive of the location of the culprit lesion (Table 17.2).
- • Cardiac biomarkers:
  - ○ Troponin: Myocardial troponin I (TnI) and troponin T (TnT) are elevated as early as 3 hours, but may stay elevated for up to 7 days.
  - ○ Creatine kinase (CK):
    - ▪ CK-MB is myocardial specific, usually elevated as early as 3 hours and peaking within 24 hours; it normalizes 2–3 days after injury. CK-MB is not routinely used in acute diagnosis of ACS.

Common infarct locations	Corresponding electrocardiographic ST changes	Suggested potential lesion location
Anterior wall	V3, V4	Left anterior descending artery (LAD)
Anteroseptal wall	V1–V4, aVR	LAD, STE in aVR suggests left main coronary
Anterolateral wall	V3–V6, I, aVL	LAD, left circumflex artery (LCX)
Lateral wall	V5, V6, I, aVL	LAD and branches including perforators and obtuse marginals
Inferior wall	II, III, aVF	Right coronary artery (RCA), LCX

(cont.)

Common infarct locations	Corresponding electrocardiographic ST changes	Suggested potential lesion location
Right ventricle (often III, aVF, associated with inferior MI)	V1, V2, II, V3R–V6R	Proximal RCA
Posterior wall	V7–V9 (with ST depression in V1–V3)	RCA, LCX

Critical Management

Critical Management Checklist

☑ Percutaneous coronary intervention (PCI)
☑ Fibrinolytics consideration if PCI unavailable
☑ Adjunctive pharmacologic therapies

Critical Management of STEMI

- Any patient with STEMI (ST-segment elevation myocardial infarction) should undergo reperfusion with percutaneous coronary intervention (PCI) within 90 minutes of presentation (ideally as soon as possible).
- Fibrinolytics should be considered for patients unable to receive PCI within 120 minutes unless there is an absolute contraindication.
  - If chosen, fibrinolytic administration should occur as soon as possible after the diagnosis of STEMI is made.
  - Alteplase, tenecteplase, and reteplase are all possible therapies.
  - Fibrinolytic inclusion criteria:
    - Patients presenting with STEMI.
    - Symptoms onset in the last 12 hours.
    - Inability to perform PCI within 120 minutes of arrival
  - Before administering fibrinolytic therapy, always review exclusion criteria.
- Other pharmacological agents include antiplatelets, antithrombins, beta-antagonists, nitrates, and morphine (see Table 17.3).
  - Antiplatelets such as aspirin have been linked to improved outcomes and should be uniformly used. The number-needed-to-treat (NNT) to save one life is approximately 42.

Table 17.3 Pharmacological agents in the treatment of acute coronary syndrome

Pharmacological agent	Example	Mechanism of action
Antiplatelets	Aspirin	Irreversibly acetylates platelet cyclooxygenase
Antithrombin	Heparin	Inhibits conversion of fibrinogen to fibrin
Beta-antagonists[a]	Metoprolol	Prevents tachycardia and increases inotropy
ACE inhibitors[b]	Lisinopril	Possibly causes a reduction in plaque rupture secondary to decreased shear force
Nitrates	Nitroglycerin	Decreases myocardial preload and afterload
GP IIb/IIIa receptor inhibitors	Eptifibatide	Inhibits the glycoprotein IIb/IIIa receptor
Thienopyridine antiplatelets	Clopidogrel	Inhibits transformation of the glycoprotein IIb/IIIa receptor
Opioid analgesics	Morphine	Reduces pain/anxiety, leading to decreased myocardial oxygen consumption
Fibrinolytics	Alteplase	Binds to fibrin and converts plasminogen to plasmin

[a] Beta-antagonists have been shown to benefit post-MI patients within 24 hours of the initial event when administered orally; early administration of IV doses does not appear to be beneficial.
[b] ACE inhibitors are also recommended within 24 hours post event, but not in the immediate treatment of ACS.

○ Anticoagulants such as heparin should also be considered.
  ▪ Either unfractionated (UF) or low molecular weight (LMW) heparin can be used; no specific data supports one over the other.
○ Beta-blockers reduce myocardial oxygen demand and decrease the potential of arrhythmia, however should be deferred to cardiology; it is not necessary to give in the emergency department (ED).
  ▪ Contraindications to beta-blockade include hypotension, cardiogenic shock, or congestive heart failure.
○ Nitrates are used to decrease pain and increase myocardial blood flow.

- They can be administered sublingually.
- Intravenous (IV) infusions should be considered if the pain persists after repeated sublingual doses.
- In patients with a right ventricular infarction (a preload-dependent condition), the use of nitrates can cause severe hypotension and should be avoided. This is often associated with an RCA lesion and bradycardia.
- Morphine can be used to decrease pain and anxiety.

Critical Management of NSTEMI and UA

- Therapy generally parallels that of STEMI.
- Immediate reperfusion is not indicated, though serial ECGs should be performed in patients with persistent symptoms to detect potential disease evolution.
- Aspirin (325 mg) should uniformly be administered.
- Therapeutic heparinization is often administered, though no mortality benefit has been linked to heparin in this setting.
- Beta-blockers can also be considered after acute management, barring any contraindications.
- Pain control can be achieved with nitrates and opioids.

Sudden Deterioration

The three most common reasons for decompensation of the ACS patient are cardiac arrhythmias, cardiogenic shock with congestive heart failure, and mechanical complications. Critical disruptions in the anatomy and function of the heart will often cause dyspnea, new murmurs, and potential hemodynamic compromise.

- **Cardiac arrhythmias:**
  - These most commonly include sinus bradycardia, sinus tachycardia, atrial and ventricular premature complexes, and non-sustained ventricular tachycardia (VT).
  - Less common but more dangerous arrhythmias include second- and third-degree heart blocks, sustained VT, ventricular fibrillation (VF), and asystole.

- ○ Antiarrhythmics – including amiodarone, procainamide, lidocaine, propranolol, or diltiazem – may be required for class-specific dysrhythmias.
- ○ Electrolyte repletion is also important in the treatment of certain dysrhythmias.
- ○ Temporary pacing may be required for symptomatic bradycardia or recurrent sinus pauses.
- **Cardiogenic shock:**
  - ○ This is caused by a decrease in ventricular function secondary to acute infarction, and exacerbated by the concomitant increased myocardial oxygen demands as the pump fails.
  - ○ Poor systolic function leads to hypotension, systemic hypoperfusion, and pulmonary congestion.
  - ○ This condition may be complicated by simultaneous valvular disease.
  - ○ The definitive intervention is emergent revascularization. Fibrinolysis is not recommended for these patients.
  - ○ Resuscitative efforts may be required in the ED prior to transport and must balance competing physiological priorities.
    - ▪ If severe **respiratory compromise** is present, orotracheal intubation may be required.
    - ▪ Managing hypotension in this setting can be challenging as both inotropic support and volume loading increase ventricular strain.
    - ▪ American Heart Association (AHA) guidelines suggest that norepinephrine, dopamine, and vasopression be used. Dobutamine is also recommended but contraindicated in patients with a systolic blood pressure less than 80 mmHg.
    - ▪ Mechanical circulatory support (MCS) devices may also be used with patients with refractory hypotension as a bridge to definitive management.
- Mechanical complications:
  - ○ Papillary muscle rupture:
    - ▪ Usually occurs 3–5 days post inferior myocardial infarction. Hypotension, pulmonary edema, and a new systolic murmur (indicative of mitral valve incompetence) are hallmarks of this condition.
    - ▪ The diagnosis is confirmed by echocardiography.
    - ▪ Medical management includes afterload reduction if possible, but the definitive management is surgical repair.
    - ▪ Patients with hypotension may require a MCS for stabilization.

- Ventricular free wall rupture:
  - Rupture may occur anytime between day 1 and day 5 post MI.
  - Usually presents with sudden-onset chest pain with resultant hypotension, tachycardia, and signs of cardiac tamponade.
  - It is diagnosed by echocardiography and requires immediate surgical treatment.
- Intraventricular septum rupture:
  - Usually occurs several days after acute infarction.
  - Associated with large anterior MI.
  - Patients present with chest pain, dyspnea, and a new systolic murmur as well as potential hemodynamic compromise.
  - Rupture causes left-to-right shunt.
  - It is diagnosed by color-Doppler flow echocardiography and requires surgical treatment.

Vasopressor of choice: Patients in cardiogenic shock post AMI suffer from a decrease in cardiac output associated with left ventricular dysfunction; in such cases, norepinephrine, epinephrine, or dobutamine can be used for circulatory support but will increase myocardial oxygen demand and risk for arrhythmia. Phenylephrine should be avoided as it increases LV afterload.

BIBLIOGRAPHY

Brady WJ, Harrigan RA, Chan TC. Acute coronary syndrome. In: Marx JA, Hockberger RS, Walls RM, et al., eds. *Rosen's Emergency Medicine: Concepts and Clinical Practice*. 7th ed. Philadelphia, PA: Mosby Elsevier, 2010.

Hollander JE, Diercks DB. Acute coronary syndromes: Acute myocardial infarction and unstable angina. In: Tintinalli JE, Stapczynski JS, Ma OJ, et al., eds. *Tintinalli's Emergency Medicine: A Comprehensive Study Guide*. 7th ed. New York, NY: McGraw-Hill, 2011.

Hollenberg SM, Parrillo JE. Myocardial ischemia. In: Hall JB, Schmidt GA, Wood LD, eds. *Principles of Critical Care*. 3rd ed. New York, NY: McGraw-Hill, 2005.

Thygesen K, Alpert JS, Jaffe AS, et al. Fourth universal definition of myocardial infarction. *J Am Coll Cardiol* 2018;72(18):2231–2264. https://doi.org/10.1016/j.jacc.2018.08.1038

18

Acute Decompensated Heart Failure

BRANDON MAUGHAN

Chapter 18:
ADHF

*Due to systolic dysfunction (impaired contractility, increased aøerload) and/or
diastolic dysfunction* (structural abnormality, impaired myocyte relaxation)

 ## Presentation

Classic: pulmonary edema, dyspnea, signs of right-sided heart failure *(hepatic congestion, JVD, dependent edema).*

Critical: respiratory distress, frothy oral secretions, chest pain, hypoxia.

 ## Diagnosis and Evaluation

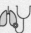

Pulmonary rales on auscultation.

CBC, CMP, BNP, cardiac enzymes, TSH, toxicology and lactate/cultures if indicated.

CXR, ECG.

POCUS may reveal B-line pattern.

 ## Management

Respiratory managment.

- ◐ *Consider NIPPV in patients maintaining their own airway.*

Cautious use of vasopressors or inotropes as needed (dobutamine, milrinone).

Preload and afterload modulation.

- ◐ *Nitrate therapy*   ◐ *ACE inhibitors*
- ◐ *Diuretics*

Treat underlying disease, if applicable, i.e., cardiac catheterization, antibiotics.

Introduction

- Heart failure (HF) is a clinical syndrome marked by elevated filling pressures to maintain acceptable cardiac output.
- Current guidelines use left ventricular ejection fraction (LVEF) to distinguish between reduced (HFrEF; LVEF < 40%), preserved (HFpEF; LVEF > 50%) and midrange ejection fractions (HFmrEF; LVEF between 40–49%).
- Beta blockers, angiotensin-converting enzyme (ACE) inhibitors, angiotensin receptor neprilysin inhibitors (ARNI), sodium-glucose transporter-2 (SGLT2) inhibitors, and cardiac resynchronization therapy, among other therapies improve outcomes in HFrEF. HFpEF management focuses on comorbidity management with recent data showing benefit from SGLT-2 inhibitor, empagliflozin.
- Acute decompensated heart failure (ADHF) is the rapid onset of new or worsening symptoms of HF (Table 18.1).
- Emergency resuscitation for most patients with hypertensive ADHF involves noninvasive positive pressure ventilation (NIPPV), IV nitrate therapy to reduce LV filling pressures, and IV loop diuretics to reduce circulating blood volume.
- Patients with hypotension and hypoperfusion in the setting of ADHF have a very poor prognosis and may warrant vasopressors as a bridge to specialized interventions such as heart catheterization, implantable cardioverter-defibrillator, or mechanical circulatory support (e.g., intra-aortic balloon pump, Impella, or ECMO).

Presentation

Classic Presentation

- ADHF classically presents with symptoms of dyspnea typically from pulmonary edema in the setting of elevated left ventricular filling pressures.
- Classic physical exam findings include pulmonary rales. Right-sided heart failure often presents with jugular venous distension (JVD), hepatic congestion, and dependent edema.
- Many cases of ADHF will present with a mixed clinical picture that includes signs and symptoms of both left- and right-sided heart failure.

Table 18.1 Etiologies of decompensated heart failure

Systolic dysfunction	Diastolic dysfunction
Impaired contractility	*Structural abnormality*
Ischemic heart disease	Ventricular hypertrophy
Dilated cardiomyopathies	Hypertrophic or constrictive cardiomyopathy
Peripartum cardiomyopathy	Constrictive pericarditis Infiltrative disease (sarcoidosis, amyloidosis)
Familial cardiomyopathy	
Myocarditis	
Alcoholic/toxic cardiomyopathy	
Chemotherapy cardiotoxicity	
Tachycardia-induced cardiomyopathy	
Stress cardiomyopathy	
Increased afterload	*Impaired myocyte relaxation*
Systemic hypertension	Myocardial ischemia or hypoxia Medications
Pulmonary hypertension	(e.g., digitalis) Hypercalcemia
Acute cor pulmonale	
Pulmonary embolism	
Aortic stenosis	
Cocaine abuse	
Medication noncompliance	
Hypervolemia (IV fluids, blood transfusion, renal failure)	

Critical Presentation

- Patients with severe ADHF may present with respiratory distress and impending respiratory failure.
- Associated clinical findings may include frothy oral secretions, diaphoresis, chest pain, and hypoxia.

- Patients who present with hypotension (SBP < 90 mmHg) have a poorer prognosis, especially if associated with clinical signs of hypoperfusion (i.e., cool and mottled extremities; altered mental status; cyanosis).
- Implantable cardioverter-defibrillators (ICDs) may be indicated for patients with ischemic or dilated cardiomyopathy and impaired systolic function (left ventricular ejection fraction < 30%).
- Cardiac resynchronization therapy (CRT) may be appropriate for patients with severe systolic heart failure and QRS interval prolongation (> 120 milliseconds).

Diagnosis and Evaluation

- **History**
  - ○ Important elements of history will include past history of cardiac dysfunction and potential causes of new cardiac dysfunction:
    - ▪ Prior history of heart disease
    - ▪ Recent weight gain or increasing edema
    - ▪ Dietary or medication noncompliance
    - ▪ Alcohol or cocaine abuse
    - ▪ Recent use of negative inotropic agents (e.g., calcium channel blockers)
    - ▪ Medication changes
- **Physical examination**
  - ○ Vital signs:
    - ▪ 90% of ADHF patients will present with systolic blood pressure that is normal (90–140 mmHg) or elevated (>140 mmHg).
    - ▪ Patients with cardiogenic pulmonary edema will typically have tachypnea and may be hypoxic.
  - ○ Patients with acute respiratory distress will often be tachycardic, although beta-blocker therapy or an underlying bradydysrhythmia may mask this.
  - ○ On examination, most ADHF patients will exhibit signs of pulmonary or peripheral vascular congestion, including pulmonary rales, diminished breath sounds in lower lung fields, jugular venous distention, and lower extremity edema. POCUS may reveal B-line pattern.
  - ○ Patients with significant valvular lesions may have corresponding murmurs on cardiac auscultation.

- Signs of impaired cardiac output and hypoperfusion (cyanosis, diaphoresis, altered mental status, oliguria) are especially worrisome due to their poor prognosis.
- **Laboratory tests**
  - A complete blood count with differential is obtained to assess for anemia or elevated white count.
  - Electrolytes are useful to evaluate for any disturbances associated with ADHF or cardiac rhythm (e.g., hyponatremia, hypokalemia, hyperkalemia, or hypomagnesemia).
  - An elevated troponin level may reflect a recent myocardial infarction (MI) causing acute heart failure, or may be caused by myocardial ischemia from ventricular strain.
  - B-type natriuretic peptide (BNP) and N-terminal pro-B-type natriuretic peptide (NT-proBNP) testing can help support or exclude a diagnosis of heart failure, although many noncardiac factors can produce elevated natriuretic peptide levels. Of note, obesity may have misleadingly/falsely low BNP levels.
  - An alcohol level or urine toxicology panel for common drugs of abuse (e.g., cocaine, amphetamines) can be sent based on clinical suspicion.
  - A TSH or T4 level can be obtained to evaluate for thyroid disease.
  - For patients with ADHF due to suspected infection or sepsis, a lactic acid level and appropriate cultures should be considered.
- **Imaging and ancillary tests**
  - Chest radiography:
    - Signs of pulmonary edema (increased interstitial markings, Kerley B lines, widened pulmonary fissures, cephalization of pulmonary vessels). See Figure 18.1 of a chest X-ray with pulmonary edema.
- ECG:
  - Evaluate for ischemia, dysrhythmias, or signs of pericardial effusion (e.g., electrical alternans).
- Echocardiography:
  - Point-of-care cardiothoracic ultrasound in the emergency department can rapidly assess for pulmonary edema (B lines), pericardial effusion (including tamponade physiology), and biventricular dysfunction, to inform clinical picture.

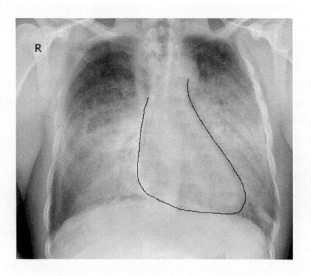

Figure 18.1 Congestive heart failure on chest X-ray.

Image courtesy of S Bhimji MD. www.ncbi.nlm.nih.gov/books/NBK554557/figure/article-19880.image.f1/ (open source)

Critical Management

- While considering the myriad causes of decompensated heart failure, the key to management in the current era is echocardiography to characterize left versus right heart failure, as this will determine next steps.
- Optimize oxygenation:
  - Sitting patients upright will improve oxygenation. Avoid recumbent or supine positioning as this will exacerbate respiratory distress.
  - Provide suctioning for frothy oral secretions.
  - Supplement oxygen as needed to maintain a saturation of ≥ 90%.
- Consider supportive respiratory adjuncts and prepare for potential respiratory deterioration:
  - For patients with moderate to severe respiratory distress who are able to maintain their airway, consider immediate noninvasive positive-pressure ventilation (NIPPV).

- NIPPV affects both preload and afterload; specifically, it drops RV preload but augments LV ejection by reducing afterload/wall stress. Though difficult to accurately predict, anticipate and prepare for relative hypotension after starting NPPV.
- Both continuous positive airway pressure (CPAP) and bi-level positive airway pressure (BiPAP) have demonstrated efficacy in patients with ADHF, particularly if initiated early.
  - Begin with a PEEP of 5 cmH$_2$O and increase incrementally until an improvement in oxygenation is seen. If BiPAP is used, the initial inspiratory pressure can be set at 10–12 cmH$_2$O and incrementally increased. The inspiratory pressure should not exceed 20 cmH$_2$O in consideration of gastric insufflation.
- Therapies to modulate preload and afterload are critical for managing ADHF.
  - Nitrate therapy reduces LV filling pressures by promoting venodilation.
    - It can be administered as sublingual tablets (0.4 mg/tablet) while intravenous (IV) access is obtained.
    - Nitrate therapy can also be given as a continuous infusion.
      - Start with 20–50 µg/minute and titrate by 20 µg/minute every 3–5 minutes until a maximum of 400 µg/minute or a MAP ≤ 65 mmHg.
    - At higher doses, IV nitrates can lower systemic vascular resistance and LV afterload, thereby improving stroke volume and cardiac output. In patients with hypertensive ADHF (i.e., SBP > 160 mmHg or MAP > 120 mmHg), a small body of literature suggests high-dose IV nitrate therapy (dose range 400–2000 ug over 1–2 minutes) in the emergency department is associated with lower rates of mechanical ventilation and ICU admission.
  - Angiotensin-converting enzyme (ACE) inhibitors decrease afterload and, in the long term, prevent ventricular remodeling.
    - Though not always given during initial assessment and stabilization, captopril can be used sublingually for immediate afterload reduction.
  - IV enalaprilat (5–10 mg) can also be used as primary or adjunctive therapy.
  - Avoid giving these drugs to patients with potential hyperkalemia, or during pregnancy.
- Diuretics, and particularly IV loop diuretics, can be used to combat the renin-angiotensin-mediated increases in circulating blood volume.

- Remember that not all patients with pulmonary edema are volume overloaded.
- In the absence of evidence of chronic volume overload, diuresis should only be initiated after other modalities of treatment – including NPPV and nitrate therapy – have been attempted. Inappropriate diuresis can lead to hypotension and acute kidney injury.
- Furosemide (40–80 mg IV), torsemide (10–20 mg IV), or bumetanide (0.5–1 mg IV) can be used as initial therapy.
- If the patient is on home diuretics, give an IV bolus dose equal to 100–200% of the home dose.

Sudden Deterioration

- Consider airway management; patients who become hypoxic, lethargic, or more confused despite NPPV should be intubated.
- Vasopressors as needed
  - Cautious use of inotropes or vasopressors to enhance cardiac output and maintain coronary filling pressure.
  - Titrate these agents to a MAP > 60 mmHg, or less if limited by signs or symptoms of cardiac ischemia.
    - Dobutamine: start IV infusion at 5–10 µg/kg/minute.
    - Milrinone: load 50 µg/kg IV over 10 minutes, then infuse 0.375–0.75 µg/kg/minute.
    - Dopamine: start IV infusion at 5–10 µg/kg/minute.
- Some patients may need specialized interventions based on their underlying disease:
  - Cardiac catheterization for ongoing ischemia.
  - Intra-arterial balloon pump or other mechanical circulatory support for cases of severe cardiogenic shock.
    - Patients with severe end-stage systolic heart failure may be considered for a left ventricular assist device (LVAD) as a bridge to heart transplant.

Vasopressor of choice: Recent data do not show clear, consistent benefit of one agent over another; personalize to individual patients hemodynamic variables.

Brandon Maughan

BIBLIOGRAPHY

Berbenetz N, Wang Y, Brown J, et al. Non-invasive positive pressure ventilation (CPAP or bilevel NPPV) for cardiogenic pulmonary oedema. *Cochrane Database Syst Rev* 2019;4(4):CD005351. https://doi.org/10.1002/14651858.CD005351.pub4

Ponikowski P, Voors AA, Anker SD, et al. 2016 ESC Guidelines for the diagnosis and treatment of acute and chronic heart failure: The Task Force for the diagnosis and treatment of acute and chronic heart failure of the European Society of Cardiology (ESC) Developed with the special contribution of the Heart Failure Association (HFA) of the ESC [published correction appears in *Eur Heart J* 2016 Dec 30]. *Eur Heart J* 2016;37(27):2129–2200. *https://doi.org/10.1093/eurheartj/ehw128*

Wang K, & Samai K. Role of high-dose intravenous nitrates in hypertensive acute heart failure. *Am J Emerg Med* 2020;38(1):132–137. https://doi.org/10.1016/j.ajem.2019.06.046

Yancy CW, Jessup M, Bozkurt B, et al. 2017 ACC/AHA/HFSA Focused Update of the 2013 ACCF/AHA Guideline for the Management of Heart Failure: A Report of the American College of Cardiology/American Heart Association Task Force on Clinical Practice Guidelines and the Heart Failure Society of America. *Circulation.* 2017;136 (6):e137-e161. https://doi.org/10.1161/CIR.0000000000000509

2013 ACCF/AHA guideline for the management of heart failure: A report of the American College of Cardiology Foundation/American Heart Association Task Force on Practice Guidelines. *J Am Coll Cardiol* 2013;62(16):e147–e239. https://doi.org/10.1016/j.jacc.2013.05.019

19

Aortic Dissection

STEFI LEE AND GREGORY HAYWARD

Chapter 19:
Aortic Dissection

 Presentation

Often severe, sudden onset chest pain, may be described as "tearing" or "sharp".

May have blood pressure differential between right and left brachial arteries.

Often hypertensive, but may be hypotensive in a proximal dissection causing heart failure.

Can present with vascular obstructive/ischemic symptoms at any organ.

May present as hemothorax.

History of risk factors such as systemic hypertension, connective tissue disorders, congenital defects, and previous cardiac procedures.

 Diagnosis and Evaluation

CTA or echocardiography are recommended diagnostic tests.

ECG to assess for ST elevations.

CXR may reveal widened mediastinum, and irregular aortic knob, and apical cap, or pleural effusion.

 Management

Transfusion and **fluid resucitation as necessary.**

Pain control.

Heart rate and blood pressure control.
- Negative inotropes (administer before vasodilators).
  + Target systolic BP 90–100 mmHg. so long as organ perfusion is maintained.
  + Beta-blockers (labetelol, esmolol) are preferred.
- Vasodilators.
  + i.e., sodium nitroprusside, nitroglycerin, nicardipine.

US to evaluate for cardiac tamponade.

ECGs to assess for MI.

Surgical consultation.

Introduction

- Aortic dissection represents the most frequent aortic catastrophe with approximately 10,000 cases annually in the United States.
- Dissection occurs with a primary tear of the intimal layer of the aorta with subsequent infiltration into the media layer, creating a false lumen which may extend the entire length of the aorta.
- Propagation of the false lumen may result in obstruction of vascular branches of the aorta, leading to end organ hypoperfusion of the brain, heart, kidneys, spine, or extremities.
- The location of injury (i.e., ascending versus descending aorta) predicts mortality and guides management decisions.

Presentation

Classic Presentation

- The majority of patients report severe sudden onset chest or back pain, described as tearing, ripping, and/or sharp.
- One-third of patients will have blood pressure differentials between left and right brachial arteries.
- Vascular obstruction and ischemia may occur at any level from compromised flow to a major branch of the aorta. This can result in syncope, stroke symptoms, acute myocardial infarction (frequently from right coronary artery compromise), mesenteric ischemia, paraplegia (from hypoperfusion of the spinal arteries), or limb ischemia.
- Patients often present hypertensive, although proximal dissection may cause aortic root dilatation and severe aortic regurgitation with ensuing heart failure, cardiogenic shock, or cardiac tamponade.
- A hemothorax (left > right) may develop in the setting of a ruptured or leaking descending aorta.
- A number of well-established risk factors exist including
  - Systemic hypertension
  - Connective tissue disorders such as Marfan syndrome, Ehlers–Danlos syndrome, vasculitides (Giant-cell or Takayasu's arteritis)
  - Congenital defects such as coarctation of the aorta, bicuspid aortic valve, annuloaortic ectasia, Turner's syndrome

- Acquired risk factors
  - Cardiac procedures including coronary catheterization, coronary stenting, aortic balloon pump placement, vascular surgery, or valve replacement
  - Infections, namely syphilis
  - Trauma
  - Cocaine
  - Third-trimester of pregnancy

Diagnosis and Evaluation

- **Electrocardiogram (ECG)** findings rarely aid in the diagnosis, though ST elevations may be present in as many as 20% of patients due to ostial coronary involvement.
- **Chest radiograph** may demonstrate widened mediastinum, an irregular aortic knob, an apical cap, or a pleural effusion.
- **Echocardiography and CT angiography** (Figure 19.1) are the most commonly used diagnostic modalities. The choice of imaging method depends on the patient's presentation, availability of equipment, and local expertise in interpretation of imaging. **Transesophageal echocardiography** can be performed at bedside, providing useful dynamic information with sensitivity and specificity > 90%. CT angiography can be rapidly performed with the added benefit of providing information about the extent of dissection, relation between true and false lumen, and compromised branches.
- **Magnetic resonance imaging (MRI)** is highly sensitive and specific, though it may be impractical in the emergency setting.
- Aortic dissections are generally classified depending on whether or not they involve the ascending aorta or aortic arch (Table 19.1).

Critical Management

Critical Management Checklist
- ☑ Massive transfusion protocol
- ☑ Cardiac monitoring and ECG for possible MI
- ☑ Ultrasound to evaluate for tamponade
- ☑ BP and HR control

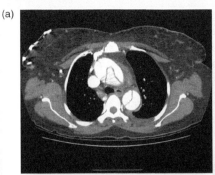

(a)

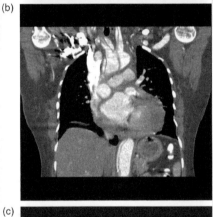

(b)

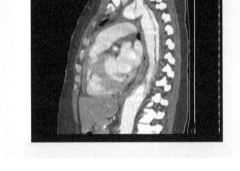

(c)

Figure 19.1 Aortic dissection diagnosed on CT angiography is visible in (a) transverse, (b) coronal and (c) sagittal views.

(Images courtesy of Amanda Holland Yang, MD.)

- Adequate IV access should be obtained in preparation for potential massive resuscitation with fluids and blood products.
- Cardiac monitoring with continuous blood pressure monitoring and electrocardiogram.
- Obtain a 12-lead ECG to rule out cardiac ischemia or infarction.

Table 19.1 Classification of aortic dissections

Stanford Classification	
Type A	Dissection involving the ascending aorta (proximal to the subclavian artery) with or without involvement of the descending aorta
Type B	Dissection of the descending aorta alone distal to the left subclavian artery
DeBakey Classification	
Type 1	Dissection of the entire aorta
Type 2	Dissection of the ascending aorta alone
Type 3	Dissection of the descending aorta alone

- In the hemodynamically unstable patient with suspected acute aortic dissection, a bedside evaluation of the aortic root with ultrasound can aid in rapid diagnosis.
- The primary goal in acute dissection (generally, less than 2 weeks duration) is to reduce the impulse or change in pressure for a given change in time ($\otimes$ pressure/$\otimes$ time)
- Aggressive early blood pressure and pain control serve as the critical interventions in acute dissection.
- Negative inotropes are prioritized to target systolic blood pressure as low as 90–100 mmHg as long as organ perfusion is maintained. After negative inotrope is started, vasodilator adjuncts can then be used to further reduce pressure.
- Beta-blockers are the initial agents of choice. They should be administered *prior* to vasodilators in order to prevent reflex tachycardia that may exacerbate shear/impulse forces.
  - **Labetalol:** Bolus 10–20 mg IV, double the dose every 10 minutes to a maximum of 80 mg/dose, *or* start a continuous infusion starting at 2–10 mg/minute IV and increase by 1 mg/minute every 10 minutes until the desired blood pressure is achieved.
  - **Esmolol:** Bolus 500 micrograms/kg IV followed by a continuous infusion starting at 25–300 micrograms/kg/minute. Titrate by 50 micrograms/kg/minute every 4 minutes.

- If necessary, vasodilators can be added after initiation of the beta-blockers.
  - **Sodium nitroprusside:** Start a continuous infusion at 1–4 micrograms/kg/minute and titrate by 0.25–0.5 micrograms/kg/minute every 2–3 minutes.
  - **Nitroglycerin:** Start a continuous infusion at 10–200 micrograms/minute and titrate by 5–10 micrograms/minute every 5–10 minutes.
  - **Nicardipine:** Start a continuous infusion at 2.5–15 mg/hour and titrate by 2.5 mg/hour every 5–10 minutes.
- Monitor for signs of end organ perfusion such as distal pulse checks, capillary refill time, mental status, and urine output.
- **Urgent surgical consultation** is indicated for emergent reparative surgery in Stanford type A dissection. Mortality increases by 50% within 72 hours for untreated type A dissection.
- **Early** surgical consultation is advised for Stanford type B dissection in the event that medical therapy alone is insufficient. Signs of this include end organ ischemia, uncontrollable pain, rapid expansion on serial imaging, and impending rupture.

Sudden Deterioration

- Sudden decompensation is mostly likely from either hemorrhagic or obstructive (i.e., tamponade) shock. Retrograde proximal dissections could migrate to cause acute aortic regurgitation (see Chapter 21 for more information).
- Maintain a low threshold for intubation with consideration for topicalized/awake approach if concerned about hemodynamic lability.
- In cases of hypotensive shock, consider acute myocardial infarction, aortic rupture, and hemopericardium.
- Pericardiocentesis should be considered but only be aimed at removing enough pericardial fluid to raise the blood pressure to an acceptable level.
- In the presence of acute myocardial infarction or stroke, aortic dissection is a contraindication to thrombolytic therapy.
- Active hemorrhagic stroke is a relative contraindication to surgery.

Vasopressor of choice: Patients with acute aortic dissection usually present with hypertension but can become hypotensive with progression of the condition. These patients will need to be aggressively resuscitated with blood products. Infusion of crystalloids and use of vasopressors such as phenylephrine and norepinephrine can be initiated as a temporizing measure but the disease is ultimately surgical in nature if vasopressors are being considered.

BIBLIOGRAPHY

Braverman AC. Aortic dissection: Prompt diagnosis and emergency treatment are critical. *Cleve Clin J Med* 2011;78:685–696.

Golledge J, & Eagle KA. Acute aortic dissection. *Lancet* 2008;372(9632):55–66.

Hagan PG, Nienaber CA, Isselbacher EM, et al. The International Registry of Acute Aortic Dissection (IRAD): New insights into an old disease. *JAMA* 2000;283(7):897–903.

Hines G, Dracea C, Katz DS. Diagnosis and management of acute type A aortic dissection. *Cardiol Rev* 2011;19:226–232.

Klompas M. Does this patient have an acute thoracic aortic dissection? *JAMA* 2002;287:2262–2272.

20

Hypertensive Emergencies

NADINE HIMELFARB

Chapter 20:
Hypertensive Emergencies

Presentation

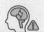

Hypertensive Crisis: SBP > 180 mmHg or DBP > 120 mmHg.

Hypertensive Urgency: Hypertensive crisis **without** evidence of acute end organ damage.

Hypertensive Emergency: Hypertensive crisis **with** evidence of acute end organ damage.

Diagnosis and Evaluation

Vital signs.

History

⊘ *Recent medication changes, recreational drug use, pre-existing conditions.*

Assess for heart failure, neurological dysfunction.

CBC, CMP, LFTs, UA.

ECG, CXR.

Consider CT to rule out aortic dissection/ICH.

Management

Administer appropriate anti-hypertensive

● *Preferably via continuous infusion, titratable, and with rapid onset.*

● *I.e., nitroprusside, nitroglycerin, labetalol, nicardipine, clevidipine, esmolol.*

● *Isolated Hypertensive Crisis: Goal is to lower MAP no more than 25%, or reduce DBP to 100–110 mmHg over 2–6 hrs.*

+ *Note: in hypertensive crisis with suspicion for eclampsia/dissection/ischemic stroke/ICH goal pressures may differ.*

Chapter 20:
Hypertensive Emergencies

📌 Remember This

- ✿ Do not use nitroprusside if intracerebral hemorrhage is suspected.

- ✿ Always consider aortic dissection in patient with hypertensive crisis and chest pain.

- ✿ Pre-eclampsia/Eclampsia: use magensium sulfate; may add labetalol/nicardipine; consult obstetrics.

| Goal SBP | 140 mmHg | Goal DBP | 90 mmHg |

Introduction

- Hypertension is defined as a systolic blood pressure (SBP) higher than 130 mmHg, or a diastolic blood pressure (DBP) higher than 80 mmHg.
- Hypertension may be essential (primary), meaning that it is not linked to an obvious underlying cause, or it may be secondary to a known etiology or other systemic disorder.
- Of people with known hypertension, 1–2% will present with an acutely elevated blood pressure referred to as a "hypertensive crisis." It is often due to factors that exacerbate a preexisting hypertension, such as medication noncompliance or substance abuse.
- Hypertensive crisis is the umbrella term that includes anyone with SBP > 180 mmHg or DBP > 120 mmHg.
  - "Hypertensive Urgency": hypertensive crisis without evidence of acute end-organ damage.
  - "Hypertensive Emergency": hypertensive crisis with evidence of acute end-organ damage. Clinical manifestations are directly related to the specific organ affected, usually the brain, heart, or kidneys (Table 20.1).

Table 20.1 Clinical manifestations of hypertensive emergencies

Hypertensive encephalopathy
Acute ischemic stroke
Acute intracerebral hemorrhage
Aortic dissection
Unstable angina/acute myocardial infarction
Acute pulmonary edema
Preeclampsia/HELLP syndrome/eclampsia
Acute renal failure

Diagnosis and Evaluation

- **History**
  - Ask for symptoms related to specific organ dysfunction:
    - Neurological symptoms: headache, altered mental status, visual changes.
    - Cardiovascular symptoms: chest pain, dyspnea.
    - Renal failure: oliguria, anuria, altered mental status, symptoms related to electrolyte abnormalities.
  - Elements of the past medical history, including coronary artery disease, prior cerebrovascular events, and renal disease should be obtained.
  - Patients should also be asked about current prescription medications for blood pressure control, as well as recent changes in their medications or dose.
  - Always consider pregnancy as a possible etiology for hypertensive symptoms in women of childbearing age.
  - Investigate potential use of recreational drugs such as cocaine, amphetamines, or phencyclidine.
- **Physical examination**
  - Confirm blood pressure measurement using an appropriately sized cuff.
  - If there is a concern for aortic dissection, the blood pressure should be taken in both upper extremities and compared for discrepancies.
  - Tachypnea and hypoxia may suggest an underlying pulmonary dysfunction or acute pulmonary edema.

○ Clinical signs of congestive heart failure such as elevated jugular venous pressure, a third heart sound, rales or B lines on lung ultrasound may also be present.

○ A full neurological examination should be performed to assess for mental status changes, focal neurological deficits, and visual changes.

- **Laboratory tests and imaging**

  ○ Complete blood count and peripheral smear to assess for hemolysis and microangiopathic anemia.

  ○ Complete serum chemistry panel to assess for renal function and presence of electrolyte derangements.

  ○ Liver panel, particularly in pregnant patients, to help rule out the HELLP syndrome (hemolysis, elevated liver enzymes, and low platelet count.)

  ○ Urinalysis with microscopic examination of the urine for presence of proteinuria, red blood cells, and/or casts.

  ○ Electrocardiogram (ECG) to look for signs of ischemia or left ventricular hypertrophy.

  ○ For patients with dyspnea or chest pain, a chest radiograph (CXR) may demonstrate pulmonary edema or mediastinal widening. If aortic dissection is suspected, computed tomography (CT) of the chest has higher sensitivity and specificity than CXR.

  ○ For patients presenting with a headache, changes in mental status, or abnormal neurological findings, a non-contrast CT of the brain should be performed to rule out an acute intracerebral hemorrhage.

Critical Management

Critical Management Checklist

☑ Identify primary pathophysiology.
☑ Choose appropriate pharmacologic antihypertensive agent.
☑ Prioritize end-organ perfusion.

- Critical management will depend on the presence of end-organ damage.
- Patients with chronically elevated blood pressure may suffer detrimental consequences if their blood pressure is lowered too quickly. Dramatic and rapid decreases in blood pressure can result in critical hypoperfusion of the brain, heart, and kidneys, resulting in ischemia or infarction.

- Correction of blood pressure in a hypertensive emergency should be via continuous infusion of medications that have a rapid onset and are both short-acting and titratable.
- The immediate goal is to reduce the mean arterial pressure (MAP) by no more than 20–25%, or to reduce the diastolic blood pressure to 100–110 mmHg within 2–6 hours. There are certain exceptions, however, and these are detailed in the "Special Considerations" section below.
- Agents should be chosen based on the specific organ(s) being damaged (Tables 20.2 and 20.3).

Table 20.2 Parenteral drugs for treatment of hypertensive emergencies

Drug	Mechanism	Initial dose	Time of onset	Duration
Nitroprusside	Arterial and venous dilator (often cited to reduce afterload/total peripheral resistance)	0.5 mcg/kg/min	Immediate	1–10 minutes
Nitroglycerin	Arterial and venous dilator (predominantly venous effect)	5–10 mcg/min (often started much higher)	Immediate	3–5 minutes
Labetalol	Alpha$_1$-, beta$_1$-, and beta$_2$- blocker	10–20 mg loading bolus followed by 0.5-2 mg/min	5–15 minutes	16–18 hours (variable)
Nicardipine	Calcium channel blocker with systemic and coronary vasodilation	5 mg/hr	Immediate	15–30 minutes
Clevidipine	Calcium channel blocker with predominantly arterial vasodilation effect)	1–2 mg/hr	2–4 minutes	5–15 minutes
Esmolol	Beta$_1$-blocker with predominant negative inotropic effect	0.5–1 mg/kg bolus followed by 50 mcg/kg/min	1–2 minutes	10–30 minutes

Table 20.3 General recommendations and considerations for specific complications of hypertensive emergency

Condition	Recommended	Considerations
Hypertensive encephalopathy	Labetalol, nicardipine, fenoldopam, clevidipine	Avoid hydralazine and nitroprusside in acute neurologic processes
Aortic dissection	Esmolol **then** nitroprusside, or nicardipine, or fenoldopam	Arterial and venodilators should be used only after negative inotrope of a beta-blocker
Acute coronary syndrome	Labetalol, or esmolol **and** nitroglycerin	Avoid hydralazine as difficult to titrate and does not offer benefit to oxygen supply/demand balance
Acute pulmonary edema	Nitroprusside or nitroglycerin	Avoid hydralazine, labetalol as difficult to titrate and does not effectively decrease preload
Preeclampsia/ eclampsia	Labetalol, nicardipine	Avoid nitroprusside, ACE inhibitors
Sympathetic crises (pheochromocytoma/ cocaine use)	Phentolamine, nicardipine, fenoldopam (consider adding a benzodiazepine)	Beta-blockers should only be used in combination with an alpha-blocker
Acute renal failure	Fenoldopam, nicardipine	Avoid nitroprusside as long-term infusion risks thiocyanate toxicity

Sudden Deterioration

- Identify key hemodynamic variables of underlying pathophysiology.
- Selection (typically) of a quick-acting, titratable agent for unstable patients (i.e., esmolol, nicardipine, labetalol, or clevidipine [specific agent per the underlying hemodynamic problem]).
- Point-of-care ultrasound and echocardiography should guide the hemodynamic intervention (e.g., aortic dissection requiring a negative inotrope or acute pulmonary edema requiring nitroglycerin).

Nadine Himelfarb

Special Considerations

Aortic Dissection

- This should always be a consideration in patients with high blood pressure and chest pain.
- Medical management involves reducing the impulse (change in pressure per unit time) on the artery. This is accomplished by first reducing inotropy so subsequent venous or arterial dilation does not incite reflex tachycardia.
  - Blood pressure control may result in a reflex tachycardia that may in turn increase shear stress. Therefore, heart rate should be controlled with a beta$_1$-blocker (cardioselective) prior to the administration of vasodilators.
  - The goal is to rapidly reduce heart rate to less than 60 beats per minute (bpm), and the SBP to 100–120 mmHg (or MAP to $<$ 80 mmHg) within 5–10 minutes.
  - Agents of choice are usually beta-blocker followed by a vasodilator. Calcium channel blockers may be used for rate control in situations where beta-blockers are contraindicated.
- Consultation for surgical management should be obtained on all patients with aortic dissection.

Acute Ischemic Stroke

- Blood pressure is commonly elevated after an ischemic cerebrovascular accident (CVA). This occurs physiologically in order to maintain cerebral perfusion pressure (CPP) in the ischemic areas of the brain.
- Lowering blood pressures during an acute CVA could cause further ischemia and damage to the brain by reducing the CPP.
- If thrombolysis is to be administered, blood pressure should be lowered to an SBP $<$ 185 mmHg and a DBP $<$ 110 mmHg.
- If thrombolysis is not a consideration, blood pressure should be lowered when the SBP $>$ 220 mmHg or the DBP $>$ 120 mmHg.

Acute Intracerebral Hemorrhage

- Patients who are hypertensive in the context of acute intracerebral hemorrhage (ICH) should have their blood pressure reduced rapidly with labetalol or nicardipine infusions (based upon AHA guidelines).
- No evidence for a specific blood pressure target currently exists for ICH. However, some sources recommend targeting an SBP of less than 140 mmHg.
- Cerebral perfusion pressure (CPP) is impacted by both mean arterial pressure (MAP) and intracranial pressure (ICP):

$$CPP = MAP - ICP$$

  - Nitroprusside is contraindicated in these patients, as direct arterial vasodilation can increase the intracranial pressure.
  - Both neurology and neurosurgical consultations should be initiated, and early invasive intracranial pressure monitoring should be considered.

Preeclampsia and Eclampsia

- Delivery of the fetus is the definitive treatment; therefore, consult Obstetrics.
- Management involves the use of magnesium sulfate and blood pressure lowering agents.
- Blood pressure must be lowered cautiously to avoid decreasing uteroplacental blood flow.
- The goal is to maintain an SBP of 140 mmHg and a DBP of 90 mmHg.
  - Blood pressure management can be achieved using intravenous labetalol or nicardipine.
  - Hydralazine is no longer recommended due to unpredictable decreases in blood pressure, duration of effect, and side effects that can mimic worsening pre-eclampsia.

BIBLIOGRAPHY

Marik PE, Rivera R. Hypertensive emergencies: An update. *Curr Opin Crit Care* 2011;17 (6):569–580.

Marik PE, Varon J. Hypertensive crises: challenges and management. *Chest* 2007;131:1949–1962.

Rodriguez MA, Kumar SK, De Caro M. Hypertensive crisis. *Cardiol Rev* 2010;18:102–107.

Unger T, Borghi C, Charchar F, et al. 2020 International Society of Hypertension Global Hypertension Practice Guidelines. *Hypertension* 2020;75:1334–1357.

21

Valvular Diseases

ERMIAS JIRRU AND ELENA KAPILOVICH

Chapter 21:
Valvular Diseases

Aortic Stenosis | **Aortic Regurgitation**

 ## Presentation

 Exertional dyspnea, pre-syncope and angina, decreased stroke volume.

 Exacerbated by tachycardia.

 Chronic: May be asymptomaticdepending on LV function and compliance.

 Angina uncommon.

 Acute: Acute decompensated HF, likely caused by underlying pathology (i.e. endocarditis).

 ## Diagnosis and Evaluation

 ECG, CXR, CBC, CMP, BNP, cardiac enzymes, culture if concern for endocarditis, consider echocardiogaphy in hemodynamically stable patient.

 May have harsh crescendo-decrescendo ejection murmur.

 May have diastolic murmur at upper right sternal border.

 Rule out aortic dissection.

 ## Management

 Maintain adequate preload and sufficient afterload; target normal heart rate.

 Maintain adequate preload;

 Reduce afterload and increase contractility; avoid atrial fibrillation.

Chapter 21:
Valvular Diseases

Mitral Stenosis	Mitral Regurgitation

 ## Presentation

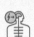 **Chronic, severe MS:** exertional dyspnea secondary to pulmonary congestion, progressive RV failure, hoarseness/dysphagia.

 Angina uncommon, exacerbated by tachycardia.

 Chronic MR: Dyspnea, AFib, CHF, systemic emboli.

 Acute MR: often caused by flail leaflet or papillary muscle rupture.

 ## Diagnosis and Evaluation

ECG, CXR, CBC, CMP, BNP, cardiac enzymes; culture if concern for endocarditis; consider echocardiography in hemodynamically stable patient.

 May have low and mumbling diastolic murmur best heard at the apex with an opening snap.

 May have early systolic or holosystolic murmur best heard at apex.

 In acute MR: murmur may be absent; consider ACS; may see rupture on echocardiogram.

 ## Management

 Avoid tachycardia and atrial **fibrillation.**

 Does not often present critically.

 Maintain rapid HR and contractility; reduce afterload.

 Consider intra-aortic balloon pump.

Introduction

- Valvular diseases are classified either as obstructing outflow (i.e., stenosis) or inadequately closing/coapting (i.e., regurgitation).
- Many mild–moderate valve lesions exist in a compensated or well-tolerated state; the tenets of hemodynamic management become particularly important in the severe or acute setting.
- As the following valvulopathies are primarily left heart-centric, the etiologies of right heart valvulopathy and failure are beyond the scope of this chapter.

Presentation

Classic Presentation

- **Aortic stenosis (AS)**
  - Classic symptoms of advancing AS are exertional dyspnea, pre-syncope and angina with an associated harsh crescendo–decrescendo ejection murmur.
  - AS can mimic or exacerbate other types of cardiac disease, including acute coronary syndrome (ACS) and acute decompensated heart failure (ADHF).
- **Aortic regurgitation (AR)**
  - Inadequate closure of the aortic valve at end-systole results in a regurgitant volume that increases LV end-diastolic volume (LVEDV).
  - It may be largely asymptomatic, depending on the function and compliance of the LV.
  - AR is associated with a diastolic murmur best heard at the upper sternal border.
  - Concomitant ventricular dysfunction can result in exertional dyspnea, ADHF, and conduction abnormalities.
  - Angina is uncommon with isolated AR.
- **Mitral stenosis (MS)**
  - Patients with MS have obstruction of flow between the left atrium (LA) and the LV, causing congestion into the pulmonary circuit.

- This results in increased pressure in the LA, the pulmonary vasculature, and the right side of the heart.
- LV function in isolated MS is largely unimpeded.
- Symptoms of MS are related to the degree of pressure gradient across the valve.
  - Mild and moderate MS are generally asymptomatic.
  - Symptoms are exacerbated by tachycardia as diastolic filling time decreases.
  - MS is associated with a "low and rumbling" diastolic murmur best heard at the apex, as well as a classic "opening snap."
- As the stenosis worsens, patients become symptomatic at rest.
  - Exertional dyspnea secondary to pulmonary congestion is the most common symptom of MS.
  - Hemoptysis.
  - Hoarseness or cough from the enlarged left atrium compressing the recurrent laryngeal nerve.
  - Dysphagia from the enlarged left atrium compressing the esophagus.
  - Malar flush or "mitral facies."
  - Progressive RV dilatation, right-sided heart failure, and pulmonary hypertension.
  - Similar to AR, chest pain is uncommon with isolated MS.

- **Mitral regurgitation (MR)**
  - *Chronic MR:*
    - Patients with chronic MR have inadequate closure of the mitral valve at end-systole with resultant regurgitant flow back into the LA.
    - It can be caused by primary valvular problems, or as a result of a dilated LV.
    - This results in increased LA volume and subsequent LA dilation.
    - MR is associated with an early systolic or holosystolic murmur best heard at the upper sternal border.
    - Chronic mild MR may be largely asymptomatic.
  - **Symptoms from isolated, chronic MR are related to both LA overload and decreases in effective cardiac output.**
    - Dyspnea.
    - Atrial fibrillation (AF) due to LA enlargement.
    - Progressive congestive heart failure (CHF) leading to right heart failure.
    - Systemic emboli.
- *Acute MR* is a medical emergency and discussed in the "Critical Presentation" section below.

Critical Presentation

- **Aortic stenosis (AS)**
  - Critical AS (aortic valve area < 0.7 cm^2/m^2) is a clinically important lesion where preload dependence in the setting of a fixed outflow tract lesion is the key point for management
  - Patients with AS are particularly sensitive to changes in cardiac output due to the pressure gradient across the aortic valve.
    - Tachycardia decreases diastolic filling time and LVEDV, effectively decreasing stroke volume.
    - Intravascular volume depletion also decreases stroke volume.
    - Therefore, hemodynamics will deteriorate without appropriate preload, making AS a "preload-dependent" condition.
- **Aortic regurgitation (AR)**
  - Chronic aortic regurgitation is rarely a critical problem.
  - Acute AR is a medical emergency caused by sudden insufficiency of the aortic valve related to various pathology: endocarditis, a perivalvular abscess, or acute aortic dissection.
  - In acute AR, the LV is unable to compensate for the dramatic and sudden increases in LVEDV.
  - Patients with acute AR will present with symptoms of acute volume overload, ADHF, or cardiogenic shock.
- **Mitral stenosis (MS)**
  - Atrial fibrillation (due to LA dilation) can cause tachycardia and hypotension.
  - Pulmonary vascular congestion via increased LA pressure causes pulmonary edema.
  - Similar to AS, symptoms of MS are exacerbated by tachycardia:
  - LVEDV decreases and cardiac output falls.
  - Thromboembolic events increase with age and the degree of stenosis.
  - 50% of mitral stenosis patients will have another, coexisting valvulopathy
- **Mitral regurgitation (MR)**
  - *Chronic MR:*
    - Critical presentations of patients with chronic MR include rapid atrial fibrillation, dyspnea, and pulmonary edema.

- Patients with chronic MR may also have a dilated LV, or decreased ventricular function which can lead to ADHF.
- *Acute MR* is a medical emergency caused by a flail leaflet or papillary muscle rupture.
  - These are often caused by endocarditis, trauma, or ACS.
  - Mitral valve failure leads to pulmonary edema and cardiogenic shock. With ventricular contraction, reverse flow substantially decreases effective cardiac output while also causing acute overload of the LA. Notably, due to the low pressure gradient between LV and LA in acute MR, a typical murmur will be difficult to discern. Up to 30–50% of patients with acute MR will have no murmur.

Diagnosis and Evaluation

- Evaluation of any valvular pathology begins with the history and physical examination, paying particular attention to whether a valvular defect has been previously noted.
- Patients with acute valvular disease will require immediate stabilization as described below.
  - If a new acute AR is discovered, the diagnosis of aortic dissection should be ruled out with a CTA or a transthoracic or transesophageal echocardiogram.
  - If a new acute MR is discovered, ACS must be considered.
    - If the ECG is unrevealing, an echocardiogram may be useful to identify a flail leaflet, vegetations, ruptured chordae tendineae, or papillary muscle rupture.
- Patients with known valvular disease should be evaluated based upon presenting symptoms.
  - The ECG may demonstrate findings of chronic structural changes from valvular dysfunction (Table 21.1).
  - A chest radiograph (CXR) is needed for patients presenting with dyspnea.
  - Basic laboratory studies – including complete blood count, chemistry, cardiac enzymes, brain natriuretic peptide (BNP), and coagulation profiles – may be helpful and should be ordered after a proper clinical assessment.

Table 21.1 Common considerations for valvular pathology

Valvular lesion	Hemodynamic considerations	Vasoactive agents of choice
Aortic stenosis	Adequate preload is key; maintain reasonable afterload to feed the coronaries at aortic root. Goal is for near-normal HR to maintain coronary perfusion	Phenylephrine classically to maintain filling pressure at aortic root but caution with too much afterload increase
Aortic regurgitation	Similar to AS, maintain adequate preload and contractility but can accept higher HR. Forward flow prioritized via chronotrope or inotrope to reduce regurgitant flow	Dobutamine or low-dose epinephrine (to avoid alpha effects)
Mitral stenosis	Diastolic filling time through the fixed lesion is key – thus, avoid tachycardia and atrial fibrillation as this will compromise filling.	Inotropes that have favorable effect in lowering pulmonary vascular resistance (e.g., milrinone)
Mitral regurgitation	Maintain rapid HR, contractility, and reduction in afterload	Dobutamine or milrinone

- ○ Blood culture and antibiotics may be indicated if endocarditis or a perivalvular abscess are suspected.
- ○ Characterization of valve dysfunction in the emergency department is not imperative if patients are hemodynamically stable.
- ○ Echocardiography should be considered in patients who are hemodynamically unstable.

Sudden Deterioration and Critical Management

- **General principles**
  - ○ Initial management should focus on acute stabilization:
    - ▪ Expectant airway management.
    - ▪ Supplemental oxygen.
    - ▪ Cardiac monitoring.
  - ○ Following stabilization, treatment should be symptom-focused.

- ○ Acute valvular dysfunction is usually secondary to a precipitating critical problem. The latter will have to be addressed as well.
- **Lesion-specific issues**
  - ○ *Aortic stenosis:*
    - ▪ Extremely sensitive to preload; keep adequate intravascular volume.
    - ▪ Consider awake/topicalized intubation; hypotension in peri-intubation setting could be catastrophic.
    - ▪ Depending on the underlying pathology, hemodynamics may be optimized by controlling the heart rate and increasing stroke volume; keep heart rate around 60 BPM and avoid atrial fibrillation.
    - ▪ AS management is complicated and requires fine balance between maintaining adequate preload and coronary perfusion (i.e., filling pressure) with a regular heart rate to promote forward flow.
  - ○ *Acute aortic regurgitation:*
    - ▪ Like acute MR, this is a true medical emergency and often presents with acute onset dyspnea from CHF.
    - ▪ Early medical management focuses on lowering LV end-diastolic pressure and increasing forward flow by reducing afterload and increasing contractility.
    - ▪ IV nitroprusside or other vasodilators can be used for afterload reduction.
    - ▪ Cardiac inotropes – such as low-dose epinephrine, dobutamine, or dopamine – can help increase contractility.
    - ▪ Avoid beta-blockers in the acute setting.
    - ▪ Unlike in MR, the use of intra-aortic balloon pumps is contraindicated since inflation of the balloon during diastole will worsen the severity of AR.
    - ▪ Treat other causes of acute AR such as infective endocarditis or aortic dissection.
    - ▪ The mainstay of treatment is early surgery to replace or repair the incompetent valve.
  - ○ *Mitral stenosis:*
    - ▪ Like AS, it may impact hemodynamics but does not often present critically.
    - ▪ Heart rate control, sinus rhythm, and mindfulness of the pulmonary vascular resistance are tenets of management.
  - ○ *Acute mitral regurgitation:*
    - ▪ This is a medical emergency, as patients typically present in acute pulmonary edema (essentially, biventricular failure) and cardiogenic shock.
    - ▪ Early medical management focuses on reducing the regurgitant volume – increasing contractility and dropping the afterload on the LV.

- If the patient is hypotensive, nitroprusside should be administered along with dobutamine.
- Intra-aortic balloon pumps are often used to increase cardiac output.
- Mild to moderate tachycardia may be beneficial as it limits the amount of regurgitation. Beta-blockers should therefore be avoided.
- Surgical management is the mainstay of treatment in most cases of acute MR.
- MR secondary to myocardial ischemia may be managed with early revascularization to restore blood flow to the papillary muscles.

Vasopressor of choice: See Table 21.1 for valve-specific hemodynamic management; generally, when two lesions require opposite management strategies, prioritize the valve lesion primarily driving the clinical decompensation.

BIBLIOGRAPHY

Carabello BA, Crawford FA. Valvular heart disease. *N Engl J Med* 1997;337:32–41.

Chandrashekhar Y, Westaby S, Narula J. Mitral stenosis. *Lancet* 2009;374 (9697):1271–1283.

Chen RS, Bivens MJ, Grossman SA. Diagnosis and management of valvular heart disease in emergency medicine. *Emerg Med Clin North Am* 2011;29:801–810, vii.

Mokadam NA, Stout KK, Verrier ED. Management of acute regurgitation in left-sided cardiac valves. *Tex Heart Inst J* 2011;38:9–19.

Stout KK, Verrier ED. Acute valvular regurgitation. *Circulation* 2009;119:3232–3241.

SECTION 5

Respiratory Emergencies

SUSAN WILCOX

22

Acute Respiratory Distress Syndrome

KATIE DICKERSON AND ELISABETH LESSENICH

Chapter 22:
ARDS

 ## Presentation

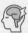
Classic Presentation:
After physiological insult (often infection), dyspnea and increased work of breathing.

Critical Presentation:
Severe dyspnea, decreasing tidal volumes and increasing respiratory rate, progressive hypoxemia.

⚠️ *Caution! May deteriorate rapidly.*

 ## Diagnosis and Evaluation

Must develop within one week of clinical insult.

Ratio of PaO_2/FiO_2 is <300 on at least 5 cm H_2O PEEP or CPAP.

Radiograph shows bilateral opacities.

Clinical findings/syndrome cannot be solely due to heart failure.

 ## Management

Address underlying cause/infection.

Prone positioning for refractory hypoxemia or P/F ratio < 150.

⊘ *Consider pulmonary vasodilators, ECMO.*

Lung-protective mechanical **ventilation in case of significant** hypoxemia or work of breathing.

⊘ *Paralyze with neuromuscular blockade if needed for ventilator synchrony.*

Sudden deterioration most often due multi-organ failure/progression of original infection.

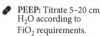 ### Lung-Protective Ventilation

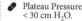

Tidal Volume:
4–8 mL/kg of ideal body weight (based upon height).

PEEP: Titrate 5–20 cm H_2O according to FiO_2 requirements.

Plateau Pressure < 30 cm H_2O.

Goal Oxygen Saturation 92–96%.

Introduction

- Acute respiratory distress syndrome (ARDS) is **severe respiratory distress of an acute and persistent nature**, caused by one or more predisposing conditions and resulting in **refractory arterial hypoxemia**.
- The pathophysiology of ARDS is characterized by **fluid build-up** within alveoli, causing **surfactant dysfunction and decreased lung compliance**
- Approximately **50% of cases are due to severe infection**, either focal (such as pneumonia) or systemic (such as sepsis). Other etiologies are listed in Table 22.1.

Presentation

Classic Presentation

- This condition can present either shortly after the patient's initial presentation in the case of a major insult to the lungs or several days after admission in patients with severe systemic illness.
- In the acute, exudative phase of ARDS, damage to the lungs causes fluid to leak across the alveolar-capillary basement membrane, causing alveolar edema and subsequent hypoxemia.
  - As a result of alveolar edema, surfactant activity is significantly compromised and lung compliance decreases.
- The acute phase of ARDS can progress to a fibrotic phase, in which case patients will exhibit continued hypoxemia, increasing dead space, pulmonary hypertension, and even greater loss of lung compliance.
- Pulmonary edema in ARDS is heterogeneous and leads to atelectatic or consolidated areas of lung interspersed with relatively unaffected regions, creating areas of intrapulmonary shunt. This results in hypoxemia that does not improve with oxygen administration alone.

Critical Presentation

- As pulmonary edema accumulates in the initial exudative phase of the disease, patients will become **dyspneic** and will demonstrate **increased work of breathing**.

Table 22.1 Etiologies of acute respiratory distress syndrome

Direct injuries to lungs	Indirect injuries
Pneumonia	
Bacterial	
Viral (including COVID)	
	Sepsis
Aspiration	
• Gastric contents	Severe trauma
• Near-drowning	• Multiple fractures
• Hydrocarbons/solvents	• Head injury
	• Burns
Smoke or toxic gas inhalation	Pancreatitis
Pulmonary contusion	Multiple blood transfusions
Embolism	
• Thromboembolism	Drug toxicity
• Fat embolism	• Salicylates
• Amniotic fluid embolism	• Hydrochlorothiazide
Oxygen toxicity	• Opiates
Reperfusion pulmonary edema	• Amiodarone
	• Cyclosporine
	• Tricyclic antidepressants
	• Chemotherapeutic agents
	Cardiopulmonary bypass
	High-altitude exposure

- Due to worsening lung compliance, **tidal volumes will decrease** and **respiratory rate will increase**. Patients will become progressively hypoxemic due to both worsening V/Q mismatch (shunt physiology).
- As above, patients may present to the ED in hypoxemic respiratory failure due to a rapidly progressive etiology, or they may present late.
- Patients **may deteriorate rapidly** during their ED course, despite appropriate therapy.

Diagnosis and Evaluation

- The diagnosis of ARDS is made clinically based on a standardized definition, easily remembered as the "4 Rs"
  - **Reason:** The syndrome must develop within one week of a known clinical insult or worsening pulmonary symptoms.
  - **R**adiograph: Chest imaging demonstrates **bilateral opacities** not fully explained by lobar collapse, nodules, or effusions. (Figure 22.1)
  - **R**ule-out volume overload/CHF: The respiratory failure is not fully explained by cardiac failure or volume overload. If a known risk factor for ARDS is not present, objective assessment such as echocardiography should be obtained to rule out hydrostatic edema.

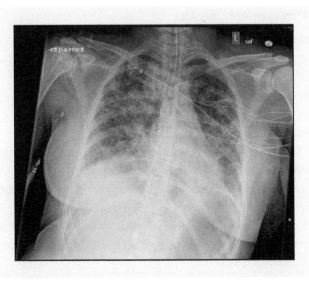

Figure 22.1 Chest radiograph of a 16-year-old girl who developed ARDS from aspiration of gastric contents, after having prolonged seizure activity with vomiting.

- $\circ$ **Ratio: PaO$_2$/FiO$_2$ ratio is < 300** on at least 5 cmH$_2$O of positive end-expiratory pressure (PEEP) or continuous positive airway pressure (CPAP).
  - It is not possible to calculate P/F ratios for patients who are on high-flow nasal cannula because the PEEP delivery is highly variable.

ARDS degree	PaO$_2$/FiO$_2$ ratio
Mild	200–300
Moderate	100–200
Severe	< 100

- **Imaging**
  - $\circ$ On a chest radiograph, ARDS looks essentially the same as cardiogenic pulmonary edema. The syndrome usually develops 4–24 hours after the appearance of radiographic abnormalities.
  - $\circ$ On CT, alveolar filling and consolidation are often seen in a heterogeneous pattern.

Critical Management

Critical Management Checklist

- ☑ Identification and treatment of underlying cause
- ☑ Mechanical ventilation if significant hypoxemia or increased work of breathing, following the "8 Ps:"
- ☑ **Proper mode of mechanical ventilation**: volume control
- ☑ **Proper volume of mechanical ventilation**: tidal volume of 4–8 mL/kg of predicted body weight
- ☑ **PEEP**: titrated 5–20 cmH2O depending on FIO$_2$ requirements
- ☑ **Plateau pressure (P$_{plat}$)**: not to exceed 30 cmH$_2$O
- ☑ **Paralysis** with neuromuscular blockade, if needed for ventilator synchrony
- ☑ **Prone positioning:** if refractory hypoxemia or P/F ratio < 150
- ☑ **Pulmonary vasodilators:** (e.g., inhaled nitric oxide or prostacyclins) if refractory hypoxemia
- ☑ **Perfusion:** veno-venous extracorporeal membrane oxygenation

- **Lung-protective ventilation** is the mainstay of management in ARDS.
  - This is done by using the **lowest possible tidal volumes, airway pressures, and oxygen concentrations**, while obtaining adequate gas exchange.
- The goal of this strategy is to support a patient's oxygenation until the inflammation and edema have cleared, while minimizing further damage due to mechanical ventilation.
- Plateau pressures, obtained via an inspiratory pause on the ventilator, represent the pressures seen by the alveoli. Elevated plateau pressures can over-distend undamaged alveoli.
  - The **goal tidal volumes are 4–8 mL/kg** of ideal body weight.
  - The **goal plateau pressures are $\leq$ 30 cmH$_2$O**.
- Alveolar hypoventilation and subsequent respiratory acidosis are acceptable, if needed, to protect the lungs with small tidal volumes and low pressures. This practice is known as "permissive hypercapnia" and targets pH > 7.2–7.3.
- **Positive end-expiratory pressure (PEEP) can stabilize damaged alveoli** and increase their surface area by **recruiting areas of atelectasis**, resulting in:
  - Improved gas exchange.
  - Reduced hypoxic pulmonary vasoconstriction.
  - Reduction in the amount of intrapulmonary shunt.
  - Reduced damage from repetitive opening and closing of atelectatic alveoli.
- **Goal oxygen saturation is 92–96%** to minimize FiO$_2$ concentrations to reduce the risk of oxygen toxicity and worsening atelectasis.
- In the ED setting, PEEP can be titrated based on required FIO$_2$ using these tables:

FiO$_2$	0.3	0.4	0.4	0.5	0.5	0.6	0.7	0.7	0.7	0.8	0.9	0.9	0.9	1.0	1.0	1.0
PEEP	5	5	8	8	10	10	10	12	14	14	14	16	18	20	22	24

- Early neuromuscular blockade with cisatracurium does not reduce mortality. However, it should be used in patients who remain dyssynchronous with the ventilator despite adequate sedation.
- In patients with refractory hypoxemia, rescue therapies may be considered.
  - Prone positioning improves oxygenation and mortality. It should be considered in patients with a PaO$_2$/FiO$_2$ < 150 despite ventilator optimization.

- Although these therapies may improve oxygenation in some patients, none have been shown to reduce mortality. There is not enough evidence to support the use of these measures on a routine basis in ARDS.
  - Inhaled nitric oxide and prostacyclin (inhaled epoprostenol) may temporarily improve hypoxemia.
  - Studies of steroids in these patients have demonstrated mixed outcomes.
  - Veno-venous (VV) ECMO may be considered in intractable cases.

Sudden Deterioration

- The most common causes for sudden decompensation are related to:
  - The respiratory system or mechanical ventilation from pneumothorax, bronchial plugging, or ET tube displacement
  - The overall state of critical illness, such as GI bleeding from a stress ulcer or septic shock from progression of the initial infection.
- Death in ARDS is most often caused by multiple organ failure rather than respiratory failure.

Vasopressor of choice: should be based on underlying etiology because isolated ARDS should not require vasopressor therapy.

BIBLIOGRAPHY

Ranieri VM, Rubenfeld GD, Thompson BT, et al. Acute respiratory distress syndrome: The Berlin Definition. *JAMA* 2012;307:2526–2533.

23

Upper Airway Emergencies

PAUL GINART AND BRIAN C. GEYER

Chapter 23:

Upper Airway Emergencies

Presentation

May vary according to severity and cause, ranging from no distress to cyanosis, altered mental status, and/or respiratory arrest.

Causes include allergic, infectious, traumatic, caustic, anatomical, and mechanical.

Caution! May deteriorate rapidly.

Diagnosis and Evaluation

 Consider This

- ✿ Ask about ACE inhibitor use or C1 esterase inhibitor deficiency.

- ✿ Determine need for intubation or surgical airway.
- ✿ Do not send pt to radiology (or anywhere other than OR) without definitive airway.
- ⚠ **Caution:** Do not use oxygen saturation as a marker of airway patency.

Imaging: CT scan, looking for evidence of swelling, mass or infection.

Labwork and history: guided by suspected underlying cause.

Chapter 23:

Upper Airway Emergencies

 Management

Securing the Airway

- If intubating, have surgical airway set up and video laryngoscopy.
- Consider use of a smaller tube.
- Consider nasal intubation.
- Consider awake intubation **to preserve airway reflexes**.
- Upper airway obstruction and high risk for hypoxemia → consider cricothyrotomy.

Use the scalpel, finger, bougie technique.

Drugs for Awake Intubation:

- *Glycopyrrolate* 4 mcg/kg 10–15 minutes pre-procedure if time permits.
- Up to 10 cc of atomized 1–4% *lidocaine* for topical anesthesia of the oropharynx.
- *Sedation with ketamine, midazolam, or remifentanil* if needed.

- Vasopressor of choice: norepinephrine (except in anaphylaxis; use epinephrine).

📌 Remember This

- Foreign body obstruction may be present: suction liquid; operating room for solid incomplete obstruction.

- Complete obstruction → subdiaphragmatic thrusts (BLS), upon loss of consciousness attempt to visualize and remove obstruction with laryngoscopy and forceps.

- No obstruction visible → Intubation.

- Visualized obstruction above vocal cords that cannot be removed → cricothyrotomy.

Paul Ginart and Brian C. Geyer

Introduction

- An upper airway emergency is the actual or impending loss of air movement through any of the structures cephalad to the mainstem bronchi.
- Representing a true life-threatening emergency, this process may be viewed as a common presentation from a diverse range of etiologies (Table 23.1).
- Treatment of upper airway emergencies requires ensuring a secure airway while treating the underlying cause.

Presentation

Classic Presentation

- Patients with upper airway emergencies may have variable initial presentations, from presenting calmly and without distress to cyanotic and obtunded.
- Patients may complain of airway symptoms such as hoarseness, shortness of breath, or speech changes. Patients may also complain of systemic symptoms such as an allergic reaction or fever.

Critical Presentation

- There is often rapid progression from benign to life-threatening symptoms, and one of the key challenges is to anticipate a patient's clinical course.
- Key warning signs of impending airway collapse include:
  - Signs of upper airway obstruction: stridor, muffled **"hot potato"** voice.
  - Difficulty managing secretions: drooling, **tripod** position, pooled secretions in posterior pharynx.
  - Signs of respiratory failure: dyspnea, tachypnea, accessory muscle use, hypoxemia.
- Patients may not demonstrate hypoxemia until late in their presentation; SpO$_2$ should never be monitored as a marker of airway patency.

Table 23.1 Differential diagnosis for upper airway emergencies

Allergic

- Anaphylaxis
- Angioedema

Infectious

- Ludwig's angina
- Retropharyngeal abscess/other deep space infections of the neck
- Peritonsillar abscess
- Epiglottitis

Traumatic and caustic

- Thermal burn
- Traumatic hematoma
- Caustic ingestion
- Inhaled toxins

Anatomical and mechanical

- Tumor/postradiation therapy changes
- Postsurgical changes
- Muscle weakness
- Congenital
- Foreign body
- Bleeding

Diagnosis and Evaluation

- The first step in the evaluation of the patient with suspected upper airway emergency is to **determine the need for emergent intubation or surgical airway, based on key warning signs, vitals, and expected clinical course.**
- If possible, a brief history should be obtained focusing on history of cancer, allergies, exposure to medications including ACE inhibitors, a family history of C1 esterase inhibitor deficiency, trauma, and recent surgery.
- A targeted physical examination should include assessment for stridor, hoarseness, urticaria, edema of skin, lips, mouth, and throat as well as a basic airway assessment for possible intubation/surgical airway including dentures, neck mobility, and cricoid evaluation
- Burns to facial skin or mouth, singed nose hairs, soot in airway should be considered high-risk features in burn patients.
- Trauma patients should be evaluated for blood in airway, facial injuries, penetrating neck injuries, and neck hematomas.
- Laboratory testing should be guided by the suspected underlying etiology.
- Imaging studies:
  - **Patients at risk for impending airway collapse should not be sent to radiology without first securing the airway.**
  - Lateral neck radiographs may demonstrate prevertebral swelling.
  - CT scan of the neck provides better anatomical detail and defines the amount and location of swelling, mass, or infection.

Critical Management

Critical Management Checklist

☑ Recognize the severity of the presentation
☑ Evaluate the need for immediate and definitive airway control
☑ Consider the differential diagnosis of the underlying etiology
☑ Secure the airway with simultaneous surgical airway setup
☑ Provide medical therapies as indicated to treat the underlying process

- Given the high-risk, time-sensitive nature of these presentations, all clinicians should be familiar with their local resources, algorithms, and airway management options prior to seeing patients.

- **Risk stratification of the patient by expected clinical course:**
  - *High-risk patients:*
    - For patients with severe anaphylaxis/angioedema, upper airway burns and signs of upper airway obstruction, **consider intubation preemptively.**
    - For trauma patients with any signs of airway involvement or "hard signs" of penetrating trauma to the neck, **consider immediate intubation.**
    - Video laryngoscopy with simultaneous surgical airway setup is recommended.
    - The high risk of airway collapse and decompensation during sedation and neuromuscular blockade must be considered in these patients.
    - The endotracheal tube should be at the smaller end of the acceptable range. (e.g., 7.0) with a back-up tube of 5.5 or smaller immediately available.
  - *Moderate-risk patients:*
    - Patients with deep space infections and upper airway tumors have lower risk for rapid evolution and acute decompensation. However, these patients may present late in their course with an impending airway obstruction.
- **Awake visualization/intubation**
  - In patients with a rapidly evolving upper airway obstruction, awake evaluation can provide invaluable information about potential complications before paralytics are administered. Paralytics should never be administered if a "cannot intubate, cannot oxygenate" situation is anticipated.
  - Giving sedation carries the risk of airway collapse during most upper airway emergencies. Optimization of local anesthesia is recommended to minimize need for sedation and to preserve airway reflexes.
  - The nasal route is usually preferred for cases mandating immediate visualization only. When planning intubation, the nasal route allows a direct passage to the vocal cords and may be easier for an awake patient to tolerate. Downsides to the nasal route include the need for reduced tube diameter and the increased risk of inadvertent extubation due to a longer pathway for the tube. Therefore, the nasal route is primarily used in cases of angioedema or when an oral mass hinders oral visualization.
  - If the patient requires immediate intubation, but not an immediate surgical airway, oral visualization/intubation is the preferred method. This may be accomplished with a flexible endoscope loaded with an endotracheal tube, or video/standard laryngoscope.

- ○ Adequate preparation – including preoxygenation, gathering appropriate staff, having desired medications drawn up, and having a detailed algorithm including back-up and surgical options – is critical prior to initiating any airway manipulation unless the patient is rapidly deteriorating.
- ○ The major steps to awake visualization/intubation are:
  - ▪ Pretreatment with glycopyrrolate (4 mcg/kg) 10–15 minutes prior (if time) to minimize secretions.
  - ▪ Topical anesthesia of oropharynx with atomized 1–4% lidocaine (can use up to 10 cc of lidocaine).
  - ▪ Sedation (+/− with ketamine, midazolam, or remifentanil as needed based on patient characteristics).
  - ▪ Airway visualization
  - ▪ Intubation
  - ▪ Postintubation management.

- **Cricothyrotomy**
  - ○ In many cases, cricothyrotomy is the definitive management technique for upper airway emergencies.
  - ○ Patients with upper airway obstruction at high risk for hypoxemia should be prepared for cricothyrotomy while the endotracheal intubation is attempted ("double setup").
  - ○ The major steps to performing a cricothyrotomy, via the scalpel-finger-bougie technique, are illustrated in Figure 23.1.
  - ○ Patients who are stable but high risk for a complicated airway can alternately undergo a surgical airway urgently in the operating room.

- **Medical therapy**
  - ○ Once the airway is secured, or for patients not immediately requiring airway intervention, medical therapy should target the underlying etiology.
  - ○ For **anaphylaxis** and **angioedema**, treat with:
    - ▪ IM epinephrine (0.3–0.5 mcg)
    - ▪ IV epinephrine (5–20 mcg bolus followed by infusion)
    - ▪ IV H_2-blockers, diphenhydramine, IV methylprednisolone, and albuterol.
    - ▪ In cases of angioedema with a known or suspected C1 esterase inhibitor deficiency, consider treatment with fresh frozen plasma or recombinant C1 esterase inhibitor.
    - ▪ For infections, treat with IV antibiotics as indicated by the underlying infection, dexamethasone, and engage consultant service swiftly.

Equiment
1. #10 scalpel
2. Bougie
3. 6.0 cuffed ET tube

1) Idenitfy the cricoidthyroid membrane with the non-domimnant hand

2) Perform a 3 cm vertical incision through the skin down to the thyroid cartilage

3) Perform a horizontal incision through the extent of the circothyroid membrane

4) Pass finger through incision to feel cartilage on the other side

5) Railroad lubricated bougie through incision preloaded with 6.0 ET tube until below sternal notch

6) Advance ET tube until cuff just enters the trachea, remove bougie, and confirm placement

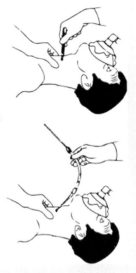

Figure 23.1 Performing a cricothyroidotomy.

Sudden Deterioration

- Sudden deterioration is the hallmark of upper airway pathology and should be expected.
- For this reason, it is **generally inappropriate to transfer patients with upper airway emergencies at risk for deterioration without a definitive airway** in place. This recommendation includes interfacility transfers, as well as intrafacility transfers to radiology or the intensive care unit. The sole exception is transport to the operating room for definitive airway management, when the ED attending deems that the benefits of management in the OR outweigh the risks of transport.

Special Circumstances

- **Foreign bodies in the airway** represent a special class of high-risk patients.

- ○ Need to rapidly distinguish complete from incomplete obstruction or esophageal foreign bodies.
- ○ Liquid and semiliquid obstructions (blood, vomit, etc.) may be cleared with suction.
- ○ Solid and poorly visualized obstructions are higher risk for poor outcomes.
- In patients with incomplete obstruction from solid material, the goal is to temporize the patient and move to the operating room for definitive management.
  - ○ Patients should be provided supplemental oxygen to prevent hypoxemia, but bag-mask ventilation should be avoided as this may worsen the obstruction.
  - ○ If the OR is not an option, the practitioner should be aware that topical anesthesia and sedation may facilitate laryngoscopy but may also result in complete obstruction (via laryngospasm or airway collapse respectively)
- Complete obstructions require immediate action to relieve the obstruction.
  - ○ In this case, basic life support techniques should be used on the conscious patient to expel the foreign body.
  - ○ Subdiaphragmatic thrusts may be applied to both the semi-upright and supine patient.
- If the patient loses consciousness or arrives unconscious:
  - ○ Immediate direct laryngoscopy should be performed to attempt removal of the obstruction using forceps.
  - ○ Cricothyrotomy is indicated if the obstruction is above the vocal cords and cannot be removed.
  - ○ If no obstruction is visible, endotracheal intubation should be performed immediately.
  - ○ Inability to ventilate the patient with subglottic obstruction indicates a tracheal obstruction. In this case:
    - ▪ Stop ventilation, deflate the cuff, replace the stylet, and advance the endotracheal tube as far as possible in an attempt to displace the obstruction into one of the mainstem bronchi.
    - ▪ Failure to ventilate at this point indicates either bilateral mainstem bronchial obstruction (which is not survivable without immediate extracorporeal membrane oxygenation) or unilateral obstruction with a contralateral pneumothorax. Thus bilateral needle or finger thoracostomies should be considered as the final salvage maneuver.

Vasopressor of choice: as indicated by circumstances. Epinephrine is first-line in anaphylaxis. Norepinephrine is appropriate for other etiologies.

BIBLIOGRAPHY

Adams JG, Barton ED, Collings J, et al., eds. *Emergency Medicine*. Philadelphia, PA: Saunders, 2008, pp. 17–30.

American Society of Anesthesiologists Task Force on Management of the Difficult Airway. Practice guidelines for management of the difficult airway: An updated report by the American Society of Anesthesiologists Task Force on Management of the Difficult Airway. *Anesthesiology* 2013;118:251–270.

Difficult Airway Society 2015 guidelines for management of unanticipated difficult intubation in adults. *Br J Anesth* 2015;115(6):827–848.

Langeron O, Amour J, Vivien B, et al. Clinical review: Management of difficult airways. *Crit Care* 2006;10:243.

Orebaugh SL. Difficult airway management in the emergency department. *J Emerg Med* 2002;22:31–48.

Walls RM, Murphy MF. *Manual of Emergency Airway Management*, 4th ed. Philadelphia, PA: Lippincott Williams & Wilkins, 2012, pp. 266–274, 377–382.

24

Asthma

IMIKOMOBONG IBIA

Chapter 24:
Asthma

Presentation

 Signs of respiratory distress, along with possible increased mucus production, acid reflux, diaphoresis, chest tightness, and prolonged expiratory phase.

 Consider the patient's asthma history (previous admissions, intubations, medication regimen, baseline PFTs).

Caution! Silent Chest
Greatly restricted air flow may lead to severe dyspnea but no audible wheeze

Diagnosis and Evaluation

 Capnography: Shark fin wave for diagnostic of bronchospasm.

 Bedside spirometry if available: Peak flow under 200 L/min indicates severe disease.

 Venous blood gas to gauge respiratory alkalosis/acidosis.

 Rule out other etiologies: Labwork, ECG, CXR.

Management

 Airway Management

- *Consider NIPPV in compliant patient protecting his/her airway, monitor closely.*
- *If NIPPV fails, intubation is required.*
- *Post-intubation is extremely tenuous and requires expert management of obstructive physiology, typically with deep sedation and neuromuscular blockade.*

 Medical Therapy

- *Albuterol, ipratropium bromide, prednisone/methylprednisolone, magnesium sulfate, epinephrine.*

Introduction

- Asthma is a chronic inflammatory disorder of the airways characterized by increased sensitivity to irritating stimuli.
- Inflammatory episodes obstruct airflow due to bronchospasm, airway edema, bronchial smooth muscle contraction, and mucous plugs, leading to recurrent episodes of wheezing, shortness of breath, chest tightness, and coughing.
- The inflammatory episodes also lead to lung hyperinflation, increased work of breathing, and ventilation–perfusion mismatch.
- A hallmark of asthma is that the inflammatory episodes are reversible.
- Asthma is extremely common, under-diagnosed, and often undertreated, leading to significant morbidity, mortality, and healthcare costs.

Presentation

Classic Presentation

- Patients present with cough, wheezing, and dyspnea. Other signs and symptoms include: increased mucous production, acid reflux, tachypnea, chest tightness, diaphoresis, accessory muscle use, and a prolonged expiratory phase.
- Key questions help risk stratify and guide management:
  - Number of prior hospital visits and admissions for asthma?
  - History of requiring intubation or ICU-level treatment?
  - Current asthma regimen?
  - Rescue medications used so far?
  - Known asthma trigger?
  - Current or recent use of systemic corticosteroids?
  - Baseline pulmonary function tests or spirometry values?

Critical Presentation

- Airflow restriction may be severe, leading to patients presenting in an upright or tripod position, with cyanosis, altered mental status, and respiratory arrest.

- **Beware of patients with suspected asthma who are not wheezing but are dyspneic.** Patients with severe disease may not have enough airflow to create a wheeze, and instead present with a **"silent chest."**

Diagnosis and Evaluation

- **Physical examination**
  - Carefully monitor heart rate, respiratory rate, blood pressure, temperature, pulse oximetry, and pain.
  - Monitor for signs of altered mental status indicating impending respiratory failure.
- **Capnography**
  - Asthma exacerbations initially produce tachypnea and a resultant low carbon dioxide level; **a normal or elevated carbon dioxide level may indicate fatigue and impending respiratory failure.**
- **Bedside spirometry**
  - If patient is able to participate, measure peak flow and/or FEV_1 (forced expiratory volume in one second) on initial assessment to evaluate severity and response to treatment. Record the best of three attempts.
  - Values can be compared to a patient's baseline and personal best.
  - Peak flow of under 200 L/minute usually represents severe exacerbation/disease.
- **Venous blood gas**
  - Can be used in addition to capnography
  - Arterial blood gas usually not necessary unless unable to accurately measure pulse oximetry
- **Chest radiography**
  - Not routinely required, but can be used to differentiate asthma from other etiologies of dyspnea including pneumothorax, congestive heart failure, and pneumonia.
- **Laboratory testing and ECG**
  - Not routinely required, but can be used to differentiate asthma from other etiologies of dyspnea.

Critical Management

- **Manage ABCs**
  - ○ *Oxygen:* Patients should be placed on supplemental oxygen therapy as needed to maintain an adequate oxygen saturation (92–96%).
  - ○ Avoid hyperoxemia.
  - ○ Patients must be monitored for signs of impending respiratory failure.
- **Medications** (see Table 24.1)
  - ○ *Inhaled beta-agonists:*
    - ▪ Inhaled albuterol is the initial rescue medication of choice.
    - ▪ Side effects include tremor, nervousness, headache, and hyperglycemia.
    - ▪ Delivered by nebulizer or metered-dose inhaler (MDI) with spacer device. In severe exacerbations, albuterol should be delivered as a continuous nebulized treatment.
  - ○ *Inhaled anticholinergics:*
    - ▪ Ipratropium bromide is an effective adjunctive therapy, addressing airway smooth muscle constriction and airway secretions.
    - ▪ Should not be used alone but has additive effect with inhaled beta-agonists.
  - ○ *Corticosteroids:*
    - ▪ Addresses the inflammatory component of the disease.
    - ▪ Administer early in treatment, as they do not take effect for a few hours.
    - ▪ There is no difference in treatment effect between enteral (prednisone) and parenteral (methylprednisone) administration; use intravenous/intramuscular route when patient is unable to take oral medications.

Table 24.1 Common medications in acute asthma management for adults

Medication	Dosing	Comments
Albuterol (nebulized)	2.5–5 mg every 20 minutes ×3 doses, then space as able	May provide continuous therapy for severe cases
Albuterol (MDI)	2–8 puffs every 20 minutes up to 4 hours, then space as able	Consider using spacer
Ipratropium bromide (nebulized)	1 mg every 30 minutes ×3 doses, then space as needed	May mix with albuterol
Ipratropium bromide (MDI)	4–8 puffs	
Epinephrine (1:1000)	0.3–0.5 mg intramuscularly, may repeat every 20 minutes ×3 doses as needed or use IV drip	
Prednisone	40–80 mg/day	For steroid burst: 40–60 mg daily
Methylprednisolone	60–125 mg/day	
Magnesium sulfate	1–2 g over 20–30 minutes	

- ○ *Epinephrine:*
  - ▪ Adjunct for patients with severe disease or those unable to tolerate inhaled therapy.
  - ▪ May produce tachycardia, arrhythmia, vasoconstriction so use with caution in patients with heart disease.
  - ▪ Intramuscular route is likely preferable as it is not sabotaged by poor skin perfusion in the setting of high sympathetic activity or shock.
  - ▪ For patients in severe status asthmaticus, can use epinephrine drip (1–15 mcg/minute).
- • *Intravenous magnesium sulfate:*
  - ○ Smooth muscle dilator that serves as adjunct for severe disease.
  - ○ Most evidence is in reducing admission for moderate asthma exacerbations.

- *Heliox:*
  - An inhaled mixture of helium and oxygen indicated only in severe asthma exacerbations.
  - Works by decreasing the density of any inhaled gas, thereby reducing the airflow resistance and work of breathing.
  - A temporary intervention intended to "buy time" while other therapies take effect.
- **Airway and ventilatory support**
  - *Noninvasive positive-pressure ventilation (NIPPV):*
    - Constant positive airway pressure (CPAP) and bi-level positive airway pressure (Bi-PAP) may be considered for patients with severe asthma.
    - NPPV requires a patent airway and patient compliance with therapy.
    - Patients receiving noninvasive positive-pressure ventilation must be carefully monitored for signs of decompensation including altered mental status, hemodynamic instability, hypercarbia, vomiting, and increased dyspnea.
    - Dexmedetomidine is an appropriate agent for easing anxiety of asthmatic patients on NIPPV; avoid benzodiazepines.
    - If noninvasive methods fail, intubation is required.
  - *Intubation:*
    - Patients with **altered mental status, severe acidosis, or hemodynamic instability should be intubated.**
    - Consider **ketamine** for induction, as this may improve bronchodilation.
  - *Ventilator management:*
    - The goal of ventilator management in the asthmatic is to oxygenate and ventilate without worsening hyperinflation, which causes barotrauma and hemodynamic instability.
    - This requires **LOW tidal volumes**, **LOW respiratory rates**, and **LONG expiratory times.**
    - Permissive hypercapnia may be required and is often well-tolerated; any pH > 7.2 is acceptable.
    - Aggressive pharmacological therapy should continue once the patient is intubated.
    - Patients may require high doses of sedation to avoid dyssynchrony; while ketamine is a useful bronchodilator, it is respiratory-sparing and thus will not help achieve ventilator synchrony; consider propofol and an opioid infusion +/− paralytic.

Sudden Deterioration

- If a patient acutely decompensates while receiving invasive or noninvasive positive pressure ventilation, consider the possibility of **pneumothorax OR intrinsic positive end-expiratory pressure (aka auto-PEEP or air trapping)**. If concern is for auto-PEEP, <u>**disconnect the ventilator circuit to allow for full exhalation.**</u> If concern is for tension pneumothorax, proceed with needle decompression and tube thoracostomy.

25

Chronic Obstructive
Pulmonary Disease

RMAAH MEMON AND ANDREW EYRE

Chapter 25:
COPD

 Presentation

Classic Presentation: Coughing, wheezing, prolonged expiratory phase, increased sputum production, respiratory distress.

May exhibit muscle wasting, weight loss, barrel chest.

Critical Presentation: Severe respiratory distress, cyanosis, AMS.

Acute COPD exacerbation may be precipitated by infection, chemical irritants, or physiological insult.

 Diagnosis and Evaluation

CXR, ECG; consider ABG and VBG.

On spirometry, FEV1:FVC < 0.7.

Labwork non specific for COPD, but can rule out other etiologies (i.e., cardiac enzymes, D-dimer).

Beware!
Altered mental status may be a sign of impending respiratory collapse.

 Management

Goal oxygen saturation:
88–92%

Chapter 25:
COPD

Pharmaceutical Interventions

- Inhaled beta agonists (albuterol preferred).

- Inhaled anticholinergics (i.e., ipratropium bromide).

- Corticosteroid.

- Antibiotics if infection is suspected.

Airway Interventions

- NIPPV can decrease work of breathing in a compliant patient, protecting his/her airway.

- If sudden deterioration, intrinsic positive end expiratory pressure (iPEEP); if suspected while intubated, briefly disconnect ventilator/BVM.

- Intubate in the case of failed NIPPV, AMS, severe acidosis, or hemodynamic instability.

  Use largest tube possible without causing damage.

Ventilator Management

Low tidal volumes.

Low respiratory rate.

Important to decrease iPEEP.

Long expiratory times.

Introduction

- Chronic obstructive pulmonary disease (COPD) is a **respiratory disease characterized by a limitation in airflow that is not fully reversible.**
- It includes chronic bronchitis and emphysema.
- Smoking is the most common risk factor for COPD. However, exposures to biofuels, air pollution, and other chemical irritants are common factors in certain areas of the world.
- It leads to alveolar damage, increased mucous production, air trapping, hyper-inflation, and airflow obstruction.
- Acute COPD exacerbations are typically caused by exposure to infection or chemical irritants.
- COPD is commonly associated with concomitant chronic conditions, including heart disease, musculoskeletal disease, cancer, and malnutrition. These conditions can impact the presentations of COPD.
- Spirometry is required to make the diagnosis, with an FEV_1 to FVC ratio of < 0.7.

Presentation

Classic Presentation

- Patients present with **coughing, wheezing, a prolonged expiratory phase, increased sputum production**, and dyspnea. Other signs may include tachypnea, accessory muscle use, pursed lip breathing, retractions, tripod position, altered mental status, cor pulmonale, right ventricular hypertrophy, subxiphoid heave, S3 or S4 heart sound, rales, and rhonchi.
- Patients with COPD may exhibit **long-term changes including barrel chest**, weight loss, and muscle wasting.

Critical Presentation

- Airflow restriction may be severe, leading to patients presenting in an upright or tripod position, with cyanosis, altered mental status, and respiratory arrest.

Diagnosis and Evaluation

- **Physical examination**
  - Monitor heart rate, respiratory rate, blood pressure, temperature, pulse oximetry, and pain.
  - Monitor for signs of **altered mental status that could indicate impending respiratory failure.**
- **Continuous pulse oximetry and capnography**
  - **A goal SpO$_2$ of 88–92% is adequate in order to avoid hyperoxemia.**
  - COPD patients tend to retain CO$_2$. On continuous waveform capnography, the plateau phase of the waveform will tend to have a sharper angle.
- **Arterial blood gas**
  - ABGs are recommended in moderate to severe exacerbations to monitor pH, PaCO$_2$ and PaO$_2$.
- **Chest radiography**
  - Recommended to evaluate for underlying etiology of a COPD exacerbation or to differentiate from other disease processes such as pneumothorax, pneumonia, CHF, or pleural effusions.
- **ECG**
  - In chronic or severe cases of COPD, may see evidence of cor pulmonale: right axis deviation, low voltage QRS complexes, right bundle branch block, right ventricular hypertrophy, and prominent P waves in the inferior leads.
- **Laboratory testing**
  - Laboratory testing in COPD is neither sensitive nor specific, but may help distinguish from other etiologies of dyspnea, especially heart failure or ACS.
  - Consider complete blood count, electrolytes, cardiac enzymes, brain natriuretic peptide, D-dimer, and medications levels.

Critical Management

Critical Management Checklist

☑ Oxygen
☑ Inhaled beta-agonists
☑ Inhaled anticholinergics

☑ Corticosteroids
☑ Antibiotics
☑ Noninvasive ventilation
☑ Intubation as needed
☑ Ventilator management

- **Manage ABCs**
  - ○ Patients should be placed on supplemental oxygen therapy as needed to maintain **adequate oxygen saturations of 88–92%.**
  - ○ **Beware of over-oxygenating** the COPD patient as this can lead to worsening ventilation–perfusion mismatch and apnea.
- **Medications** (Table 25.1)
  - ○ *Inhaled beta-agonists:*
    - ▪ Inhaled albuterol is the **initial rescue medication of choice.**

Table 25.1 Common medications for acute COPD management in adults

Medication	Dosing	Comments
Albuterol (nebulized)	2.5–5 mg every 20 minutes ×3 doses, then space as able	May provide continuous therapy for severe cases
Albuterol (MDI)	2–8 puffs every 20 minutes up to 4 hours, then space as able	Consider using spacer
Ipratropium bromide (nebulized)	1 mg every 30 minutes ×3 doses, then space as needed	May mix with albuterol
Ipratropium bromide (MDI)	4–8 puffs	
Prednisone	40 mg/day	No benefit to more than 5–7 days
Methylprednisolone	60–125 mg/day	
Levofloxacin	500–750 mg PO or IV daily	
Ceftazidime	1 g IV every 8–12 hours	
Azithromycin	500 mg PO or IV, then 250 mg daily	

- Common side effects include tremor, nervousness, palpitations, headache, and hyperglycemia.
- Delivered by nebulizer or metered-dose inhaler (MDI) with spacer device.
○ *Inhaled anticholinergics:*
    - Ipratropium bromide is an effective therapy and treats airway smooth muscle constriction and airway secretions.
    - Although previously suggested to be more effective than beta2-agonists in acute COPD, recent data suggests that anticholinergics should be used as adjuncts in most cases.
○ *Corticosteroids:*
    - Systemic corticosteroids are critical in COPD exacerbations to address the inflammatory component of the disease.
    - **Administer early in treatment as they do not take effect for hours**. There is no difference between enteral and parenteral administration.
    - There is no benefit to high-dose steroids.
    - Most patients should be treated with 40 mg of prednisone for 5 days.
○ *Antibiotics:*
    - For most moderate/severe COPD exacerbations, if there is any evidence of bacterial infection (fever, increased or new purulent sputum production, new opacity on chest radiograph), it is appropriate to start antibiotics with coverage for common respiratory pathogens.
    - **Common antibiotic classes include macrolides and fluoroquinolones.**
- **Airway and ventilatory support**
○ *Noninvasive positive pressure ventilation (NIPPV):*
    - NIPPV may be considered for certain patients with moderate to severe COPD exacerbations.
    - NIPPV decreases the work of breathing, but requires a patient to have a patent airway and be compliant with the therapy.
    - Patients receiving NIPPV must be carefully monitored for signs of decompensation including altered mental status, hemodynamic instability, worsening hypercarbia, vomiting, and increased dyspnea.
    - **If noninvasive methods fail, the patient will require intubation.**
○ *Intubation:*
    - Patients with **altered mental status, severe acidosis, or hemodynamic instability should be intubated.**
    - If intubation is required, use the **largest tube possible** that will not cause damage to decrease airway resistance during mechanical ventilation.

○ *Ventilator management:*
  ▪ The goal of ventilator management in the COPD patient is to oxygenate and ventilate without causing barotrauma and hemodynamic instability.
  ▪ This requires **LOW tidal volumes (6–8 mL/kg PBW), LOW respiratory rates (8–10 bpm)**, and **LONG expiratory times (I:E ratio of 1:4 and greater).**
  ▪ Permissive hypercapnia may be required and is often well-tolerated; any pH > 7.2 is acceptable.
  ▪ Pharmacological therapy should continue once the patient is intubated.

Sudden Deterioration

- As with asthmatics, if a patient acutely decompensates while receiving invasive or noninvasive positive pressure ventilation, consider the possibility of **pneumothorax OR intrinsic positive end-expiratory pressure (aka auto-PEEP or air trapping).** If concern is for auto-PEEP, **disconnect the ventilator circuit to allow for full exhalation.** If concern is for tension pneumothorax, proceed with needle decompression and tube thoracostomy.

BIBLIOGRAPHY

Global Initiative for Chronic Obstructive Lung Disease. Global Strategy for the Diagnosis, Management, and Treatment of Chronic Obstructive Lung Disease. Available from: https://goldcopd.org/wp-content/uploads/2019/12/GOLD-2020-FINAL-ver1.2-03Dec19_WMV.pdf [last accessed February 16, 2023].

26

Massive Hemoptysis

AMAR DESHWAR AND ELISABETH LESSENICH

Chapter 26:
Massive Hemoptysis

 ## Presentation

History of pulmonary or cardiovascular injury or disease.

May begin as minor and rapidly progress to massive with features of active hemorrhage and respiratory failure.

 ## Diagnosis and Evaluation

Obtain a focused history in attempt to uncover underlying cause.

Exclude other sources of bleeding (i.e., GI or ENT).

Labwork: Sputum culture, CBC, BMP, coagulation studies, type and screen, LFTs, and blood gasses.

Imaging: Chest CTA.

 ## Management

Airway management
- Position patient in lateral decubitus, position with culprit lung down.
- Use an 8.5 or greater ET tube to facilitate later bronchoscopy.
- Consider selective intubation into the non-injured lung.

Transfuse blood products as needed and reverse coagulopathy.
- If vasopressor still indicated, use norepinephrine.

Locate, control, and treat underlying bleeding.
- Locate: Bronchoscopy or CTA.
- Control and Treat: anticoagulation reversal (if applicable), via bronchoscopy: cold saline irrigation, topical administration of vasoconstrictive agents/ coagulant, endobronchial balloon tamponade.
- Treat: Bronchial artery embolization is often **definitive, surgery in some cases, address underlying cause.**

Introduction

- Hemoptysis is the expectoration of blood from the respiratory tract that originates from below the vocal cords.
- The definition of what is considered "**massive hemoptysis**" has evolved. Previously proposed volumes of blood ranged anywhere from 200 to 1000 mL over 24 hours. Recently there has been a shift toward considering as "massive" any hemoptysis that causes clinical consequences of respiratory failure, airway obstruction or hypotension.
- Common etiologies of massive hemoptysis are listed in Table 26.1.
- Massive hemoptysis is a medical emergency, as patients can die from:
  - **Asphyxiation** due to flooding of the alveoli with blood (most common).
  - Intractable hypoxemia from **ventilation–perfusion mismatch.**
  - Exsanguination from massive hemorrhage (least common).
- Fewer than 5% of hemoptysis cases are massive. Despite advances in diagnosis and management, mortality estimates range between

Table 26.1 Common causes of massive hemoptysis

Bronchitis
Bronchiectasis
Aspergilloma
Tumor
Tuberculosis
Lung abscess
Emboli
Coagulopathy
Autoimmune disorders
Arterial venous malformation
Alveolar hemorrhage
Mitral stenosis
Pneumonia

13–18%. Mortality correlates with amount of blood expectorated, rate of bleeding, and the underlying pulmonary reserve.

- **Anatomy**
  - ○ **Bronchial arteries branch** from the thoracic aorta or intercostal arteries, and supply oxygenated blood to the lung parenchyma.
    - ▪ These arteries are at systemic pressure, may bleed profusely, and are the source of massive hemoptysis in 90% of cases.
  - ○ **Non-bronchial systemic collaterals** (originating off the thoracic aorta, subclavian, brachiocephalic), and are the source in 5% of cases.
  - ○ **Vessel injury** from inflammation (arteritis), trauma, bronchiectasis, or erosion from an adjacent malignancy can result in massive hemorrhage.
  - ○ **Pulmonary arteries** carry large volumes of deoxygenated blood from the right ventricle across the pulmonary capillary bed and return oxygenated blood via the pulmonary veins.

This is a low-flow system and infrequent cause of truly massive hemoptysis.

Presentation

Classic Presentation

- Worldwide, tuberculosis (TB) is the most common cause of massive hemoptysis. In the United States, patients frequently have a history of pulmonary disease or smoking, cancer, prior hemoptysis, immunosuppression, cardiac disease, or coagulopathy/anticoagulant use.
- Patients may present with a sentinel bleed, with only a small amount of initial hemoptysis.

Critical Presentation

- The clinical course of these patients can be difficult to predict, as small amounts of hemoptysis may suddenly become massive.
- Patients may present to the ED in extremis with active hemorrhage and respiratory failure.

Diagnosis and Evaluation

- **Focused history and physical examination**
  - One must exclude bleeding from nonpulmonary source, such as a GI (hematemesis) or ENT (epistaxis) etiology. Expectorated material that is foamy, purulent, or has an alkaline pH suggests a lower respiratory source rather than GI source.
  - One should inquire about prior episodes of hemoptysis, known etiology of hemoptysis, and the location of the lesion, if known.
  - History of cancer, pulmonary disease, or smoking should be obtained. A history of anticoagulant use or other coagulation disorders should be determined.
- **Laboratory tests**
  - All patients should have complete blood count, prothrombin time and partial thromboplastin time, electrolytes, arterial blood gas, liver function tests.
  - Rapid type and cross-matching of blood should be performed.
  - When obtainable, sputum samples should be sent for bacterial, fungal, and mycobacterial cultures.
- **Imaging studies**
  - Chest radiography may be helpful in identifying infiltrates, lymphadenopathy, or cavitary/mass lesions. However, the sensitivity is < 50%, so a negative film still warrants further imaging.
  - If the patient does not have active bleeding and is stable enough to go to radiology, a **CT angiography of the chest** may aid in identifying an underlying etiology and potential therapeutic target for interventional radiology. Notably, bronchiectasis, lung abscess, pulmonary artery aneurysm, pulmonary embolism, and mass lesions are difficult to detect by bronchoscopy but can be identified by CT angiography of the chest.

Critical Management

Critical Management Checklist

☑ Rapidly assess the patient's airway, breathing, and circulation.
☑ Establish and maintain airway patency,
☑ Transfuse blood products as needed for resuscitation and reversal of coagulopathy.

☑ Localize the source of bleeding
☑ Position patient with suspected bleeding lung down
☑ Early consultation with pulmonary, interventional radiology, and
   thoracic surgery services as indicated
☑ Control the bleeding (i.e., bronchoscopy, angiography or surgery)
☑ Definitive treatment of underlying source of bleeding

- **Prompt airway assessment and management**
  - If emergent intubation is indicated due to hypoxemia, poor gas
    exchange, hemodynamic instability, or ongoing hemoptysis, a large
    single lumen endotracheal tube of 8.5 mm or greater will allow for
    optimal diagnostic and therapeutic bronchoscopy.
  - **Unilateral lung ventilation** by selective intubation into the
    mainstem bronchus of the nonbleeding lung can minimize spillage
    of blood to the unaffected lung. This can be done under visual
    guidance via bronchoscopy. Alternatively, a gum elastic bougie can
    be used by rotating its tip left or right into the non-bleeding
    mainstem bronchus. Finally, if the left lung is the culprit lung, the
    endotracheal tube can be blindly advanced into the right mainstem.
  - An endobronchial blocker is a device placed bronchoscopically that
    may also be used to isolate the bleeding area from the rest of the
    lung parenchyma. Placement of these advanced tracheal and
    bronchial devices requires an experienced operator.
  - For refractory hypoxemia and hemodynamic instability, ECMO can be
    considered as a temporary bridge to stabilize oxygenation. Note that
    ECMO often requires anticoagulation and may exacerbate bleeding.
- **Resuscitation**
  - At least two points of large-bore IV access (18-gauge or larger)
    is imperative.
  - Blood product transfusion should be initiated for those who are
    coagulopathic, anemic, or bleeding rapidly.
- **Patient positioning**
  - If the bleeding site is known, immediately place the patient in lateral
    decubitus position with the **culprit lung down** in order to protect
    the nonbleeding lung.
- **Localize source of bleeding**
  - The initial diagnostic procedure, **flexible bronchoscopy** can be
    performed at the bedside. Localizing the bleeding requires

visualization of active bleeding, though this may not always be successful. Blood can be suctioned and lavaged to clear the airway.
○ Rigid bronchoscopy provides benefits of greater suctioning and superior visualization but is typically reserved for the operating room and has less access to distal airways.
○ When bronchoscopy is nondiagnostic or if bleeding continues, **CT angiography of the chest** should be performed to localize bleeding and allow for therapeutic embolization.
- **Control the bleeding**
  ○ *Medical therapies:*
    ▪ While the patient is being prepared for more definitive diagnostics and management, inhaled TXA may help to reduce bleeding volume.
    ▪ Reversing coagulopathy should be tailored to the individual patient's relevant anticoagulation history.
  ○ *Bronchoscopic techniques:*
    ▪ Techniques to control hemorrhage include irrigation with **cold saline** (causing local vasoconstriction); topical administration of **vasoconstrictive agents** (epinephrine or vasopressin) or topical coagulant; **endobronchial balloon tamponade**; electrocautery; and **unilateral lung ventilation.**
  ○ *Bronchial artery embolization:*
    ▪ Embolization may be a first-line treatment in many cases.
    ▪ This is often a definitive treatment and has replaced the need for emergent surgery in many patients. It is used primarily for hemorrhage involving bronchial circulation.
    ▪ In patients requiring surgical treatment, prior embolization can stop or slow bleeding, which reduces operative risk.
  ○ *Surgical techniques:*
    ▪ Uncontrollable, unilateral massive hemoptysis refractory to bronchoscopy and angiographic embolization should be evaluated promptly by a thoracic surgeon for potential lung resection.
    ▪ Relative contraindications to surgery include severe or diffuse underlying pulmonary disease and active TB. Every effort should be made to stabilize patient and reduce bleeding before surgery as perioperative mortality is much higher with active bleeding.
    ▪ Definitive therapy for massive hemoptysis includes treatment of the underlying cause.

Sudden Deterioration

- If the patient has worsening respiratory distress, intubate the patient to protect the airway.
- If the patient becomes hemodynamically unstable due to exsanguination, transfuse blood products through a large-bore IV or central access, reverse any coagulopathy that exists, and consider vasopressors as needed.
- For sudden, severe hemoptysis requiring emergent intubation, it is essential to mobilize multiple resources simultaneously and prepare a "double setup" for possible cricothyrotomy.

Vasopressor of choice: give blood products first, then initiate norepinephrine if needed.

BIBLIOGRAPHY

Davidson K, & Shojaee S. Managing massive hemoptysis. *Chest* 2020;157(1):77–88.

Radchenko C, Alraiyes AH, & Shojaee S. A systematic approach to the management of massive hemoptysis. *J Thorac Dis* 2017;9(Suppl 10):S1069.

27

Pulmonary Embolism

KATHRYN OSKAR AND LIZA GONEN SMITH

Chapter 27:
Pulmonary Embolism

 ## Presentation

Presentation may vary; suspect with worsening dyspnea, chest pain, syncope, hypoxemia, or unexplained hypotension.

Presence of risk factors: Age 40+, hypercoaguable state (*i.e., trauma, cancer, prolonged immobilization, hormonal contraceptives, thrombophilia*).

Patient may have evidence of DVT (leg pain/swelling).

Critical Presentation: Right heart failure, systemic hypotension, PEA.

 ## Diagnosis and Evaluation

ECG: non-specific changes (e.g., sinus tachycardia).

US: Echocardiography may show signs of right ventricular strain; US of lower extremity may show DVT.

Labwork: D-dimer (non-specific), troponin and BNP for risk stratification.

CXR: Non-specific, but may rule out other etiologies.

CT pulmonary angiography is diagnostic.

---------- Chapter 27: ----------
Pulmonary Embolism

 Management

Airway management and hemodynamic monitoring.

Pressor of choice: norepinephrine.

Judicious fluid administration if PE with right heart strain is suspected.

Initiate anticoagulation.

Consider thrombolysis or thrombectomy in high-risk, unstable patients.

High Risk PE:

Leads to sustained hypotension (SBP < 90 mmHg of decrease of 40 mmHg sustained for 15 min).

Intermediate Risk PE:

Biomarker or imaging evidence of right ventricular dysfunction.

IV Thrombolysis

In hemodynamically unstable, high-risk PE.

In case of sudden deterioration.

Consider in accordance with thrombolysis contraindications.

Alteplase 15 mg bolus, then 85 mg over 2 hrs if indicated.

In cardiac arrest: *Alteplase 50 mg bolus, then 50 mg over 2 hrs.*

*Dosing varies amongst recent trials.
Refer to institutional guidelines.

Introduction

- Acute pulmonary embolism (PE) carries a high risk of morbidity and mortality and has a wide spectrum of severity, from incidental diagnosis in an asymptomatic patient to sudden refractory shock and cardiovascular collapse.
- Although the exact incidence remains uncertain, it is estimated that approximately 600,000 patients are diagnosed with PE annually in the United States, with mortality rates as high as 30% for patients with hemodynamic instability at presentation.
- A **high-risk** PE is one associated with hypotension or bradycardia. An **intermediate-risk** PE has evidence of RV strain, either by imaging or biomarkers (troponin or BNP). All others are **low-risk** PEs.
- The diagnosis of PE is often complicated by presentations that can be subtle, atypical, or confounded by another coexisting disease.

Presentation

Classic Presentation

- Suspect PE in any patient with new or worsening dyspnea, chest pain (particularly pleuritic or atypical chest pain), syncope, hypoxemia, or unexplained hypotension.
- Suspicion must be heightened in patients with a higher risk for venous thromboembolism (Table 27.1), as about 79% of patients diagnosed with acute PE have evidence of deep vein thrombosis (DVT), such as pain or swelling in their legs.
- Fever, tachypnea, and tachycardia are common but nonspecific findings.

Critical Presentation

- With significant clot burden, **right heart strain** can develop, with right ventricular dilation and hypokinesis in turn causing clinical signs of right heart such as jugular venous distention and hypotension.
- Right heart failure leads to impaired left ventricular filling, causing tachycardia and systemic hypotension.

Table 27.1 Risk factors for venous thromboembolism

Age > 40 years

History of venous thromboembolism

Prolonged immobilization, including long air or ground travel
Cancer

Trauma or major surgery
Obesity

Pregnancy

Hormonal contraceptives or hormonal replacement therapy

Acute illness or inflammatory diseases (such as inflammatory bowel disease)
Genetic or acquired thrombophilia

- Factor V Leiden

- Lupus anticoagulant

- Antiphospholipid antibody syndrome

- Antithrombin III deficiency

- Protein C or protein S deficiency

- Pulseless electrical activity (PEA) is the most common rhythm in cardiac arrest caused by obstructive PE.

Diagnosis and Evaluation

The evaluation for suspected PE is tailored to the level of the clinician's suspicion for this diagnosis based on the patient's history, physical examination, and risk factors.

- **ECG**
  - ECG changes in PE are usually the result of acute pulmonary hypertension, manifesting as tachycardia, symmetric T wave inversion in the anterior leads (V_1–V_4), the nonspecific McGinn–White $S1Q_3T_3$ pattern, P-wave pulmonale, and right bundle branch block.
- **Chest radiography**
  - Chest X-ray is rarely diagnostic for PE, but can identify alternative diagnoses.
  - **"Hampton's hump,"** a pleural-based, wedge-shaped area of infiltrate, can be seen in pulmonary infarction and is suggestive of PE.

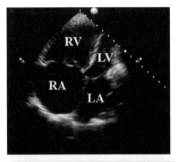

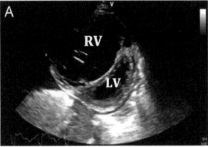

Figure 27.1 (a) RV dilation appreciated on apical four chamber view. (b) "D-sign" from elevated RV pressure resulting in septal flattening and bowing into LV.

- ○ **"Westermark's sign,"** unilateral lung oligemia, is a rare radiographic manifestation of a large PE.
- **Ultrasonography**
  - ○ Point of care cardiac ultrasonography may show signs of right ventricular strain in the presence of intermediate-risk PE.
    - ▪ **Dilated right ventricle:** RV size greater than LV on apical four chamber view, D-sign on parasternal short axis view (Figure 27.1). Patients may have a chronically dilated RV in the setting of COPD or pulmonary hypertension, making this finding sensitive but not specific.
    - ▪ **McConnell's sign:** RV free wall akinesis with sparing of the apex. This finding is more suggestive of acute RV strain rather than chronic.
    - ▪ Tricuspid annular plane systolic excursion **(TAPSE)** ≤ **16mm** is consistent with RV dysfunction and is an independent risk factor for mortality.
  - ○ Absence of cardiac ultrasound findings does not rule out the presence of PE.
  - ○ Lower extremity venous ultrasonography may show DVT. If DVT is present in a patient with suspected PE, anticoagulant therapy can be initiated before further testing.

Table 27.2 Canadian (Wells) prediction score for suspected acute pulmonary embolism

Symptoms of deep-venous thrombosis – 3.0
PE as likely as or more likely than alternative diagnosis – 3.0 Heart rate > 100 beats/minute – 1.5
Immobilization or surgery in previous 4 weeks – 1.5
Previous DVT or PE – 1.5 Hemoptysis – 1.0
Cancer – 1.0
Total score
< 2 – low pretest probability
2 to 6 – moderate pretest probability
> 6 – high pretest probability

- **Laboratory tests**
  - **D-dimer** assay, which detects the presence of fibrin degradation products, can be used as a screening test for the presence of thromboembolic disease.
    - Positive screens are nonspecific, as this test can become positive in many inflammatory states including trauma, infection, or other acute illness.
    - If a patient is deemed to have low-to-moderate clinical probability for PE estimated by clinical prediction rules (Table 27.2), a negative D-dimer test (< 500 ng/mL or < 10 ng/mL x patient age in years) can preclude the need for further evaluation and imaging studies.
    - Patient with negative PE rule-out criteria (PERC) have < 2% chance of PE and do not require D-dimer testing (Table 27.3).
  - **Troponin** and **brain natriuretic peptide (BNP)** levels can risk-stratify patients with confirmed diagnosis of PE, but are not diagnostic tools.
    - Elevated BNP and troponin have independently been associated with increased risk of adverse outcome and death in acute PE.
- **Pulmonary imaging**
  - If the clinical probability for PE is high or the D-dimer screen is positive in a patient suspected to have PE, perform **CT pulmonary angiography** (Figure 27.2) or ventilation–perfusion (V/Q) scintigraphy if CT is contraindicated.

Table 27.3 Pulmonary Embolism Rule-Out Criteria (PERC Rule)

Low pretest probability based on clinical estimate plus all of the following must be true:
Age < 50 years
Pulse rate < 100 beats/min
Oxygen saturation > 94%
No hemoptysis
No unilateral leg swelling
No recent major surgery or trauma
No prior PE or DVT
No hormone use

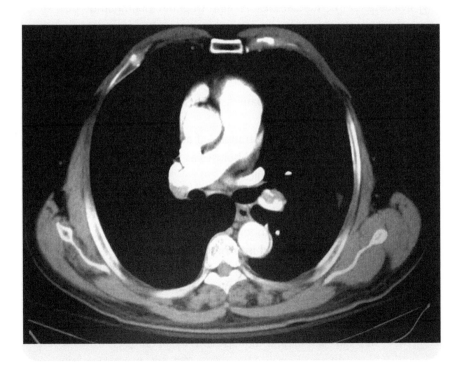

Figure 27.2 Computed tomography angiography of the chest showing a pulmonary embolism.

- ○ In pregnant patients, use shared decision making and additional clinical decision tools, such as the YEARS algorithm, when choosing whether to obtain a CT scan.
- ○ Magnetic resonance angiography has insufficient sensitivity for the diagnosis of PE.

Critical Management

Critical Management Checklist

☑ Recognize the diverse possible presentations of PE
☑ Risk-stratify stable patients
☑ Test with D-dimer, or CT scan as indicated
☑ Promptly resuscitate hypoxemic or hemodynamically unstable patients
☑ Consider lysis or thrombectomy in hemodynamically unstable patients with high-risk PE
☑ Evaluate for intermediate risk PE with troponin, brain natriuretic peptide, and echo
☑ Initiate anticoagulation

- **Manage ABCs**
  - ○ Consider intubation for patients with severe hypoxemia refractory to high-flow oxygen.
  - ○ Judicious volume administration – if acute PE with RV strain is suspected, avoid large fluid boluses as they can further dilate the RV and worsen hemodynamics.
  - ○ Initiate vasopressor support with norepinephrine.
  - ○ If a central line is indicated, this should be placed before starting anticoagulation or thrombolysis.
- **Risk-stratify high-risk and intermediate-risk PEs**
  - ○ High risk PE entails sustained hypotension (SBP < 90 mmHg or decrease of 40 mmHg for 15 minutes), bradycardia, or pulselessness.
  - ○ Intermediate risk PE shows evidence of right heart dysfunction via biomarkers or imaging:
    - ▪ Troponin I > 0.4 ng/mL (or troponin T > 0.1 ng/mL).
    - ▪ Brain natriuretic peptide (BNP) > 90 pg/mL or N-terminal pro-BNP > 500 pg/mL.

- ECG changes with a new right bundle-branch block, anteroseptal ST elevation or depression, or anteroseptal T-wave inversion.
  - Echocardiography demonstrating right ventricular dilation or hypokinesis.
- **Anticoagulation**
  - Patients diagnosed with PE should be started on anticoagulation unless otherwise contraindicated to prevent clot propagation.
  - Start patients with high clinical probability of PE on anticoagulation therapy while awaiting diagnostic confirmation.
  - **Intravenous unfractionated heparin** may be the best initial choice in unstable patient who might need to undergo procedural intervention.
    - Initial bolus dose of 80 IU/kg IV (up to 5000 IU) followed by continuous infusion of 18 IU/kg per hour to target activated thromboplastin time 1.5–2.5 times normal value.
  - **Oral factor Xa inhibitors** such as apixaban and rivaroxaban are noninferior to enoxaparin/warfarin with decreased significant bleeding.
    - Apixaban 10 mg twice daily x 7 days then 5 mg twice daily afterward.
    - Rivaroxaban 15 mg twice daily x 3 weeks then 20 mg daily afterward.
  - **Dabigatran,** oral direct thrombin inhibitor, approved for treatment of PE after 5–10 days of parenteral anticoagulation.
  - Subcutaneous **low-molecular weight heparin** (LMWH) or **fondaparinux** (preferred in patients with history of heparin-induced thrombocytopenia) can be initiated as bridging therapy to a vitamin-K antagonist if creatinine clearance > 30.
    - **Enoxaparin (LMWH)**: 1 mg/kg subcutaneously twice daily.
    - **Warfarin:** daily oral dosing to achieve a target international normalized ratio (INR) of 2.0–3.0.
  - **Pregnancy:** anticoagulant of choice is LMWH.
  - **Cancer:** anticoagulant of choice is LMWH though apixaban, rivaroxaban, edoxaban, and dabigatran can also be used.
  - Patients diagnosed with PE in the setting of a major contraindication to anti-coagulation should be considered for inferior vena cava filter **(IVC filter)** placement to prevent further embolic burden from reaching the lungs.
  - **Most hemodynamically stable patients with PE will recover completely with anticoagulation therapy alone.**

- **Consider need for thrombolysis**
  - ○ Intravenous thrombolysis is associated with reduced mortality in hemodynamically unstable (high-risk) PE. Data do not support routine systemic thrombolysis in intermediate-risk PE.
    - ▪ First, consider absolute and relative contraindications to systemic thrombolysis (Table 27.4).
    - ▪ Give **alteplase 15 mg bolus followed by 85 mg over 2 hours** if indicated.
    - ▪ In a cardiac arrest due to suspected PE, **alteplase 50 mg bolus can be given followed by 50 mg over 2 hours**.
  - ○ **Catheter-directed thrombolysis,** percutaneous mechanical thrombectomy, or surgical thrombectomy may be warranted for unstable patients, particularly those with large clot burden on imaging, persistent hypoxemia, shock index (HR/SBP) > 1.0, or relative contraindication to systemic thrombolysis.
  - ○ Many healthcare facilities are adopting pulmonary embolism response teams (**PERT**). This multidisciplinary approach brings together medical, surgical, and endovascular specialists to collaboratively pursue most appropriate treatment. If available, activate PERT early for intermediate and high-risk PE if available.

Sudden Deterioration

- If a patient with known or highly likely PE becomes pulseless, give IV thrombolysis as part of resuscitation.
- The most common cause of respiratory and hemodynamic deterioration is sudden increase in clot burden or worsening of RV dilation (e.g., large volume fluid bolus).
- If hypotension develops, consider inotrope/pressor support and thrombolysis.
- Intubation may be necessary to improve oxygenation/ventilation and establish control of the airway, but is very hemodynamically perilous for patients with RV failure and should be done with caution and pressor support.
- Activate PERT or consult appropriate specialty services early for consideration of more advanced therapies.

Table 27.4 Systemic thrombolysis contraindications

Absolute:

Prior intracranial hemorrhage

Recent traumatic brain or face injury (confirmed radiographically) *

Recent brain or spinal cord surgery

Recent ischemic stroke (< 3 months prior)

Known arteriovenous malformation

Known intracranial neoplasm

Known ischemic stroke in the last 3 months

Known bleeding diathesis

Active bleeding (excluding menstrual)

*does not include syncope with mild head trauma

Relative:

Recent ischemic stroke (> 3 months prior)

Recent major surgery (not brain/spine; < 3 weeks prior)

Recent internal bleeding (< 3 weeks prior)

Recent puncture of non-compressible vessel

Platelets < 100

Oral anticoagulants

Age > 75 years

Dementia

Pregnancy or < 1 week postpartum

Vasopressor of choice: norepinephrine.

BIBLIOGRAPHY

Giri J, Sista A, & Weinberg I. Interventional therapies for acute pulmonary embolism-current status and principles for the development of novel evidence: a scientific statement from the American Heart Association. *Circulation* 2019;140(20): e774–e801.

SECTION 6

Gastrointestinal Emergencies

CASSIDY DAHN

28

Gastrointestinal Bleeding

JOEL MOLL, ROBERT TIDWELL, AND ROBERT ADAMS

Chapter 28:
GI Bleed

Upper GI Bleed:

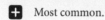 Most common.

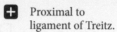 Proximal to ligament of Treitz.

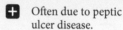 Often due to peptic ulcer disease.

Presentation

 Hematemesis ("coffee grounds" emesis), melena (dark, tarry stools).

 May also see hematochezia in large or brisk UGIB.

 Critical Presentation: signs of shock.

Diagnosis and Evaluation

 CBC, coagulation studies, type and screen, CMP, cardiac enzymes.

BUN/Cr ratio > 30 suggestive of UGIB.

 CXR to exclude free air (perforation).

Management

 Airway management and hemodynamic support.

Transfuse as necessary.

 Correct coagulopathies and reverse anti-coagulants.

 High-dose proton pump inhibitor.

 Consider balloon tamponade in massive hematemesis.

 Variceal: cephalosporin /flouroquinolone, consider octreotide.

 Consult GI, surgery, IR as needed.

Chapter 28:
GI Bleed

Lower GI Bleed:

 Distal to ligament of Treitz, often due to diverticular disease.

 ## Presentation

Hematochezia
(bright red blood per rectum).

Critical Presentation:
signs of shock.

 ## Diagnosis and Evaluation

CBC, coagulation studies, type and
screen, CMP, cardiac enzymes.

Consider, CTA to localize source.

 ## Management

Airway management
and hemodynamic
support.

🔘 *Transfuse as necessary.*

Correct coagulopathies
and reverse
anti-coagulants.

Consult GI, surgery,
IR as needed.

Introduction

- **Upper gastrointestinal bleed (UGIB)**
  - UGIB is bleeding proximal to the ligament of Treitz (esophageal, gastric, or duodenal source).
  - More common than lower gastrointestinal bleeding (approximately 70% of GIB).
  - **Most common cause is peptic ulcer disease.**
  - Common etiologies are listed in Table 28.1 (in order of frequency).
  - Varices result from increased portal resistance and blood flow. They can cause upper or lower GI bleeds, and have a higher mortality than nonvariceal bleeding, with up to 30% mortality during the first variceal bleed episode.
- **Lower gastrointestinal bleed (LGIB)**
  - LGIB is bleeding distal to the ligament of Treitz.

Table 28.1 Common etiologies of upper gastrointestinal bleed

Adult patients
Gastric and/or duodenal ulcers
Esophagogastric varices
Severe or erosive gastritis/duodenitis
Severe or erosive esophagitis
Portal hypertensive gastropathy
Angiodysplasia (also known as vascular ectasia)
Mallory-Weiss syndrome
Mass lesions (polyps/cancers)
No lesion identified (10–15% of patients)
Pediatric patients
Stress gastritis or ulcer
Esophagitis
Peptic ulcer disease
Mallory-Weiss tear (associated with vomiting)

Table 28.2 Common etiologies of lower gastrointestinal bleed

Adult patients

Diverticulosis

Ischemia

Anorectal (hemorrhoids, anal fissures, rectal ulcers)

Neoplasia (polyps and cancers)

Angiodysplasia

Postpolypectomy

Inflammatory bowel disease

Radiation colitis

Other colitis (infectious, antibiotic-associated, ischemic, colitis of unclear etiology)

Small bowel/upper GI bleed

Pediatric patients

Infectious/allergic colitis

Anorectal fissure

Inflammatory/infectious enteritis/colitis

Neonate: Consider necrotizing enterocolitis, malrotation/volvulus, Hirschsprung, coagulopathy, Meckel's diverticulum, or intussusception

- ○ Less common than UGIB (approximately 30% of GIB).
- ○ LGIB has lower mortality rate than UGIB.
- ○ **Most common cause is diverticular disease.**
- ○ Often self-limited, although can be massive.
- ○ Common etiologies are listed in Table 28.2 (in order of frequency).
- **Differential diagnosis considerations**
  - ○ Oropharyngeal or nasopharyngeal bleeding.
  - ○ Black stools: iron or bismuth (Pepto-Bismol), but will be guaiac negative.
  - ○ Bright red stools or emesis: red foods including wine, beets.
  - ○ False-positive guaiac tests: certain fruits (cantaloupe, grapefruit, figs), uncooked vegetables, red meat, methylene blue, chlorophyll, iodide, cupric sulfate, bromides; however, any positive test should be assumed positive until proven otherwise

○ False-negative guaiac test: dry stools, low pH, antacids, antioxidants (e.g., high-dose vitamin C); use of hemoccult developer and card on gastric contents will cause false-negative due to the pH. (Use separate gastroccult developer and card.)

Presentation

Classic Presentation

- **Upper gastrointestinal bleed**
  ○ Presentation: hematemesis, coffee-ground emesis, and/or melena.
  ○ **Hematemesis:** more easily recognized as "coffee grounds;" usually signifies higher risk of active bleeding.
  ○ **Melena:** dark, tarry stools. Usually suggests a minimum loss of 100–200 mL of blood from UGI tract. Dark color is due to the partial digestion of blood and indicates blood that has been present in the GI tract for 12–14 hours.
- **Lower gastrointestinal bleed**
  ○ Presentation: bright red blood per rectum (BRBPR), also known as **hematochezia**.
  ○ Caveat: large (usually > 1 L) or brisk UGIB may present with BRBPR or hematochezia as well. **Approximately 10–15% of hematochezia is due to UGIB.**
- In addition, patients may present with symptoms/signs of associated comorbidities (e.g., encephalopathy due to liver disease, dyspnea due to blood loss, etc.).

Critical Presentation

- Higher severity of disease is indicated by:
  ○ **Signs of shock** such as hypotension, resting tachycardia, altered mental status (AMS), decreased urine output (UOP), cool skin, syncope, orthostasis. Note that change in pulse with posture is more sensitive than hypotension, but medications may mask or blunt changes (e.g., beta-blockers).
  ○ **Elderly patient** with more than two comorbidities, recurrent hemorrhage, or ischemic chest pain.

- **Variceal bleed:** suspect if history or stigmata of liver disease, cirrhosis, excessive alcohol use.
- **Aorto-enteric fistula:** suspect if there is a history of aortic graft surgery. This should prompt immediate surgical consultation and – if stable – urgent CT of abdomen with IV contrast.
- Hematemesis or hematochezia in the setting of UGIB, both associated with higher mortality and suggest a significant bleed.
- **Glasgow-Blatchford Score > 6:** this tool can help risk-stratify patients.

Diagnosis and Evaluation

- **Vital signs**
  - **Hypotension, tachycardia, tachypnea, or signs of inadequate perfusion can indicate hemorrhagic shock and require immediate treatment.**
- **History**
  - Ask about history that may be significant for peptic ulcer disease, liver disease, diverticular disease, use of anticoagulation, aortic surgery, etc.
  - Associated risk factors for *peptic ulcer disease:*
    - Non-steroidal anti-inflammatory drugs (NSAIDs), anticoagulants, glucocorticoid, or aspirin use
    - *Helicobacter pylori* infection
    - Critical illness
    - Gastric acid production
- **Physical**
  - **Assess hemodynamic status immediately.**
  - Abdominal examination: ascites, surgical scars, pain/tenderness suggesting acute abdomen (e.g., rebound and guarding).
  - Check for stigmata of liver disease (e.g., encephalopathy, gynecomastiatia), bruising suggestive of anticoagulant use or thrombocytopenia.
  - Consider rectal examination if diagnostic uncertainty: Evaluate stool (melena vs BRBPR), hemorrhoids, anal fissures, anorectal mass.
- **Nasogastric aspiration and lavage**
  - Uncertain utility and evidence for need in acute setting
  - Procedure may cause false-negative and false-positive results.

- ○ May be useful for risk stratification in high-risk patients.
- ○ Higher risk procedure among patients with esophageal varices as etiology of GIB.
- **Laboratory testing**
  - ○ *Complete blood count:*
    - Hemoglobin/hematocrit (Hgb/Hct) may not initially reflect extent of acute blood loss during active bleeding.
    - **Suspected or confirmed significant blood loss or hemodynamic instability are indications for transfusion despite initial hemoglobin.**
    - Initial Hct < 30% for UGIB portends worse prognosis.
  - ○ *Coagulation profile (PT/PTT/INR) and fibrinogen in patients with liver disease:*
    - Initial elevated INR from underlying liver disease portends worse outcomes.
    - Caveat: Neither coagulation studies nor platelet count are affected by antiplatelet agents, direct thrombin inhibitors, or Xa inhibitors.
  - ○ *Type and screen/type and cross:*
    - For critical patients or high-risk GIB, be sure to have blood preemptively prepared by the blood bank.
  - ○ *Chemistries:*
    - BUN/creatinine ratio > 30 without kidney injury suggests UGIB. (Digested blood is a source of urea.)
    - Use chemistries to evaluate for associated comorbidities such as renal failure or liver disease.
  - ○ *Cardiac enzymes:*
    - Use cardiac enzymes and ECG to evaluate for signs of cardiac stress and to evaluate for other etiologies. (E.g., abdominal pain could be the only symptom of a myocardial infarction.)
- **Glasgow-Blatchford score**
  - ○ Uses patient's vital signs, blood analysis results, and clinical presentation to establish score.
  - ○ **Adult** patients with **UGIB** may be considered for discharge with outpatient follow-up if patients have **all the following**:
    - Overall score 0 (some new evidence suggests ≤ 1 may be safe)
    - Normal Hgb (> 13 g/dL for men or 12 g/dL for women)
    - SBP ≥ 110 mmHg
    - Pulse < 100 beats/minute
    - BUN < 18.2
    - No melena, syncope, heart failure, or liver failure

- **Differentiating UGIB from LGIB**
  - *UGIB is suggested by*
    - History of UGIB or peptic ulcer disease risk factors
    - Melanic stool on examination
    - BUN/Cr ratio > 30
    - Younger age
  - *LGIB is suggested by*
    - History of LGIB, hemorrhoids, diverticular disease
    - Clots in stool
    - Hematochezia + hemodynamic instability may suggest UGIB
    - Older age

Critical Management

Critical Management Checklist

- ☑ Secure airway (if massive hematemesis or risk for aspiration)
- ☑ Establish large bore IV access
- ☑ Resuscitate with blood products as needed (PRBCs, FFP, PLTs, CRYO)
- ☑ Correct coagulopathies and reverse anticoagulants
- ☑ High-dose proton pump inhibitor
- ☑ Consider balloon tamponade in massive hematemesis (Blakemore/Minnesota/Linton tubes)
- ☑ Variceal: start cephalosporin/fluoroquinolone and consider octreotide
- ☑ UGIB: obtain CXR to exclude free air (perforation)
- ☑ LGIB: if stable, obtain CTA abdomen/pelvis to localize source
- ☑ Consult gastroenterology, surgery, interventional radiology as appropriate

- **All patients**
  - Large-bore IV access for volume resuscitation: short > 18G peripheral IVs. *Remember, due to greater length and smaller size of lumen, multilumen central lines are significantly slower and not the best for volume resuscitation!*
  - Secure the airway if indicated.
  - Type and cross for blood products.
  - **Blood product resuscitation:**
    - **PRBCs** for significant active bleeding, unstable hemodynamics, or HGB < 7
    - **FFP** for significant active bleeding, unstable hemodynamics, or INR > 2

- **PLTS** for every six rounds of resuscitation or PLTS < 50k
- **CRYO** as part of your institutional protocol or FIB < 150
- **Massive transfusion protocols are essential for mitigating mortality related to significant bleeding by ensuring early and balanced transfusion, reducing further coagulopathy due to transfusion of high volume of crystalloid or only red cells.**
  - Correct **coagulopathies**:
    - Consider indication for the patient's anticoagulation and weigh the risk of further bleeding before reversing anticoagulation.
    - Consider antifibrinolytic agents (e.g., TXA) in the setting of massive bleeding, though evidence is mixed.
    - **Warfarin, Xa inhibitors, or liver disease:** Consider fresh frozen plasma (FFP) or prothrombin complex concentrate (PCC).
    - **Heparin:** consider protamine.
    - **Dabigatran:** consider idarucizumab or PCC.
    - **Thrombocytopathia**: consider DDAVP for uremic platelet dysfunction or anti platelet agents.
  - Consult for bleeding control (GI for endoscopy, interventional radiology, surgery).
  - Admission to appropriate level of care. Patients with unstable vital signs, brisk bleeding, or elevated Glasgow-Blatchford Score are appropriate for ICU level of care.

Management Specifics for Upper Gastrointestinal Bleed

- Consider proton pump inhibitors (PPIs)
- H_2-receptor antagonists have not been shown to have the same reduction in rebleeding or transfusion requirements as PPIs.
- Consider metoclopramide to promote gastric motility and help improve visualization during endoscopy.

Variceal Bleeding

- **Prophylactic antibiotics** (usually third-generation cephalosporin or fluoroquinolone) to prevent spontaneous bacterial peritonitis due to higher risk of bacterial translocation during acute GIB.
- Decrease splanchnic blood flow (limited evidence supporting use):
  - **Octreotide**: bolus and infusion
  - **Vasopressin**: bolus and infusion.

- Insertion of balloon-tamponade device (e.g., Blakemore/Minnesota/Linton) tube to tamponade bleeding varices.
- Transjugular intrahepatic portosystemic shunt (TIPS):
  - Placement of stent from portal vein to hepatic vein to decrease pressure in the portal system.
  - Usually placed by interventional radiology.
  - Can act as a bridge to liver transplantation in the setting of severe or recurrent bleeding.

Management Specifics for Lower Gastrointestinal Bleed

- There are fewer evidence-based therapies for LGIB than for UGIB.
- Angiography can identify the site in 40% of LGIB, but must be actively bleeding (usually indicated by hemodynamic instability or continued transfusion requirement).
- Alternate localization strategies include tagged RBC scan, capsule endoscopy, or push enteroscopy for stable patients.
- Sigmoidoscopy/colonoscopy is helpful for stable patients and has the potential benefit of also being therapeutic.
- Surgical intervention is required more commonly in LGIB than UGIB.

Sudden Deterioration

- Secure the airway if indicated
  - If possible, resuscitate prior to intubation with blood products and vasopressors as needed.
  - Place large bore nasogastric tube prior to intubation and suction gastrointestinal contents.
  - Administer promotility agents (e.g., metoclopramide) prior to intubation.
  - Prepare double suction setups.
  - Direct laryngoscopy is often preferred due to risk of video laryngoscopy contamination by blood.
  - Intubate patient with head of bed elevated.
  - Be prepared to transition to surgical airway.
  - Consider reduced-dose sedative (e.g., ketamine) and higher-dose paralytic depending on degree of shock.

- ○ Anticipate need for further resuscitation and/or vasopressors following induction and transition to positive pressure.
- If hemoptysis was incorrectly labeled as hematemesis, then consider intubation of patient and ventilation with hemorrhaging lung in dependent position.
- Initiate massive transfusion for patients with active bleeding and hemodynamic instability.
- For continued hypotension despite massive transfusion, maintain MAP > 65 with vasopressors.
- Always consider hypocalcemia as a cause of refractory hypotension in patients receiving significant PRBCs.
- In the setting of massive hematemesis, consider placement of Blakemore/Minnesota tube to tamponade bleeding varices.
- Check chest X-ray to assess for development of free air, requiring surgical intervention.
- Emergent consultation for control of bleeding source.

Special Circumstances

- **Aortoenteric fistula**
  - ○ Suggested by a **history of aortic graft** (at any time).
  - ○ The fistula usually involves the lower duodenum or jejunum.
  - ○ **Emergent, early surgical consultation** is needed (esophagogastroduodenoscopy or colonoscopy will not visualize these areas and will not be therapeutic).
- **Liver disease**
  - ○ Manage as presumed variceal bleeding.
- **Jehovah's Witnesses**
  - ○ It is unlawful to transfuse if the patient expressly forbids it; document the patient's wishes carefully.
  - ○ Manage shock and critical illness according to standard protocols.
  - ○ Experimental use of hemoglobin substitutes is not yet approved by the FDA.
  - ○ Most other treatment options (i.e., erythropoietin, factor VIIa) are not helpful in the short term for acute bleeding.
  - ○ Some patients will accept fractions of whole blood (e.g., albumin) or transfusions.

BIBLIOGRAPHY

Barkun AN, Almadi M, Kuipers EJ, et al. Management of nonvariceal upper gastrointestinal bleeding: Guideline recommendations from the International Consensus Group. *Ann Intern Med* 2019;171(11):805–822. https://doi.org/10.7326/M19-1795

Chavez-Tapia NC, Barrientos-Gutierrez T, Tellez-Avila F, et al. Meta-analysis: Antibiotic prophylaxis for cirrhotic patients with upper gastrointestinal – an updated Cochrane review. *Aliment Pharmacol Ther* 2011;34(5):509–518. https://doi.org/10.1111/j.1365-2036.2011.04746.x

Gong EJ, Hsing LC, Seo HI, et al. Selected nasogastric lavage in patients with nonvariceal upper gastrointestinal bleeding. *BMC Gastroenterol* 2021;21(1):113. https://doi.org/10.1186/s12876-021-01690-z

HALT-IT Trial Collaborators. Effects of a high-dose 24-h infusion of tranexamic acid on death and thromboembolic events in patients with acute gastrointestinal bleeding (HALT-IT): An international randomised, double-blind, placebo-controlled trial. *Lancet* 2020;395(10241):1927–1936. https://doi.org/10.1016/S0140-6736(20)30848-5

Kamboj AK, Hoversten P, Leggett CL. Upper gastrointestinal bleeding: Etiologies and management. *Mayo Clin Proc* 2019;94(4):697–703. https://doi.org/10.1016/j.mayocp.2019.01.022

Laine L, Jensen DM. Management of patients with ulcer bleeding. *Am J Gastroenterol* 2012;107(3):345–360; quiz 361. https://doi.org/10.1038/ajg.2011.480

Tayyem O, Bilal M, Samuel R, et al. Evaluation and management of variceal bleeding. *Dis Mon* 2018;64(7):312–320. https://doi.org/10.1016/j.disamonth.2018.02.001

29

Abdominal Aortic Aneurysms

PAYAL MODI AND NATHANIEL OZ

Chapter 29:
AAA

 ## Presentation

May present as asymptomatic (found on routine imaging), symptomatic (often abdominal or lower back pain), or, most often, ruptured.

Ruptured AAA: Severe, abrupt "tearing" abdominal or back pain.

May or may not see classic triad of hypotension, pain, and pulsatile abdominal mass.

 ## Diagnosis and Evaluation

Stable vital signs are falsely reassuring; in event of rapid deterioration suspect aneurysm rupture.

Labwork: CBC, type and screen, coagulation studies.

Imaging: US may be used for screening, but CT is most accurate and preferred to rule out rupture.

 ## Management

Airway management.

Hemodynamic monitoring.

Blood transfusions and norepinephrine as needed.

Expedite surgery **for definitive** management of rupture.

Introduction

- **Abdominal aortic aneurysm** (AAA) refers to aortic dilatations of > 3 cm.
- True AAA is a localized dilatation of the aorta caused by weakening of the aorta wall involving all three layers (intima, media, and adventitia).
- False aneurysms or pseudoaneurysms typically occur at sites of vessel injury that allows blood to leak out from the arterial lumen while remaining enclosed by adventitia or surrounding soft tissue.
- 90% of aortic aneurysms occur in the descending aorta, most commonly infrarenally.
- **Aortic dissection is *not* the same as AAA.** In dissection, blood enters the media of the aorta and splits the aortic wall.
- AAA causes 15,000 deaths annually in the United States.
  - Screening and early intervention has improved death rates; mortality is 1–2% for elective repair of AAAs.
  - **Mortality is as high as 90% in ruptured aneurysms and 50% for those who receive emergency surgery.**
  - Rupture risk is related to the size of the AAA as detailed in Table 29.1.
- Risk factors for the development of an AAA are listed in Table 29.2.

Presentation

Asymptomatic

- AAA may be identified from screening patients with risk factors or as an incidental finding on abdominal imaging.

Table 29.1 Abdominal aortic aneurysm size and risk of rupture

AAA diameter (cm)	5-year risk of rupture (%/year)
< 4.0 cm	0%
4.0–4.9 cm	0.5–5%
5.0–5.9 cm	3–15%
6.0–6.9 cm	10–20%
7.0–7.9 cm	20–40%
≥ 8.0 cm	30–50%

Table 29.2 Risk factors for abdominal aortic aneurysm

Male sex (6:1)

Age older than 50 years

History of atherosclerotic disease

Family history of AAA in first-degree relative
Smoking (90% of AAA)

Hypertension
Hyperlipidemia

Previous aortic aneurysm
End-stage syphilis

Mycotic infections (immunosuppression, IV drug use, syphilis)

Symptomatic

- In AAA, pain is usually described as abdominal or lower back.
- Atypical presentations include pain in the chest, thigh, inguinal area, or scrotum.
- Presentation of inflammatory aneurysms may also include systemic signs such as fever or weight loss.
- Less common but critical presentations of AAA include:
  - Extremity ischemia due to thromboembolism from within the aneurysm.
  - Complete aortic occlusion
  - Disseminated intravascular coagulation (DIC)
  - Aortic fistulization:
    - Aortoenteric fistulas at the duodenum can present as upper or lower GI bleeding.
    - Aortovenous fistulas to the inferior vena cava can present as high-output heart failure with lower-extremity edema, dilated superficial veins, decreased peripheral blood flow, and renal insufficiency with hematuria.

Ruptured

- Rupture is often the first presentation of patients with AAA and is usually experienced as severe abdominal or back pain.

- This pain is severe or abrupt in onset and characterized as a ripping or tearing.
- Any patient with these symptoms and a known AAA is at risk for imminent rupture.
- The **classic triad is hypotension, pain, and pulsatile abdominal mass,** though this occurs in only 50% of patients.
- **Hypotension is the least consistent** part of the triad, occurring in as few as 33% of patients.
- Stable vital signs can be falsely reassuring as these patients can deteriorate rapidly.
- Bleeding can lead to hemorrhagic shock with hypotension, altered mental status, syncope, and death.

Diagnosis and Evaluation

- **Physical examination**
  - Physical examination may be unremarkable and cannot be used to rule out AAA.
  - Signs of rupture:
    - Periumbilical ecchymosis (Cullen's sign)
    - Flank ecchymosis (Grey–Turner's sign)
    - Vulvar or scrotal hematomas (Bryant's sign).
  - **Complete peripheral vascular examination should be performed.**
- **Diagnostic tests**
  - *Laboratory tests:*
    - No specific laboratory study can diagnose an AAA.
    - In mycotic aneurysms, blood cultures can be positive and reveal the etiology of the infecting agent.
  - *Abdominal radiography:*
    - Although abdominal radiography is not preferred, imaging may show calcification of the aortic wall.
  - *Ultrasound:*
    - **Ultrasound (US) is the preferred method of screening and has 100% sensitivity.**
    - Point of care US can be used to evaluate an unstable patient with a potential AAA, obviating the need to send the patient to radiology.
      - The entire abdominal aorta must be visualized for diagnosis.

- Patients with a normal diameter abdominal aorta are unlikely to have an AAA.
- US is limited by obesity, bowel gas, and abdominal tenderness.
  - **US is not sensitive enough to rule out AAA *rupture*.**
    - Free intraperitoneal or retroperitoneal blood in the presence of other clinical symptoms may be suggestive of rupture.
  - The biggest limitation of US is operator expertise.
- *Computed tomography (CT):*
  - CT can determine the presence, location, and size of an AAA with 100% accuracy.
  - IV contrast is not always necessary to identify AAA or hemorrhage from a rupture.
  - The crescent sign (layering blood within aorta) indicates an impending rupture.
  - During rupture, blood is frequently seen as retroperitoneal fluid adjacent to the aneurysm.
  - CT can detect aneurysmal retroperitoneal hemorrhage with higher sensitivity than other imaging modalities.
- *Magnetic resonance imaging (MRI):*
  - MRI is minimally invasive and, when combined with magnetic resonance angiography (MRA), can provide excellent details for the preoperative evaluation of AAAs.
  - MRI has 100% sensitivity in detecting aneurysms, and successfully identifies the proximal and distal extent of the aneurysms, the number and origins of renal arteries, and the presence of inflammation.
  - The use of MRI is not realistic for unstable patients due to the length of time required to obtain the images.

Critical Management

Critical Management Checklist

- ☑ Establish access with at minimum two large bore IVs
- ☑ Ensure continuous hemodynamic monitoring
- ☑ Perform bedside abdominal aortic US
- ☑ Immediately involve vascular surgery and prepare for transfer to OR for intervention and repair
- ☑ Obtain CT imaging at discretion of surgical consultants

☑ Respond to hypotension as needed with packed red blood cells or massive transfusion as needed

☑ Avoid over-transfusion or inducing hypertension (may propagate bleeding)

☑ Consider norepinephrine as first-line agent for patients requiring vasopressors

- Hemodynamically unstable patients should have standard resuscitative measures while preparing for transfer to the operating room.
  - **Shorter ED to OR times have increased likelihood of survival.**
  - **Diagnostic testing should be kept to a minimum** and not delay transfer to the OR.
- Symptomatic patients with known AAA should be evaluated by vascular surgery regardless of the AAA size.
- **Surgical management**
  - Ruptured AAA is fatal unless treated surgically.
  - The vascular surgeon may choose to repair via open approach with laparotomy or endovascular technique.
    - Open AAA repair requires direct access to the aorta through an abdominal or retroperitoneal approach.
    - Endovascular aneurysm repair (EVAR) involves gaining access to the lumen of the aorta, usually via femoral artery cutdown or percutaneously and placing a graft.
- Nonemergent treatment and monitoring
  - Nonemergent management is summarized in Table 29.3.
  - AAAs greater than 5 cm are at greatest risk for rupture and should be referred to a vascular surgeon for prompt evaluation (outpatient evaluation only if asymptomatic).

Table 29.3 Nonemergent treatment and monitoring

Asymptomatic AAA size	Monitoring
3–4 cm	Annual ultrasound
4–4.5 cm	Ultrasound every six months
> 4.5 cm	Refer to vascular surgeon
>5.5 cm	Surgery indicated

- ○ In patients with a small AAA, reduction of the expansion rate and rupture risk can be attempted with smoking cessation, blood pressure control, and beta blockade.
- **Complications of repair**
  - ○ *Infection:*
    - Infection can disrupt the anastomosis between native artery and the graft, leading to leakage of blood and pseudoaneurysm formation.
    - Subtle signs of graft infections include low-grade fever, abdominal or back pain.
    - Patients may also present in florid septic shock due to bacteremia.
    - CT should be performed to evaluate possible infection. Findings consistent with graft infection include fluid or gas collections adjacent to the graft.
  - ○ *Fistulization*
    - **Aortoenteric fistula (AEF) is a true surgical emergency.**
      - ☐ An AEF must be considered in any patient with occult or massive GI bleeding and history of abdominal aortic surgery.
      - ☐ In an unstable patient, diagnostic testing may be averted in lieu of emergent laparotomy or angiography.
      - ☐ In a stable patient, upper endoscopy and/or CT may be useful diagnostic adjuncts.
    - Aortocaval fistula:
      - ☐ Spontaneous aortocaval fistula is rare and occurs in only 4% of all AAA.
      - ☐ Physical signs may be subtle or vague. The presence of low back pain, machinery-like abdominal murmur, and high-output cardiac failure unresponsive to medical treatment should raise the suspicion.
      - ☐ Preoperative diagnosis is crucial, as adequate preparation is needed because of the massive bleeding during surgery.
      - ☐ Successful treatment depends on management of perioperative hemodynamics as well as control of bleeding from the fistula.
  - ○ *Endoleak*
    - Defined as a failure of the graft following EVAR resulting in persistent blood flow into the aneurysmal sac. These are classified into five categories depending on location of the leak.
    - Patients with suspected endoleak may be evaluated with CT and/or angiography.
    - Any patient suspected of having an endoleak should be evaluated by vascular surgery; many patients will require surgical reintervention.
  - ○ *Graft Migration*
    - Common indication requiring surgical reintervention.

- Defined as equal to or greater than 10 mm of caudal migration.
- Potential complications of graft migration include endoleak, aneurysm expansion, and rupture.
  - *Ischemia*
    - This is a frequent complication of EVAR resulting from thromboembolism, dissection or graft malposition leading to obstruction of aortic branches.

Sudden Deterioration

- In patients with suspected symptomatic AAA, **sudden deterioration almost certainly indicates an aneurysm rupture.**
- In the absence of immediate intervention, hemorrhagic shock will lead to death in more than 90% of patients.
- In the event of hemodynamic collapse, initiate massive transfusion of PRBCs and FFP via rapid blood delivery devices (e.g., Belmont or Level One).
- Notably, **if patient requires ACLS, survival is unlikely.**

30

Fulminant Hepatic Failure

AQSA SHAKOOR, DANIELLE WALSH, AND DESIREE ROGERS

Chapter 30:
Fulminant Hepatitis

*Not to be confused with acute or chronic liver failure or decompensated cirrhosis

 ## Presentation

May be vague, elusive, and vary by cause
Causes include drug-induced, infectious, vascular, pregnancy-related, and/or metabolic.

Maintain a high index of suspicion.

 ## Diagnosis and Evaluation

Lab work: CMP, LFT, toxicology, urine studies (including 24-hour copper), infectious and immune markers, hematologic and coagulation studies, lipid panel.

Notable markers of hepatic failure:

Elevated: PT, AST/ALT/ALP/GGT, high ammonia, total bilirubin.

Decreased: Albumin.

Imaging: Abdominal ultrasound, CT brain, MRI abdomen with and without contrast.

 ## Management

Multisystem Support

- First line vasopressor: *norepinephrine.*
- Maintain normocapnia.
- Goal blood glucose 120–200 mg/dL.
- Correct coagulopathy.
- Initiate RRT early if indicated.

👁 Consider This

- ✿ In case of acetaminophen overdose, give N-acetylcysteine as soon as possible.
- ✿ In sudden deterioration, consider infectious causes.

Remember This

- ✿ Close neurological monitoring is imperative to recognize cerebral edema.

  | *Goal ICP < 20 mmHg* | *Goal CPP> 60 mmHg* |

  Goal Na+ 145–155 mmol/L

Introduction

- **Fulminant**, or acute, **hepatic failure** is defined as severe hepatocyte dysfunction resulting in rapid elevation of aminotransferases, encephalopathy, coagulopathy, and multi-organ failure in an otherwise healthy individual without pre-existing liver disease.
- Acute liver failure (ALF) has an incidence of 1–2/100,000 people in the United States or approximately 3,000–6,000 cases per year with **nearly 30% of patients requiring a liver transplantation.**
- **ALF** is fundamentally different and **should not be confused with acute or chronic liver failure** or decompensated cirrhosis as the etiology of ALF is the most important determinant of transplant-free survival (Table 30.1).

Etiology

Presentation

See Figure 30.1.

Table 30.1 Etiologies of acute hepatic failure

Drugs	Acetaminophen, carbon tetrachloride, sulfonamides, tetracyclines, cocaine, isoniazid, NSAIDs, rifampicin, disulfiram, valproic acid
Infectious	Hepatitis A/B/D/E, Cytomegalovirus, Epstein-Barr Virus, Adenovirus, Herpes Varicella Zoster, Herpes Simples Virus
Vascular	Budd-Chiari Syndrome, right heart failure, shock liver, veno-occlusive disorder
Pregnancy	HELLP syndrome, acute fatty liver of pregnancy, galactosemia
Metabolic/ Miscellaneous	Wilson's disease, Reye syndrome, Tyrosinemia, hereditary fructose intolerance, Amanita phalloides, autoimmune hepatitis, primary graft failure of transplanted liver

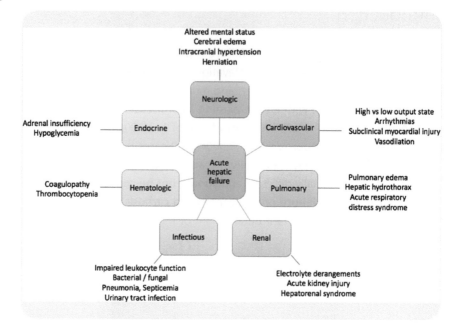

Figure 30.1 Presentation of acute hepatic failure.

Diagnosis and Evaluation

Recognition of hepatic injury may be delayed, particularly in hyperacute cases where jaundice is minimal and the presenting symptoms include confusion or agitation. **A high index of suspicion must be maintained**. Diagnostic work-up is below (Table 30.2).

Critical Management

Critical Management Checklist

☑ Evaluate airway and need for intubation (typically for grade III or higher encephalopathy)

☑ Establish access with two large bore IVs

☑ Correct coagulopathy if associated with proven or suspected bleeding

☑ Neurologic monitoring and frequent assessment for worsening cerebral edema

☑ Assess need for N-Acetylcysteine early if there is suspicion that ALF is secondary to drug ingestion.

Table 30.2 Diagnostic workup of acute hepatic failure

Chemistry	Acetaminophen level, albumin, alkaline phosphatase, alpha-1 antitrypsin level, alpha-1antitrypsin phenotype, ALT, AST, ammonia level, amylase, beta hCG, bilirubin, ceruloplasmin, cholesterol, comprehensive metabolic panel, ethanol level, GGT, lactic acid, LDH, lipase, magnesium, phosphorus, serum copper, uric acid
Hematology/ Coagulation	Antithrombin III activity assay, CBC, D-dimer, factor V, VII, VIII, fibrin monomer assay, fibrinogen, INR, PT, PTT, TEG, thrombin-antithrombin complexes
Immunology	Alpha fetoprotein (AFP) tumor marker, anti-nuclear Ab screen (ANA, IgG), anti-smooth muscle Ab, mitochondrial M2 Ab IgG
Urine studies	Urine creatinine, urine sodium, 24-hour urine copper level, urine drug screen, urinalysis
Imaging	Abdominal ultrasound, CT brain without contrast, CXR, MRI abdomen with and without contrast, transthoracic ultrasound
Microbiology/ Infectious disease	Anti-CMV Ab, CMV Ab (IgM, IgG), Coxsackie B virus Ab, EBV Ab, Hep A Ab (total and IgM), HBV panel, Hep C Ab, Hep E (pregnancy/recent travel), HSV DNA by PCR, HIV Ag/Ab, RPR
Other	EKG

Acetaminophen Toxicity

- The **leading cause of ALF in developed countries and responsible for 45.7% of cases in the United States**.
- Many patients may not have detectable levels of the compound at time of presentation, making clinical history paramount.
- The Rumack-Mathews nomogram (Figure 30.2) is a validated tool to determine risk of hepatotoxicity **within 24 hours** of acetaminophen ingestion. The **treatment or 150 line** (150 mg/mL concentration at 4 hours) was used in the US National Multicenter Open Study of Oral N-Acetylcysteine (NAC) for the Treatment of APAP Overdose and is the treatment line most commonly used in the United States.

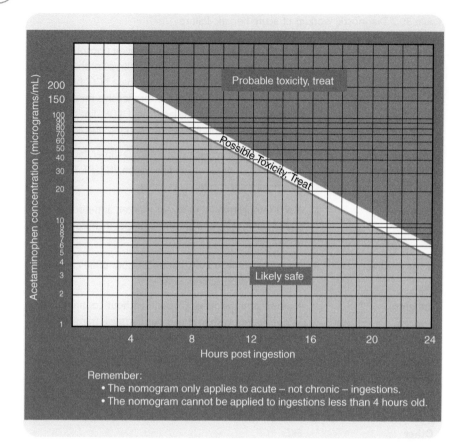

Figure 30.2 The Rumack-Mathews nomogram.

Acetaminophen Dosages

- Therapeutic range: 5–20 mcg/mL.
- Potentially toxic/critical value: > 150 mcg/mL measured 4 hours after the dose.

Management of Acetaminophen Toxicity

- Gastrointestinal (GI) decontamination
  - Treatment with activated charcoal (AC), 1 g/kg (maximum dose 50 g), if presentation within 2 hours of ingestion.

- Should not be administered to patients who are encephalopathic or are unable to protect their airway unless intubated.
- **N-acetylcysteine (NAC)**
  - Indicated for **all Acetaminophen levels** where toxicity is possible.
    - **Almost 100% effective if given within 8 hours post-ingestion** and may even be beneficial late after ingestion.
  - The 20-hour intravenous (IV) protocol is the most commonly used in practice
    - Loading dose of 150 mg/kg over 60 minutes.
    - Next, administer a 4-hour IV infusion at 12.5 mg/kg per hour (total 50 mg/kg).
    - Followed by a 16-hour IV infusion at 6.25 mg/kg per hour (total 100 mg/kg).
    - The **infusions SHOULD be continued beyond the 20 hours for patients with large ingestions or ongoing elevations in serum transaminases at the clinician's discretion.**
- Anaphylactoid reaction
  - Non-IgE mediated **anaphylactoid reaction** has been described with IV NAC administration.
  - This is typically abated with a **decrease in infusion rate**, antihistamine administration, and supportive care. However, with severe reactions, the infusion should be stopped. Consider restarting the infusion at a lower rate once symptoms improve.

Neurologic Complications

Surveillance

- **Frequent neurological checks.**
  - Worsening hepatic encephalopathy may be **due to progression to cerebral edema. Risk for cerebral edema is based on West Haven criteria grading system (Table 30.3).**
- Minimize sedation to avoid confusing drug effects with clinical deterioration.
  - If needed, choose shorter acting agents.
  - Consider avoiding agents that have significant hepatic metabolism.

Table 30.3 West Haven criteria for hepatic encephalopathy

Grade 1	Euphoria or anxiety, trivial lack of awareness, shortened attention span, impaired performance of addition
Grade 2	Lethargy or apathy, minimal disorientation, inappropriate behavior, subtle personality change, impaired performance of subtraction
Grade 3	Confusion, disorientation, semi-stuporous, responsive to verbal stimuli
Grade 4	Coma

- Imaging:
  - Consider CT scan to evaluate for cerebral edema and rule out other causes of altered mental status; however, remember that a **normal scan does NOT rule out cerebral edema**.

Hepatic Encephalopathy Grading System

- Ultrasound assessment of **optic nerve sheath diameter** (ONSD) may be useful as a surrogate for increased intracranial pressure in patients with high-grade hepatic encephalopathy (ONSD > 6 mm suggests elevated ICP > 20 mmHg)
- Herniation is unlikely with ammonia levels <150 µM/L.
- Unlike with chronic hepatic failure, lactulose has not been proven to have any long-term benefit in acute fulminant hepatic failure.
- Strongly consider intubation and intracranial pressure monitoring in patients with Grade 3 or 4 encephalopathy.

Management of Cerebral Edema/Elevated Intracranial Pressure (ICP)

- **Goals ICP < 20 mmHg** and **cerebral perfusion pressure (CPP) > 60 mmHg** (CPP = MAP − ICP).
  - Even if no ICP monitoring is available, manage grade 3–4 encephalopathy as if ICP is elevated.
- Basic management:
  - Intubation if not protecting airway or concern for progressive, high-grade encephalopathy

- ○ Position head of bed at 30–45°.
- ○ Keep head in midline position to allow jugular venous drainage.
- ○ Eliminate suctioning and lying patient supine for turns.
- ○ Consider specific treatments to prevent elevated ICP during intubation.
    - ▪ Maintain **normocapnia.**
    - ▪ Consider premedication with fentanyl (2–3 mcg/kg) or topicalization with lidocaine to attenuate ICP excursions during laryngoscopy
- ○ Correct hyponatremia and target Na 145–155 mmol/L.
- ○ Control fever and seizures.
- Osmotic therapy:
    - ○ Indicated for severe intracranial hypertension defined as sustained ICP > 20–25 mmHg for > 5–10 min.
    - ○ Mannitol
        - ☐ Avoid when serum osmolality > 320 mOsm/L OR with renal failure (risk of renal toxicity).
    - ○ Hypertonic saline with **goal Na 145–155 mmol/L.**
        - ☐ Often preferred over mannitol
        - ☐ No diuretic properties or renal toxicity

Cardiovascular Complications

Circulatory Dysfunction

- Presents as **vasodilatory shock with hyperdynamic circulation**.
    - ○ Frequently develop severe vasoplegia (low systemic vascular resistance resulting in low MAP and high cardiac output).
- Treatment:
    - ○ Treat hypovolemia with crystalloid; consider albumin as well.
    - ○ **Norepinephrine as first-line vasopressor.**
    - ○ Vasopressin is a useful adjunct in these patients and should be added early.
    - ○ Consider a higher target MAP target (> 70) to increase cerebral perfusion and maintain renal perfusion.
        - ▪ Discontinue diuretics and antihypertensives.
    - ○ Consider stress dose steroids for refractory hypotension.

Respiratory Complications

Respiratory Insufficiency

- High-flow nasal cannula is preferred over noninvasive ventilation when mental status is questionable.
- Should patients require high PEEP in moderate–severe ARDS, be cognizant of risk of increased ICP and reduced venous return.
- **Avoid hypercapnia** as this can worsen ICP.

Hepatic Hydrothorax

- Medical management includes diuretics and salt restriction.
- Thoracostomy tube can be considered in patients requiring increasing respiratory support.

Gastrointestinal Complications

- ALF is a hypercatabolic state and enteral nutrition over parenteral nutrition should be implemented if there are no contraindications for enteral feeding.
- Stress ulcer prophylaxis may be appropriate even in non-intubated patients.

Hypoglycemia

- Target serum **blood glucose 120–200 mg/dL.**
  - Bolus dextrose 50%, 50 mL via IV push as needed.
  - If glucose is persistently low, initiate low-volume infusion of D5W, D10W, or D20W as needed and titrate rate to goal blood glucose; consider more concentrated formulations (i.e., D10 or D20) to limit the amount of free water infused to avoid hyponatremia which could worsen cerebral edema.
  - Check blood glucose every 30 minutes until the goal is reached.

Renal Complications

Renal Failure

- Renal failure occurs in up to 50% of patients with ALF. Early initiation of continuous renal replacement therapy (CRRT) has been associated with improved outcomes.
- Indications for renal replacement therapy:
  - Hyperkalemia (> 8 mmol/L with EKG changes).
  - Fluid overload or pulmonary edema unresponsive to diuretic therapy.
  - Severe metabolic acidosis (pH < 7.15).
  - Blood urea nitrogen (BUN) concentration > 35.7 mmol/L or worsening hepatic encephalopathy.
  - Kidney Disease Improving Global Outcomes (KDIGO) stage 3 AKI or greater.

Hepatorenal Syndrome (HRS)

- Type I represents an acute, more severe form of renal dysfunction while Type II is a slower and less severe **form of renal dysfunction.**
- **Liver transplant is currently the best therapy for HRS.**
- The diagnosis of HRS is not always clear, and technical diagnostic criteria entail a trial of albumin as well as abstinence from diuretics and beta blockade for several days; maintain suspicion early on and consider empiric treatment.
- Empiric treatment for HRS:
  - Albumin
  - Consider vasopressors to maintain MAP > 70: norepinephrine first-line, vasopressin second-line.
  - +/− Octreotide.

Management of Coagulopathy

Correction of coagulopathy in acute liver failure depends on the clinical suspicion for acute bleeding.

- Significant active hemorrhage
  - Consider viscoelastic testing, including **thromboelastography (TEG) or ROTEM**, to help determine coagulation balance, as INR itself is an unreliable metric in acute liver failure many patients may actually be paradoxically thrombophilia.
  - Attempt to target goals of:
    - ☐ Platelet count > 50,000
    - ☐ Fibrinogen levels > 150 mg/dL
    - ☐ Appropriate level of hemoglobin (Hg) > 7g/dL.

Patients without Acute Bleeding

- Vitamin K may be administered for elevated INR; FFP is not indicated without clinical bleeding.
- Maintain platelet count > 10,000,

Venous Thrombosis Prophylaxis

- DVT prophylaxis should be administered as there is a tendency towards thrombosis even with elevated INRs.
- Utilize intermittent pneumatic compression stockings in addition to chemical DVT PPX.

Infectious Complications

- The presence of **hepatic encephalopathy and > 2 SIRS criteria** are significant predictors of bacteremia.
- Empiric broad spectrum antibiotic administration should be provided in patients with ALF who have signs of SIRS, refractory hypotension, or unexplained worsening grade of hepatic encephalopathy.

Transplant Indications

Liver transplantation is the only definitive treatment for ALF and should be considered in patients with persistent or worsening hepatic failure or patients experiencing life-threatening extra-hepatic organ dysfunction.

- Due to the complexity and time sensitive nature of transplantation evaluation, **consultation with a transplant hepatologist or a referral to a transplant center should be made as soon as possible for patients in ALF.**
- While there are multiple criteria for transplantation in ALF, it is generally best to involve hepatologists and/or dedicated transplant center consultation as opposed to speculating regarding patient viability.
- As a point of reference, absolute contraindications to liver transplant are relatively few and include active malignancy, uncontrolled sepsis or septic shock, significant comorbid conditions, and patients considered otherwise moribund. Relative indications including age, ALF etiology, substance use, and psychosocial support vary by center.

Sudden Deterioration

- In patients with ALF, sudden mental status deterioration is almost always secondary to worsening cerebral edema or herniation. Secure the airway and treat cerebral edema early and aggressively.
- For hypotension refractory to fluid resuscitation, start vasopressors with Norepinephrine as first-line agent.
- Keep infection high on your differential in patients with acute deterioration. Pan-culture and treat empirically with broad spectrum antibiotics.

Special Circumstances

- Advanced extracorporeal therapies are at the forefront for management of ALF refractory to medical therapy. The MARS and PLEX systems are available at specialized centers and may be utilized for patients with worsening clinical deterioration with standard of care therapies described above. Molecular Adsorbent Recirculating System (MARS) is a specialized liver dialysis system that utilizes a combination of albumin-based dialysate in conjunction with CRRT (or conventional hemodialysis) and a charcoal filter to facilitate removal of albumin-bound toxins from circulation. It is used for cases of severe, refractory ALF and may decrease severity of hepatic encephalopathy while improving systemic perfusion.

BIBLIOGRAPHY

Paugam-Burtz C, Levesque E, Louvet A, et al. Management of liver failure in general intensive care unit. *Anaesth Crit Care Pain Med* 2020;39(1):143–161. https://doi.org/10.1016/j.accpm.2019.06.014

31

Acute Mesenteric Ischemia

JEFFREY N. SIEGELMAN AND SOTHIVIN LANH

Chapter 31:
Acute Mesenteric Ischemia

 ## Presentation

Presence of risk factors (*esp. 50+ years of age, cardiovascular disease, hypercoagulable states, and hypoperfusion*).

Severe, acute non-specific abdominal pain with pain out of proportion to exam.

In case of any suspicion, consult surgery as soon as possible.

 ## Diagnosis and Evaluation

Non-specific lab values.

CT angiography without oral contrast
May see pneumatosis intestinalis, thickened bowel walls, dilated bowel loops, and/or evidence of infarction/thrombosis.

Negative CT and high suspicion may warrant angiography or diagnostic laparotomy.

 ## Management

Fluid resuscitation and broad-spectrum antibiotics.

NG tube.

Hemodynamic monitoring.

Pre-op lab work to expedite surgery.

Heparin if no contraindications.

Surgery!

Introduction

- **Mesenteric ischemia** is a generic term referring to hypoperfusion of the intestines. It can be either acute or chronic and is caused by several different etiologies. The blood supply to the abdominal organs is listed in Table 31.1.
- It is a rare but life-threatening vascular emergency, occurring with increasing frequency (0.1% of all hospital admissions) and with mortality rates between 60% and 80%.
- It affects primarily those older than 50 years with systemic and cardiovascular disease.
- The acute form is more common and results in rapid intestinal ischemia, infarction/necrosis, sepsis, and death. Splanchnic vascular insufficiency in chronic ischemia can also threaten bowel viability.
- Small bowel ischemia is much more common than ischemic colitis.
- Despite advances in diagnostic testing, **survival has not significantly improved**, largely due to the **difficulty of making a timely diagnosis**.
- **Pathogenesis**
  - Critical threshold of hypoperfusion leads to intestinal villi ischemia, release of endothelial factors, inflammatory cells, oxygen free radicals, and intraluminal bacteria proliferation.
  - Watershed areas of intestinal vascular supply are at highest risk.
    - Necrosis/infarction may be seen as early as **10–12 hours after onset.**
    - Untreated intestinal ischemia can lead to intestinal gangrene, bowel perforation, diffuse peritonitis, septic shock, cardiac depression, multi-system organ failure, and death.
- **Etiology**
  - *Mesenteric arterial embolism (MAE)*
    - The most common, accounting for 50% of cases.

Table 31.1 Arterial supply to abdominal organs

Arterial supply	Target organs
Celiac	Esophagus, stomach, proximal duodenum, liver, gallbladder, pancreas, and spleen
Superior mesenteric artery	Distal duodenum, jejunum, ileum, colon to the splenic flexure
Inferior mesenteric artery	Descending colon, sigmoid, and rectum

- Median age is 70 years, and it is more common in women than men.
- Most mural thrombi originate from cardiac source and often lodge in a branch of the superior mesenteric artery (SMA) .
  - *Mesenteric arterial thrombosis (MAT)*
    - Accounts for 15–25% of cases.
    - Almost always associated with **severe atherosclerosis**, prompting thrombus formation in the SMA.
    - Consequently, patients often have preceding symptoms of chronic mesenteric ischemia:
      - **Intestinal angina:** postprandial abdominal pain that occurs due to inability to augment blood flow that normally is needed after eating.
    - Cachexia and malnutrition.
    - Perioperative mortality ranges 70–100%, with frequent delay in diagnosis
  - *Nonocclusive mesenteric ischemia (NOMI)*
    - NOMI accounts for 20–30% and can occur in all ages of critically ill hospitalized patients.
    - Occurs in diseases that lead to cardiovascular dysfunction (shock, sepsis, burns, trauma, pancreatitis, etc.) with **low cardiac output** or **use of vasopressors** resulting in splanchnic vasoconstriction.
  - *Mesenteric venous thrombosis (MVT)*
    - The least common form, accounting for only 5% of cases.
    - Associated with hypercoagulable states, inflammatory conditions, and trauma.
    - Often occurs in younger patients and causes milder symptoms
    - Venous congestion leads to bowel edema, which can severely limit blood supply.
  - **Key risk factors**
    - Key risk factors for mesenteric ischemia are listed in Table 31.2.

Presentation

Classic and Critical Presentation

- Diagnosis should be considered in those **older than 50 years** or younger with other risk factors, presenting with nonspecific abdominal pain and risk factors for the disease.

Table 31.2 Key risk factors for subtypes of mesenteric ischemia

Etiology	Key risk factors
Mesenteric arterial embolism	• Cardiac disease: recent myocardial infarction, **ventricular aneurysm**, valvular disease, infective endocarditis • **Cardiac arrhythmias**, particularly atrial fibrillation • Vasculature: **aortic atherosclerosis, aortic aneurysm**, aortic instrumentation or surgery
Mesenteric arterial thrombosis	• **Peripheral vascular disease** • Low cardiac output states • Advanced age
Nonocclusive mesenteric ischemia	• **Severe cardiovascular disease**: heart failure, cardiogenic shock, peripheral vascular disease, arrhythmias • Hypoperfusion: **shock**, severe burns • Drugs: vasoconstrictive medications, **cocaine/methamphetamine** use • Chronic renal insufficiency/hemodialysis
Mesenteric venous thrombosis	• Hypercoagulable states: **inherited thrombophilia** and acquired thrombophilia (e.g., **malignancy**, oral contraceptives) • **Abdominal inflammatory conditions**: diverticulitis, pancreatitis, inflammatory bowel disease • **Splenectomy** and other abdominal trauma • Other: portal hypertension, abdominal mass, history of venous thromboembolism

- The physician must have a high index of suspicion as the history may be difficult to obtain.
- Acute onset of severe, poorly localized abdominal pain.
- May exhibit **pain out of proportion to the examination**.
- History of prior embolic event or personal or family history of DVT/PE.
- Commonly causes diarrhea due to cathartic stimulus of ischemia.
- Gross or occult GI bleeding if ischemia has been present for several hours.

Table 31.3 Presentation of the subtypes of mesenteric ischemia

Mesenteric arterial embolism	Mesenteric arterial thrombosis	Nonocclusive mesenteric ischemia	Mesenteric venous thrombosis
• Appears ill	*Acute*	• Critically ill patient with worsening clinical picture or failure to thrive	• Insidious presentation (1–2 weeks)
• Tachycardia	• Similar to MAE		• Nonspecific abdominal pain
• Acute unrelenting abdominal pain	*Subacute*		• Diarrhea
• Nausea/vomiting	• Postprandial pain		• Vomiting
• Frequent bowel movements	• Weight loss		
	• Nausea		

- Peritonitis is a late finding and indicates severe bowel ischemia and necrosis.
- Clinical presentations of the subtypes of mesenteric ischemia are listed in Table 31.3.

Diagnosis and Evaluation

- **Laboratory work**
  - Nonspecific, but may reveal the following:
    - Leukocytosis with left shift
    - Hemoconcentration
    - Lactic acidosis (though neither sensitive nor specific for mesenteric ischemia)
    - Elevated CPK and hyperkalemia may also be present

- **Imaging**
  - ○ *Abdominal radiography:*
    - ▪ May assess for other possible diagnoses or complications (i.e., obstruction and perforation), especially if patient is too unstable for CT scan, though abnormal findings are noted only 20% of the time.
    - ▪ May show a dynamic ileus, thumb-printing or thickening of bowel loops, pneumatosis, or late finding of free air or air in the portal venous system.
  - ○ *CT-angiography (CTA):*
    - ▪ Contrast-enhanced multi-detector CT **without** oral contrast is now the **most commonly used test** to diagnose acute mesenteric ischemia.
    - ▪ Recent meta-analysis has shown sensitivity of 82.8–97.6% and specificity of 91.2–98.2% comparable with conventional angiography.
    - ▪ May show thickened bowel walls, dilated bowel loops, pneumatosis, air in the portal system, infarction, or arterial or venous thrombosis. **See Figure 31.1**.
  - ○ CTA may also identify alternative etiology if AMI is ruled out.
  - ○ If CTA is completely normal but there is a high index of suspicion, further angiography or surgical consultation (for diagnostic laparotomy) is recommended.

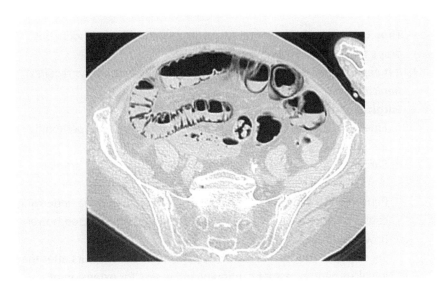

Figure 31.1 Pneumatosis intestinalis.

Pneumatosis intestinalis CT LF Darmischaemie.jpg © Hellerhoff Source: (https://commons.wikimedia.org/wiki/File:Pneumatosis_intestinalis_CT_LF_Darmischaemie.jpg). (CC BY-SA 3.0)

○ *Angiography:*
  ▪ **Gold standard** – though invasive, not readily available, and rarely employed.
  ▪ Angiography has been largely replaced by CTA, but it is used if there is diagnostic uncertainty.
  ▪ Both diagnostic and potentially therapeutic.

Critical Management

Critical Management Checklist

☑ Establish IV access and begin fluid resuscitation with crystalloid products
☑ Establish hemodynamic monitoring and support
☑ **Consult general or vascular surgery emergently if high suspicion**
☑ Place NG tube for GI decompression
☑ Prepare blood and check coagulation factors, preoperative laboratory studies
☑ Discontinue medications with vasoconstrictive properties as able
☑ Begin broad-spectrum antibiotics
☑ Start heparin therapy if there are no contraindications

- **Time is bowel** – 50% survival when diagnosed within 24 hours but drops to less than 30% after 24 hours.
- *It is imperative to remember that this diagnosis almost always requires surgical repair.*
- **Surgical management**
  ○ Emergent laparotomy is indicated, especially if signs of peritonitis are present.
  ○ Surgery is generally the standard of care for mesenteric arterial embolism and thrombosis.
  ○ Performed to determine the extent of damage, to find the underlying cause, to revascularize viable bowel, and to resect infarcted bowel.
  ○ Bowel is often left in discontinuity.
  ○ Second-look procedures are often performed 24–48 hours after the initial surgery to restore continuity and assess for extension of ischemia. This also ensures that at-risk or ischemic bowel is not used for the final anastomosis.

Table 31.4 Management of the subtypes of mesenteric ischemia

Mesenteric arterial embolism	Mesenteric arterial thrombosis	Nonocclusive mesenteric ischemia	Mesenteric venous thrombosis
Embolectomy, then distal bypass graft	Bypass graft or stenting	Treat the underlying cause	Depends on extent of ischemia
Resect necrotic bowel	Resect necrotic bowel	Fewer surgical options	Difficult for surgical management if diffuse thrombosis
		Papaverine	Mild ischemia: treat with anticoagulation
		Resect necrotic bowel	Severe ischemia: treat with bowel resection of necrotic segments

- **Novel treatments**
  - ○ Glucagon drips may decrease vasospasm.
  - ○ Papaverine, a phosphodiesterase inhibitor that reduces mesenteric vasoconstriction, can be directly infused into the SMA during angiography.
- **Subtype management**
  - ○ Specific management for each subtype of mesenteric ischemia is listed in Table 31.4.

Sudden Deterioration

- Hemodynamically unstable patients should be sent immediately to the OR for emergent exploratory laparotomy.
- Findings of ischemic bowel on abdominal plain film, such as pneumatosis intestinalis (see Figure 31.1), should prompt emergency surgery consultation prior to CT.

Vasopressor of choice: norepinephrine, only used if absolutely necessary.

32

The Surgical Abdomen

SARAH FISHER AND CARLA HAACK

Chapter 32:
Surgical Abdomen

 Presentation

Acute abdominal pain, may be accompanied by referred pain and **non-specific symptoms like weakness, nausea, and vomiting.**

 Diagnosis and Evaluation

Thorough history to determine location and characterization of pain, mode of onset, associated symptoms, and duration/frequency of symptoms.

Labwork: CBC, BMP, urine pregnancy, coagulation studies and type and screen if surgery is anticipated.

Abdominal physical exam.

Imaging: CXR, US, and/or CT.

✿ *Use water-soluble contrast if perforation or obstruction is suspected.*

 Management

Airway management and hemodynamic monitoring.

Fluid resuscitation.

Surgical consultation and pre-op preparations.

Symptom relief with analgesics/antiemetics.
⊘ *Consider opioids.*

If signs of sepsis, administer antibiotics early.

NG tube for decompression in the case of ileus or bowel obstruction.

In case of rapid deterioration, re-assess, consider bedside imaging, and consult surgery.

Introduction

- Abdominal pain is the most common reason for emergency department visits and is a leading cause of hospital admissions in the United States.
- **Acute abdominal pain** is defined as sudden-onset pain lasting < 7 days, due to a wide spectrum of causes that range from benign to life threatening.
- When the need for surgical intervention is suspected, prompt involvement of appropriate consultants is essential.

Presentation

Classic and Critical Presentations

- Characterization of the pain is essential; some use the PQRST mnemonic (Table 32.1).
- Understanding of the following pathophysiology will help differentiate sources:
  - Autonomic nerves (sympathetic and parasympathetic) innervate the abdominal **viscera**; pain is often described as dull, crampy, or aching and is often poorly localized.
  - Somatic nerves (spinal nerves) innervate the parietal **peritoneum**, and transmit sharp and severe, localizable signals.
- The **location** and **characterization** of the pain can help focus the differential diagnosis of abdominal pain (see Figure 32.1).
- **Referred pain** is pain at a site (or sites) distant from the initiating organ due to a shared neural origin with another body organ, such as right shoulder pain due to biliary colic or back pain due to pancreatitis.

Table 32.1 Descriptors of pain (PQRST)

P2	Palliating and Provoking factors
Q	Quality (i.e., dull, sharp, stabbing, throbbing)
R2	Radiation, Referral
S	Severity
T	Temporal factors (time, mode of onset, duration, progression, previous episodes)

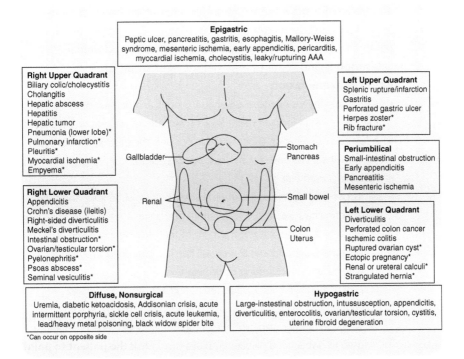

Epigastric
Peptic ulcer, pancreatitis, gastritis, esophagitis, Mallory-Weiss syndrome, mesenteric ischemia, early appendicitis, pericarditis, myocardial ischemia, cholecystitis, leaky/rupturing AAA

Right Upper Quadrant
Biliary colic/cholecystitis
Cholangitis
Hepatic abscess
Hepatitis
Hepatic tumor
Pneumonia (lower lobe)*
Pulmonary infarction*
Pleuritis*
Myocardial ischemia*
Empyema*

Left Upper Quadrant
Splenic rupture/infarction
Gastritis
Perforated gastric ulcer
Herpes zoster*
Rib fracture*

Periumbilical
Small-intestinal obstruction
Early appendicitis
Pancreatitis
Mesenteric ischemia

Right Lower Quadrant
Appendicitis
Crohn's disease (ileitis)
Right-sided diverticulitis
Meckel's diverticulitis
Intestinal obstruction*
Ovarian/testicular torsion*
Pyelonephritis*
Psoas abscess*
Seminal vesiculitis*

Left Lower Quadrant
Diverticulitis
Perforated colon cancer
Ischemic colitis
Ruptured ovarian cyst*
Ectopic pregnancy*
Renal or ureteral calculi*
Strangulated hernia*

Diffuse, Nonsurgical
Uremia, diabetic ketoacidosis, Addisonian crisis, acute intermittent porphyria, sickle cell crisis, acute leukemia, lead/heavy metal poisoning, black widow spider bite

Hypogastric
Large-instestinal obstruction, intussusception, appendicitis, diverticulitis, enterocolitis, ovarian/testicular torsion, cystitis, uterine fibroid degeneration

Labels: Stomach, Pancreas, Gallbladder, Renal, Small bowel, Colon, Uterus

*Can occur on opposite side

Figure 32.1 Location and differential diagnosis of acute abdominal pain.

- **Acute-onset pain > 6 hours in a previously healthy patient is often due to a surgical condition.**

Diagnosis and Evaluation

- **History and physical characteristics**
  - A thorough history will generally narrow the differential diagnosis.
    - **Duration of symptoms**, **mode of onset** (gradual and insidious versus sudden), and **associated symptoms** (nausea, vomiting, anorexia, changes in bowel habits, fatigue, rash) should be noted.
    - Change over time should be noted: the transition from poorly described vague abdominal pain to persistent sharp discomfort specific to an area of the abdomen, such as occurs in appendicitis, often signifies the worsening of an intra-abdominal process.
  - **Past medical and surgical histories** and **medication usage** may harbor clues (e.g., prior abdominal surgery may suggest adhesions as

an etiology for bowel obstruction) or rule out potential diagnoses (e.g., prior cholecystectomy in the setting of right upper quadrant pain). The use of steroids may blunt response to abdominal catastrophes and requires a higher index of suspicion.

○ **Physical examination**

- Assess the patient overall, including vital signs and demeanor. Remember the use of beta blockade medications may blunt or prevent tachycardia.
- A focused examination should include not only the gastrointestinal system but also the cardiovascular and respiratory systems.
- *Abdominal examination:*
  □ Inspect the abdomen for surgical scars, bulges, pulsations, and other abnormalities (i.e., skin discoloration, petechiae).
  □ Observe the respiratory movement of the abdomen; in cases of peritonitis, the abdominal wall will barely move due to muscle rigidity, which can be localized or generalized.
  □ Auscultate for bowel sounds, bruits, and abnormal pulsations.
  □ Begin the palpation portion of the examination gently, progressing slowly to deeper palpation. (Remember that the stethoscope can be used to distract and palpate simultaneously.) **Ask the patient to point with one finger to the area that is most painful, and begin palpating the abdomen far away from that point.**
  □ Involuntary guarding (physiological contraction of the abdominal wall) denotes an underlying inflammatory process (i.e., peritonitis), which can be localized or generalized.
  □ Muscular rigidity, the extreme of involuntary guarding, can be absent in cases of chronic deconditioning, the severely decompensated patient, or the elderly.
  □ Inguinal hernia exam is an important component for all patients with abdominal pain.
  □ Rectal and/or pelvic examinations should be performed in appropriate patients.

○ **Laboratory testing**

- Results of a selected test should be anticipated to *alter the management plan*; otherwise that test should not be ordered.
- Initial bloodwork including a **hematocrit** and **electrolytes** should be checked.
- The **white blood cell count (WBC),** while useful, is not particularly sensitive or specific, as WBCs can be elevated in a variety of nonsurgical conditions, and normal or low in surgical conditions.

- In patients with concern for sepsis and/or intra-abdominal catastrophe, a blood gas with **base deficit** and **lactic acid** should be checked and can be used to trend the resuscitation.
- **Coagulation studies** and a **type and screen** are generally necessary tests for the patient with acute abdominal pain of suspected surgical etiology. Cross-matched blood should be requested in select patients.
- All females of child-bearing age with an abdominal complaint should have a urine pregnancy test.
○ **Radiological testing**
  - Abdominal plain films are rarely diagnostic, although they may identify air–fluid levels (suggestive of a bowel obstruction or ileus), volvulus, renal or ureteral calculi, and occasionally free intraperitoneal air.
  - The initial test of choice to identify free intraperitoneal air from a perforated viscus is the **upright chest radiograph**. For patients who cannot sit upright, consider a lateral decubitus radiograph.
  - **Ultrasound** should be considered for suspected biliary (acute cholecystitis) and gynecological etiologies of acute abdominal pain (tubo-ovarian abscess, ectopic pregnancy).
  - **Computed tomography (CT)** has largely supplanted plain film radiology in many centers, but concerns of cost and the risk of ionizing radiation require judicious use of this modality.
    ☐ When considering abdominal and pelvic CT, the suspected diagnosis should guide the use of IV and oral contrast. Many emergency departments have established protocols to guide the use of contrast.
    ☐ *Water-soluble* oral contrast should be used in cases of suspected obstruction or perforation.
    ☐ The interpretation of findings on CT (or any test) should match the story painted by the history and physical examination. Otherwise, reevaluate the patient.

Critical Management

Critical Management Checklist
☑ Establish IV access and begin fluid resuscitation with crystalloid products
☑ Establish hemodynamic monitoring and support
☑ Appropriate surgical consultation (early if high suspicion for a surgical abdomen)

☑ Prepare blood and check coagulation factors, preoperative laboratory studies

☑ Place NG tube for GI decompression (if ileus or bowel obstruction)

☑ If signs of sepsis, initiate broad-spectrum antibiotics early

☑ Provide appropriate symptom relief with analgesia and antiemetics

☑ Prepare blood and check coagulation factors, preoperative laboratory studies

- **The unstable patient**
  - As with the stable patient, a well-formulated differential diagnosis based on careful history and physical examination will guide the plan of care far better than a "shotgun" approach of imaging and laboratory tests.
- **Resuscitation** must begin concurrently with the diagnostic modalities.
  - **Intubation** may be necessary for airway protection.
  - **Large-bore intravenous access** should be secured and judicious fluid resuscitation with correction of electrolyte abnormalities initiated.
  - **Nasogastric decompression** is beneficial in patients with generalized ileus or small bowel obstruction and should accompany intubation when abdominal catastrophe is suspected.
  - A **Foley catheter** can be placed to monitor fluid status and guide resuscitation.
  - Hypothermia should be corrected with **warming blankets** and **heated fluids**.
  - **Frequent reassessment** of hemodynamics and acid–base status is necessary.
  - An unstable patient should *never* be transported to the radiology suite without a physician.
- **Pain control**
  - **Early and appropriate opioid administration** is recommended.
  - Historically, some clinicians have cautioned against the use of analgesia in the patient with an "acute abdomen" out of concern that opioids would mask presenting symptoms and confound timely diagnosis. Over the past decade, multiple prospective, randomized, controlled trials have failed to show that early analgesia administration impairs diagnostic accuracy.

- **Preparation for the OR**
  - Patients with an acute abdomen requiring surgical correction should be treated in similar fashion as the unstable patient.
  - Appropriate fluid resuscitation should be given (via large-bore intravenous access), and electrolyte abnormalities should be corrected.
  - In addition to a type and screen, **cross-matched blood** should be available for the operating suite in cases in which the degree of operative intervention is unknown (i.e., the patient with large amounts of free intraperitoneal air, as opposed to the stable patient with early appendicitis).

Sudden Deterioration

- **Acute changes in patient presentation, hemodynamics, or laboratory values should prompt immediate reassessment and heighten suspicion for intra-abdominal catastrophe**
  - Bedside re-evaluation of the patient is necessary
  - Imaging modalities such as bedside ultrasound and upright chest radiograph should be performed in favor of CT studies that require transport until the patient is stabilized.
  - Critical management (as above) may be necessary.
  - Surgical consultation, if not already performed, should be strongly considered.

Special Circumstances

- **Special populations**
  - A higher index of suspicion for abdominal catastrophe is necessary in situations in which the history is compromised or in which the physical examination is altered or unreliable.
  - Some patients, including **children, developmentally delayed, or obtunded individuals** (from illness or drugs) cannot give a reliable history.
  - **Patients with spinal cord injuries** and impaired sensation often present in a delayed fashion.

- ○ **Pregnancy** displaces the abdominal viscera and alters the presentation of common illnesses.
- ○ **The elderly or immunosuppressed** may not experience symptoms in the same way as most adults.
- ○ **Morbid obesity** hinders physical examination.
- ○ **Chronic or high-dose steroid use may mask or diminish abdominal pain**.

33

Abdominal Compartment Syndrome

SARAH FISHER AND CARLA HAACK

Chapter 33:
Abdominal Compartment Syndrome

Increased pressure within the abdominal cavity ≥ 20 mmHg associated with new organ dysfuncton

 Presentation

Signs: Decreased cardiac output, decreased CPP, decrease in pulmonary compliance (increase in peak airway pressures in ventilated pts), oliguria, and/or bowel ischemia/necrosis.

History of precipitating factor/cause (i.e. hemorrhage, inflammation, ascites, burns, sepsis).

 Diagnosis and Evaluation

Measure IAP with a urinary catheter in supine patient (at end-expiration).

✿ *Normal IAP: 0–5 mmHg, may increase to 15 mmHg after uncomplicated surgical procedures.*

 Management

Airway, hemodyamic, and IAP monitoring.

If cause is expected to resolve, use analgesia, sedation, and pharmacological paralysis.

Definitive treatment is decompressive laparotomy.

✿ *No consensus on exactly when to intervene.*

Careful fluid resuscitation: in euvolemic patients, favor pressors (norepinephrine) over more fluids.

CVP and PCWP are not reliable measures in the setting of IAP.

Introduction

- **Abdominal compartment syndrome (ACS)** is defined as increased pressure within the abdominal cavity $\geq$ 20 mmHg associated with *new* organ dysfunction or failure.
- **ACS is a surgical emergency.**
- Increased intra-abdominal pressure (IAP) from fluid or gas accumulation compromises the respiratory and cardiovascular systems and decreases perfusion to abdominal organs.
- Sources of increased IAP include:
  - hemorrhage (traumatic or iatrogenic)
  - inflammation (peritonitis, pancreatitis)
  - hollow viscus perforation
  - ascites
  - systemic sources (capillary leak and bowel edema from sepsis, burns, or massive fluid resuscitation).
- ACS can be primary (resulting from an intra-abdominal process), or secondary (due to bowel edema from aggressive fluid resuscitation or sepsis) and can occur in patients whose abdomen has not been surgically altered.
- IAP measurements > 25 mmHg are often associated with significant organ dysfunction requiring surgical decompression, **but there is not a universal threshold value applicable to all patients**.
- IAP is influenced by respiration, body mass index, position, and severity of illness. In the critically ill hypotensive patient, even slight increases in IAP may compromise abdominal perfusion, leading to further clinical decline.

Presentation

Classic and Critical Presentations

- **Neurological**
  - Increased IAP **decreases cerebral perfusion pressure** due to decreased cardiac output (CO) and hypotension and increased thoracic pressure with functional obstruction of cerebral venous outflow.

- **Cardiovascular**
  - Increased IAP directly compresses the vena cava, **decreasing venous return and cardiac output (CO)**, which increases systemic venous congestion and edema. The diaphragm bulges upward, displacing the heart and compromising diastolic filling, which further decreases CO.
- **Respiratory**
  - The cephalad displacement of the diaphragm **decreases pulmonary compliance**, leading to segmental alveolar collapse and subsequent ventilation/perfusion mismatch. In patients on ventilators, an **increase in peak airway pressures** will be observed in addition to increased difficulty in ventilating overall. The increase in thoracic pressure artificially increases central venous pressure (CVP) and pulmonary capillary wedge pressure (PCWP), compromising the value of these markers for guiding resuscitation.
- **Renal**
  - Direct compression of the kidneys combined with decreased vascular inflow and outflow can create **oliguria** and compromise renal function even in the setting of maintained hemodynamics.
- **Gastrointestinal**
  - Direct compression within the abdominal cavity **decreases splanchnic blood flow** leading to bowel ischemia and necrosis. This also contributes to the formation of bowel edema, which in turn increases IAP.
- **Musculoskeletal**
  - **Musculoskeletal dysfunction**, both within the abdominal wall and in the extremities, is also observed as a result of decreased CO, global ischemia, and reperfusion injury.

Diagnosis and Evaluation

- The most efficient way to recognize and treat ACS is by recognizing and correcting predisposing factors before ACS occurs.
- In the closed abdomen, the gold standard approach to measuring IAP uses a urinary bladder catheter ("**bladder pressures**") with the patient in **full supine position and, if on mechanical ventilation, with neuromuscular blockade.**

- ○ Normal IAP ranges from 0–5 mmHg, with IAP after uncomplicated surgical procedures ranging between 3–15 mmHg.
  - ○ A maximum of 20–25 mL of sterile saline is injected into the catheter, which is then clamped and connected to a transducing device.
  - ○ The pubic symphysis is used as the zeroing point on a supine patient.
  - ○ Time should be allowed for the detrusor muscle of the bladder to accommodate the volume before the pressure is measured.
  - ○ IAP should be measured at end expiration.
- IAP may be artificially elevated by abdominal wall contraction (such as *in an awake patient* or in situations of inadequate analgesia), body habitus (obesity), or patient positioning (raising the head of the bed). In intubated patients, pharmacological paralysis enhances the accuracy of IAP measurements and provides therapeutic benefit.

Critical Management

- **Early recognition** of risk factors and delaying definitive abdominal wall closure remains the best therapy for ACS. In cases in which the abdominal wall is already closed or the decompression is inadequate, timely intervention can be life-saving.
- Any patient suspected of having ACS should have frequent measurements of IAP after optimizing conditions for measurement (see above).
- The definitive treatment for a patient with ACS is **decompressive laparotomy**.
- There is some evidence to support the use of percutaneous decompression using a diagnostic peritoneal lavage catheter as an alternative treatment prior to decompressive laparotomy.
- There is **no standard consensus on when to intervene.** The decision is made based on clinical judgment, presence of end-organ failure, and serial measurements of IAP.
- Aggressive **fluid resuscitation** predisposes to third-spacing, bowel edema, and subsequent worsening of IAP. A patient should be resuscitated to the degree to which volume is indicated, but upon reaching euvolemia, pressors should be favored over crystalloid. In trauma patients and other select groups, consider the use of blood products and colloids over crystalloids.

- **CVP and PCWP are unreliable** in the setting of increased IAP.
- If the underlying insult causing ACS is expected to resolve within a relatively short time period, temporizing measures other than surgical decompression can be adopted. **Liberal analgesia** and **sedation** as well as **pharmacological paralysis** are adjunct measures that may decrease abdominal wall tension. Paracentesis and renal replacement therapy can be used in appropriately selected patients (e.g., cirrhosis) to normalize fluid balance.

Sudden Deterioration

- **ACS can occur even in the already decompressed abdomen**, often due to an abdominal closure system that is too tight.
- Re-examine the patient and re-measure the IAP to assess for worsening pressures and need for possible surgical decompression.
- Monitor the peak airway pressures and tidal volume delivery on all ventilated patients to ensure appropriate minute ventilation and avoid respiratory acidosis.
- Norepinephrine is the first-choice vasopressor.

SECTION 7

Renal Emergencies

KARI GORDER

34

·······

Acid–Base Interpretation

PETER G. CZARNECKI AND CHANU RHEE

Introduction

- Acid–base disturbances are common in critically ill patients, and correct interpretation is crucial to proper management. The arterial blood gas (ABG) is the gold standard for determining acid–base status.
- **Acidemia** refers to a pH ≤ 7.35.
- **Alkalemia** refers to a pH ≥ 7.45.
- **Acidosis** refers to a process that increases hydrogen ion concentration.
- **Alkalosis** refers to a process that decreases hydrogen ion concentration.
- Patients are either acidemic or alkalemic, but can have multiple simultaneous acid–base disturbances.
- The major buffering system at physiologic pH is the bicarbonate buffer system, in which carbonic acid is the conjugate acid, and bicarbonate the conjugate base. Carbon dioxide diffuses easily across biological membranes, and thus, across all physiologic compartments, and is eliminated through alveolar gas:

$$HCO_3^- + H^+ \rightleftarrows H_2CO_3 \rightleftarrows H_2O + CO_2$$

- Normal values from an ABG are pH of 7.36–7.44, $[HCO_3^-]$ of 21–27 mM, $PaCO_2$ of 35–45 mmHg, and pO_2 of 80–100 mmHg.

- The pH, $PaCO_2$, and pO_2 are measured directly, while the $[HCO_3^-]$ is calculated from the Henderson-Hasselbalch equation.
- **Venous blood gases (VBG)** are increasingly being used for convenience. Compared to an ABG, the VBG pH is lower by approximately 0.02–0.04, the $PaCO_2$ is higher by 3–8 mmHg, the $[HCO_3^-]$ concentration is 1–2 mM higher, and the pO_2 is not useful. In general, VBG values correlate well with ABGs, but periodic correlation with ABGs should be performed if serial VBGs are used.

Basic Approach for Arterial Blood Gas Interpretation

Step 1: Look at the pH and $PaCO_2$ to determine the primary disorder. The calculated HCO_3^- should be examined to ensure proper interpretation:
  ○ Low pH with low HCO_3^- = Metabolic acidosis
  ○ Low pH with high $PaCO_2$ = Respiratory acidosis
  ○ High pH with low $PaCO_2$ = Respiratory alkalosis
  ○ High pH with high HCO_3^- = Metabolic alkalosis

Step 2: Determine if the appropriate compensation is present (based on formulas specific to each disorder). Remember that compensation never fully corrects the pH (see Table 34.1).

Step 3: If the degree of compensation is not appropriate, determine whether multiple disorders are present.
  ○ Metabolic acidosis or alkalosis:
    ▪ $PaCO_2$ lower than expected = concomitant respiratory alkalosis.
    ▪ $PaCO_2$ higher than expected = concomitant respiratory acidosis.
  ○ Respiratory acidosis or alkalosis:
    ▪ pH lower than expected = concomitant metabolic acidosis.
    ▪ pH higher than expected = concomitant metabolic alkalosis.

Step 4: If a metabolic acidosis is present, determine whether it is an anion-gap metabolic acidosis. If an anion-gap metabolic acidosis is present, calculate the delta-delta gap (see below) to assess for concomitant derangements.

Step 5: If normal pH, consider other possibilities:
- High $PaCO_2$ and high HCO_3^- suggests respiratory acidosis + metabolic alkalosis.

Table 34.1 Compensation formulas for primary acid–base disorders

Primary disorder	Expected compensation
Metabolic acidosis	1. Expected $PaCO_2 = 1.5 \times [HCO^-] + 8 \pm 2$ (**Winter's formula**) 2. Alternatively, the $PaCO_2$ should be approximately $HCO_3^- + 15$
Metabolic alkalosis acidosis	$PaCO_2 = 0.7 \times [HCO_3] + 20 \pm 5$ Respiratory 1. Acute: ↓pH by 0.08 for every ↑10 $PaCO_2$ 2. Chronic: ↓pH by 0.03 for every ↑10 $PaCO_2$
Respiratory alkalosis	1. Acute: ↑pH by 0.08 for every ↓10 $PaCO_2$ 2. Chronic: ↑pH by 0.03 for every ↓10 $PaCO_2$

- Low $PaCO_2$ and low HCO_3^- suggests respiratory alkalosis + metabolic acidosis.
- Normal $PaCO_2$ and HCO_3^- but elevated anion gap suggests anion gap metabolic acidosis + metabolic alkalosis.
- Normal $PaCO_2$, HCO_3^- and anion gap suggests no acid–base disturbance, or non-anion-gap acidosis + metabolic alkalosis.

Metabolic Acidosis

Presentation

Classic Presentation

- Symptoms depend on the severity and etiology of the underlying acidosis and are often nonspecific: e.g., altered mental status, weakness, nausea, and abdominal pain.
- **Hyperkalemia** is often present due to intracellular shifting of H^+ into cells and consequential extracellular shifting of K^+.
- **Kussmaul respirations** are classically associated with diabetic ketoacidosis (DKA), and refer to rapid, deep breathing.

Critical presentation

- Extreme acidemia leads to neurological dysfunction (severe obtundation, coma, and seizures) as well as cardiovascular complications (arrhythmias, decreased cardiac contractility, arteriolar vasodilation, and decreased responsiveness to catecholamines). Profound hypotension and shock can result, which in turn propagate acidosis.

Diagnosis and Evaluation

History and physical examination

- History and physical examination are generally helpful to reveal the etiology of the acidosis (e.g., a patient with a history of DKA who presents with nausea, weakness, and signs of dehydration).

Diagnostic tests

- Obtain a **basic metabolic panel** including other electrolytes, **an ABG**, and other basic tests to investigate the etiology of the acidosis.
- Calculate the anion gap ($Na^+ - [Cl^- + HCO_3^-]$). The expected anion gap is $2.5 \times$ [Albumin].
- If an elevated anion gap (AG) is present, check the **delta-delta gap (ΔΔ)** to evaluate for secondary metabolic derangements.
- Introduction of a foreign acid should widen the anion gap by the same degree to which it reduces the serum bicarbonate concentration. In a pure anion-gap acidosis, the ΔΔ is therefore close to 1. In a coexisting non-gap acidosis, the $[HCO_3^-]$ is reduced by a larger extent than by the difference in AG. In a coexisting metabolic alkalosis, reduction in serum $[HCO_3^-]$ is lesser than the difference in AG.
- $ΔΔ = ΔAG/Δ[HCO_3^-]$ (AG − Expected AG)/(24 − HCO_3^-).
  - ΔΔ < 1 = simultaneous non-AG acidosis
  - ΔΔ 1–2 = pure AG metabolic acidosis
  - ΔΔ > 2 = simultaneous metabolic alkalosis.
- If an anion-gap acidosis is present, check serum ketones, lactate, and BUN (Table 34.2).
- If unrevealing, consider toxin screen and serum osmolality to check osmolal gap.
  - Osmolal gap (OG) = measured osmoles − calculated osmoles ($2 \times [Na^+] +$ Glucose/18 + BUN/2.8).

Table 34.2 Etiologies of anion-gap acidosis

Lactic acidosis – common and feared cause of metabolic acidosis in critically ill patients. Degree of elevation correlates with mortality

- **Type A lactic acidosis** (impaired systemic perfusion/oxygenation) – shock (any type), severe hypoxemia, severe anemia

- **Type B lactic acidosis** (no impaired system perfusion/oxygenation)

Type B1 (systemic processes): liver and/or renal dysfunction (decreased clearance of lactate), seizures, hypothermic shivering, severe exercise, severe asthma exacerbation, ischemic bowel (increased production of lactate), malignancy, diabetic ketoacidosis **Type B2 (drugs)**: metformin, isoniazid, linezolid, HIV meds, cyanide, carbon monoxide

Type B3 (congenital/inborn errors of metabolism) Ketoacidosis – diabetic ketoacidosis, alcoholic ketoacidosis, starvation ketoacidosis

Renal failure – decreased excretion of organic anions (phosphates, sulfates, urate)

Ingestions – methanol, ethylene glycol, salicylates, toluene

- ○ OG > 10 suggests ingestion leading to unmeasured osmoles. The major ingestions that cause an elevated OG include various alcohols (ethanol, methanol, ethylene glycol, acetone, isopropyl alcohol), formaldehyde, paraldehyde, and diethyl ether. However, smaller ingestions can be missed and serum volatiles screen should also be checked if high suspicion.
- If a **non-anion gap acidosis** is present, a history is most useful; Causes of non-anion gap acidosis are listed in Table 34.3.
  - ○ If history is unrevealing, check **urine anion gap** = Urine Na^+ + Urine K^+ – Urine Cl^-.
  - ○ Urine anion gap, like the serum anion gap, is actually a surrogate for unmeasured ions, in this case NH_4^+ (which is excreted with Cl^-).
  - ○ The normal renal response to acidemia is to increase ammonium excretion.
  - ○ A **negative urine anion gap** suggests increased renal NH_4^+ excretion consistent with diarrhea, type II renal tubular acidosis (RTA), or dilutional acidosis.
  - ○ A **positive urine anion gap** suggests impaired renal NH_4^+ consistent with type I or IV RTA or chronic kidney disease.

Table 34.3 Etiologies of non-anion-gap acidosis

Diarrhea – due to loss of sodium bicarbonate. Most common cause of non-AG acidosis

Dilutional – from rapid infusion of saline that lacks bicarbonate and contains an excess of chloride. Normally causes no more than a mild metabolic acidosis

Renal tubular acidosis

- Type I (distal): impaired distal H^+ secretion. Severe acidosis, positive urine anion gap, associated hypokalemia. *Etiologies:* idiopathic, familial, medications (amphotericin B, lithium), Sjögren syndrome, renal transplantation, obstructive uropathy, sickle cell anemia, rheumatoid arthritis

- Type II (proximal): impaired proximal HCO_3^- reabsorption. Moderate acidosis, negative urine anion gap, associated hypokalemia. *Etiologies:* idiopathic, familial, multiple myeloma, medications (ifosfamide, tenofovir, acetazolamide), amyloidosis, heavy metals, renal transplantation, vitamin D deficiency, paroxysmal nocturnal hemoglobinuria

- Type III: rare autosomal recessive syndrome with features of both distal and proximal RTA.

- Type IV (hypoaldosteronism): decreased ammonium excretion. Mild acidosis, positive urine anion gap, associated hyperkalemia. *Etiologies:* chronic kidney disease (most often diabetic nephropathy), NSAIDs, calcineurin inhibitors, ACE inhibitors/ARBs, potassium-sparing diuretics (spironolactone, eplerenone, amiloride), TMP-SMX, primary adrenal insufficiency, heparin

Acetazolamide – carbonic anhydrase inhibitor causes impaired HCO – reabsorption

Hyperalimentation (TPN) – NH_4Cl and amino acids metabolized to HCl

Ureteral diversion – i.e., ureterocolonic fistula. Urinary Cl^- absorbed by colonic mucosa in exchange for HCO_3^-, leading to increased GI loss of HCO_3^-

Pancreatic fistula – HCO_3^--rich fluid excreted into and lost in the intestines

Posthypocapnia – patients with preexisting, prolonged respiratory alkalosis have compensatory decrease in HCO_3^-. If respiratory alkalosis resolves rapidly (i.e., with sedation and mechanical ventilation), underlying non-anion-gap acidosis will be "unmasked"

Critical Management

- The most important step is to identify and treat the underlying etiology.
  - Type A lactic acidosis suggests shock and tissue hypoxia, from hypoperfusion or fluid maldistribution.

- ○ Diabetic ketoacidosis is treated with volume resuscitation and insulin. Alcoholic and starvation ketoacidosis are treated through restoration of glycolytic metabolism, with dextrose, insulin, thiamine and aggressive potassium and phosphorus replacement.
- ○ Methanol and ethylene glycol ingestions are treated with fomepizole and/or urgent hemodialysis. Salicylate intoxication requires urgent hemodialysis.
- ○ Metformin-associated lactic acidosis requires urgent hemodialysis.
- Anion-gap acidoses from pyroglutamate (5-oxoproline) in the context of prolonged acetaminophen intake, from propylene glycol containing injection solutions (diazepam, lorazepam, phenytoin, phenobarbital etc.), and from other rare pharmacological therapies (thiosulfate, benzoate, phenylacetate etc.) are uncommon in the emergency medicine setting, but sometimes recognized in chronically critically ill inpatients.
- Potassium levels should be followed carefully, as initial hyperkalemia will normalize or shift to hypokalemia once acidosis is corrected.
- Critically ill patients with metabolic acidosis often require intubation and mechanical ventilation for airway protection, hemodynamic instability, etc.
  - ○ Intubating patients with metabolic acidosis is quite risky as respiratory compensation must be maintained to prevent worsening acidemia
- Alkaline therapy with intravenous sodium bicarbonate is controversial; if used, it should only be done as a temporizing measure in those with severe acidosis, defined as a pH of < 7.10–7.15. The theoretical benefits of raising cardiac output and blood pressure and increasing responsiveness to catecholamine vasopressors are unproven in lactic acidosis. Restoration of adequate tissue perfusion in type A lactic acidosis or reversal of ketoacidosis of any cause is sufficient to normalize the anion gap acidosis, while additionally administered bicarbonate remains in the system.
- Potential risks of sodium bicarbonate include paradoxical worsening of intracellular acidosis and volume and/or sodium overload. Physiologic $NaHCO_3$ solution has very little buffering capacity in a high volume, but may be used as resuscitation fluid in volume avid conditions. $NaHCO_3$ from 50 mL ampoules contain 1 M solution with a much larger buffering capacity per unit volume; however, the solution is highly hyperosmolar and represents a significant sodium load (comparable to 5–6% NaCl).

Finally, all administered bicarbonate converts to CO_2 which needs to be eliminated through alveolar exhalation. In patients with obstructive airway disease or high dead space fraction, in whom the minute ventilation cannot be increased, addition of bicarbonate may lead to further elevation of $PaCO_2$ and worsening respiratory acidosis.

- Metabolic buffering capacity may be provided by hemodialysis or continuous renal replacement therapy (CRRT), while preserving volume net neutrality. It therefore has an important role not only in anion-gap acidosis from intoxications by dialyzable agents, but also in certain cardiogenic shock conditions (RV failure with diuretic resistant oliguria) in which acidosis correction and even to negative volume balancing is required.

- An alternative to sodium bicarbonate is THAM (Tris-(hydroxymethyl-) aminomethane; tromethamine), a non-bicarbonate buffer. In contrast to sodium bicarbonate, THAM buffers protons without generating CO_2, making it useful in patients with coexisting metabolic and respiratory acidosis. However, protonated THAM needs to be eliminated by the kidneys or by renal replacement therapy and must be used cautiously in patients with renal failure.

Metabolic Alkalosis

Presentation

Classic Presentation

- Similar to metabolic acidosis, symptoms are nonspecific and usually related to the underlying etiology.
- Signs of volume depletion are present in many patients with contraction alkalosis or protracted vomiting.

Critical Presentation

- Although not as common as severe metabolic acidosis, severe alkalemia can be equally devastating.
- **Neurological symptoms** include altered mental status, coma, and seizures.
- **Cardiovascular symptoms** include increased risk of arrhythmias and arteriolar vasoconstriction, which can cause decreased coronary blood flow.
- Alkalemia can also induce hypokalemia, hypocalcemia, and hypophosphatemia.

Diagnosis and Evaluation

History and Physical Examination

- History and physical examination are generally revealing for patients in the Emergency Department (e.g., multiple episodes of emesis with signs of dehydration). The same applies to critically ill inpatients on the Intensive Care Unit, in whom often prolonged NG suctioning is the leading cause for metabolic alkalosis.

Diagnostic Tests

- Urine chloride: a urine Cl^- < 20 suggests saline-responsive etiology (conditions in which chloride is lost). A urine Cl^- > 20 suggests saline-resistant etiology (see Table 34.4).
- Blood pressure: hypertension with a saline-resistant metabolic alkalosis suggests hyperaldosteronism.

Table 34.4 Etiologies of metabolic alkalosis

Saline-responsive (urine Cl^- < 20)

- GI losses of H^+: vomiting, nasogastric tube suctioning

- Contraction alkalosis from diuresis (extracellular fluid contracts around a fixed amount of HCO^-)

- Posthypercapnia: patient with preexisting, chronic respiratory acidosis develops compensatory increase in HCO; over time; rapid correction of respiratory acidosis to a "normal" $PaCO_2$ (usually with mechanical ventilation) "unmasks" compensatory metabolic alkalosis

Saline-resistant (urine Cl^- > 20)

- Hyperaldosteronism: *primary* (Conn syndrome) = aldosterone-secreting adenoma; *secondary* = exogenous mineralocorticoids, Cushing syndrome, renovascular disease

- Hypokalemia: induces a shift of K^+ out of cells and H^+ into cells, and intracellular acidosis in renal tubular cells promotes H^+ secretion and HCO – reabsorption

- Exogenous alkali load (i.e., intravenous sodium bicarbonate)

- Bartter syndrome (defective NaCl reabsorption in ascending loop of Henle)

- Gitelman syndrome (defective NaCl cotransporter in distal tubule)

Critical Management

- The cornerstone for most patients with **saline-responsive metabolic alkalosis** is correction of volume depletion with isotonic sodium chloride.
- In patients with concurrent hypokalemia, potassium repletion will improve alkalosis due to transcellular H^+/K^+ exchange. For patients with metabolic alkalosis in whom saline administration is contraindicated (i.e., CHF patients who require diuresis), potassium repletion is still useful. Acetazolamide can help correct both alkalosis and fluid overload.

Respiratory Acidosis

Presentation

Classic Presentation

- Mild to moderate compensatory hypercapnia, especially when chronic, usually has minimal symptoms, but patients may be anxious or complain of dyspnea.

Critical Presentation

- As hypercarbia worsens, patients become progressively confused, somnolent, and obtunded ("CO_2 narcosis"). Elevated $PaCO_2$ leads to cerebral vasodilation and can cause papilledema.
- **Cardiovascular complications** of acute hypercarbia include tachycardia/arrhythmias and hypertension (mediated by sympathetic nervous system hyperactivity), pulmonary vasoconstriction, and exacerbation of right heart dysfunction.
- Other manifestations are those of severe acidemia, regardless of etiology, and include neurological and other cardiovascular complications (seizures, vasodilation, hypotension).

Diagnosis and Evaluation

- History and physical examination may be revealing (e.g., COPD with chronic CO_2 retention), but most patients will warrant a drug and

Table 34.5 Etiologies of respiratory acidosis

CNS depression: sedating medications (opiates, benzodiazepines), CNS pathology or trauma

Lower airway obstruction: COPD, asthma

Upper airway obstruction: laryngospasm, laryngeal edema, tracheal stenosis, obstructive sleep apnea, foreign body

Chest wall disorders: severe kyphoscoliosis, flail chest, ankylosing spondylitis, pectus excavatum

Neuromuscular disorders: Guillain–Barré, myasthenia gravis, poliomyelitis, amyotrophic lateral sclerosis, muscular dystrophy, diaphragmatic dysfunction, botulism

Obesity-hypoventilation syndrome

Lung parenchymal disease (i.e., pneumonia, pulmonary edema, interstitial lung disease): usually causes hypoxia, tachypnea, and respiratory alkalosis, but may progress to muscle fatigue and respiratory acidosis

toxicology screen, chest radiograph, and sometimes neuroimaging if routine studies are nondiagnostic. Table 34.5 lists causes of respiratory acidosis.

Critical Management

- If medications are a suspected culprit, or the etiology is unclear, reversal (e.g., with naloxone for opiate overdose or flumazenil for benzodiazepines) is warranted.
- Noninvasive positive-pressure ventilation with BiPAP can be useful in those with mild to moderate respiratory acidosis with a quickly reversible condition. The evidence of benefit for BiPAP is strongest for moderate to severe COPD exacerbations, in which mortality is clearly decreased; benefit is also seen with pulmonary edema, although effect on mortality is less clear. BiPAP also appears to be useful for asthma exacerbations, and some cases of pneumonia.
- If severe acidemia is present, or the patient is obtunded, intubation may be indicated.

Respiratory Alkalosis

Presentation

Classic Presentation

- Arespiratory alkalosis is most commonly due to hypoxemia leading to hyperventilation
- Dyspnea and anxiety will often be apparent.

Critical Presentation

- **Acute hypocapnia** can cause cerebral vasoconstriction, leading to confusion, dizziness, syncope, and seizure.
- Respiratory alkalosis causes an increase in binding of calcium to albumin, and many of the symptoms of severe respiratory alkalosis are due to hypocalcemia (e.g., paresthesias, perioral numbness, and tetany). Hypokalemia and hypophosphatemia may also occur due to intracellular shifts.
- Other critical symptoms are those of severe alkalemia, including systemic and coronary vasoconstriction, and arrhythmias.

Diagnosis and Evaluation

- Assess for causes of tachypnea (e.g., fever, anxiety). Table 34.6 lists causes of respiratory alkalosis.
- In patients with hypoxemia, chest radiography is warranted to evaluate for pulmonary pathology.
- Serum chemistries should be checked (importantly potassium, calcium, and phosphorus).

Critical Management

- Treatment is primarily directed at correcting the underlying disorder and managing hypoxemia (if present) as respiratory alkalosis itself is rarely life threatening. Careful attention should be paid to calcium, potassium, and phosphate levels.

Table 34.6 Etiologies of respiratory alkalosis

Hypoxia (leading to hyperventilation; most common cause)

Psychiatric conditions: anxiety, pain

CNS disorder (tumor, trauma, stroke, infection/inflammation; focal lesions of the brainstem)

Fever

Medications: salicylates (mixed metabolic acidosis and respiratory alkalosis), methylxanthines, progesterone, nicotine

Pregnancy (due to progesterone excess)

Hyperthyroidism liver failure

Sepsis

Iatrogenic (mechanically ventilated patients)

Sudden Deterioration

- Acute changes in any patient with an acid–base disorder require a rapid reevaluation of the patient's mental status and vital signs, as well as repeat ABG determination.
- If the patient is mechanically ventilated, note any recent ventilator setting changes that might explain a change in CO_2 levels.
- Mechanically ventilated patients emergently hemodialyzed for intoxications causing (anion-gap) metabolic acidosis are at risk for profound iatrogenic respiratory alkalosis, if ventilator settings are not continuously adjusted during the dialysis treatment course. Initial high minute ventilation is indicated, in order to provide respiratory compensation, but reductions in tidal volume and/or respiratory rate are necessary, while the dialysis treatment eliminates the offending agent and increases serum bicarbonate concentration.

BIBLIOGRAPHY

Cooper DJ, Walley KR, Wiggs BR, et al. Bicarbonate does not improve hemodynamics in critically ill patients who have lactic acidosis: A prospective, controlled clinical study. *Ann Intern Med* 1990;112:492.

Gray A, Goodacre S, Newby D, et al. Noninvasive ventilation in acute cardiogenic pulmonary edema. *N Engl J Med* 2008;359:142–151.

Hoste EA, Colpaert K, Vanholder RC, et al. Sodium bicarbonate versus THAM in ICU patients with mild metabolic acidosis. *J Nephrol* 2005;18:303.

Maletesha G, Singh NK, Bharija A, et al. Comparison of arterial and venous pH, bicarbonate, PCO_2 and O_2 in initial emergency department assessment. *Emerg Med J* 2007;24(8):569.

Ram FS, Picot J, Lightowler J, et al. Noninvasive positive pressure ventilation for treatment of respiratory failure due to exacerbations of chronic obstructive pulmonary disease. *Cochrane Database Syst Rev* 2004;1:CD004104.

35

Common Electrolyte Disorders (Sodium, Potassium, Calcium, Magnesium)

CHRISTINE K. CHAN AND JOHN E. ARBO

Chapter 35:
Electrolyte Disorders

Hyponatremia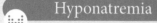

Hypernatremia

Common Etiologies

 SIADH, psychogenic or primary polydipsia.

 Diabetes insipidus, patients **with limited mobility/fluid** intake or impaired thirst mechanism.

Associated Lab Value

 Serum Na < 135 mEq/L.

 Serum Na > 150 mEq/L.

Critical Presentation

 Headache, encephalopathy, seizures, respiratory arrest.

 Rapid increases in Na may present with confusion or seizure.

Principles of Management

 Determine duration, degree of hyponatremia, and severity of symptoms to guide treatment.

 If there are seizures or AMS, administer 100 mL 3% saline bolus.

 Unless clearly severe/acute hyponatremia, exercise caution in raising sodium > 8 mEq in 24 hours.

 Determine volume status **and replace free water deficit.**

 Take care not to lower the Na level by no more than 0.5 mEq/hour.

Chapter 35:
Electrolyte Disorders

Hypocalcemia	Hypercalcemia

 Common Etiologies

 Hypoparathyroidism, hepatic/renal disease, vitamin D **deficiency, calcium** sequestration/precipitation.

 Hyperparathyroidism, malignancy, familial hypocalciuric hypercalcemia, vitamin D excess, thiazide diuretics, calcium antacids.

 Associated Lab Value

 Serum Ca < 8.5 mg/dL.

Corrected for low albumin: iCa < 4.5 mg/dL.

 Serum Ca: Mild 10.5–12.0 mg/dL, Moderate 12.0–14.0 mg/dL, Severe > 14.0 mg/dL.

 Critical Presentation

 Ionized Ca < 2.0 mg/dL may present with tetany, arrythmia, papilledema, psychiatric manifestations.

 Serum Ca > 14.0 mg/dL may present with delirium, abdominal pain, osteopenia nephrolithiasis, hypertension bradycardia, and must be treated regardless of symptoms.

 Principles of Management

 Measure serum and ionized calcium, albumin, PTH, phosphate, magnesium, vitamin D, renal function.

 ECG, conitnuous cardiac monitoring.

 Replete magnesium if necessary.

 If severe, administer IV calcium.

 Measure serum and ionized calcium, albumin, PTH, PTHrP, phosphate, magnesium, vitamin D, renal function.

 ECG, continuous cardiac monitoring.

 Fluid administration.

 Administer calcium-lowering medications.

 Consider hemodialysis for Ca >18 mg/dL or severe symptoms.

Chapter 35:
Electrolyte Disorders

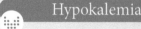 Hypokalemia   Hyperkalemia

 Common Etiologies

 Consider renal losses, GI losses, transcellular shift, decreased intake, plasma-pharesis.

 Consider impaired excretion, transcellular shift, hypoaldosteronism, excess intake, or hemolysis of blood sample.

 Associated Lab Value

 Serum K < 3.5 mEq/L.

 Serum K > 5.5 mEq/L.

 Critical Presentation

 Below 2.5 mEq/L may present as muscle weakness, rhabdomyolysis, vomiting, arrhythmia, impaired renal function.

 Severe hyperkalemia may present as arrhythmias, weakness in the extremities, flaccid paralysis.

 Principles of Management

 For severe hypokalemia, administer KCl.

 ECG, ensure continuous cardiac monitoring.

 Correct magnesium and pH disturbances.

 Administer furosemide and insulin with D50.

 For hyperkalemia > 7 OR if ECG changes, administer calcium.

 ECG, ensure continuous cardiac monitoring.

Chapter 35:
Electrolyte Disorders

Hypomagnesemia | Hypermagnesemia

Common Etiologies

 Consider GI losses (pancreatitis, PPIs, diarrhea, small bowel syndrome), renal losses (alcohol, diuretics), other medications, diabetes, hypercalcemia.

 Renal insuffiiciency, excessive intake or administration.

Associated Lab Value

 Severe: Serum Mg < 1.0 mg/dL.

 Severe: Serum Mg > 4.0 mg/dL.

Critical Presentation

 Prolonged QT, QRS widening, tachyarrythmia, tremor, convulsions, delirium, coma.

 Bradyarrythmia, slowed AV conduction, pumonary edema, absent deep tendon reflex, lethargy, encephalopathy, apnea.

Principles of Management

 24-hour urine Mg excretion level may help differentiate etiology.

 Replete Mg, ECG, ensure continuous cardiac monitoring.

 Stop all sources of Mg.

 ECG, ensure continuous cardiac monitoring.

 In hemodynamic instability, administer calcium gluconate, IV fluids, and loop diuretics.

Disorders of Sodium Regulation

Introduction

- Serum sodium (Na) concentration is mediated by free water intake, circulating levels of antidiuretic hormone (ADH), and renal filtration of sodium.
- **Hyponatremia** is defined as serum sodium level of < 135 mEq/L and is due to an excess of total body water compared to total body sodium content, and often involves an imbalance of the hormone vasopressin (antidiuretic hormone, ADH). This can occur in hypovolemic, euvolemic, and hypervolemic states.
- **Hypernatremia** is defined as a serum sodium level of > 150 mEq/L, and is due to a deficit of free water relative to sodium. Since most people are able to respond to their thirst stimulus, hypernatremia is typically seen in patients with limited mobility or impaired thirst mechanisms. Hypernatremia can also occur in diabetes insipidus, defined as a loss of free water due to a deficiency or insensitivity to ADH.

Hyponatremia

Presentation

Classic Presentation

- Signs and symptoms of mild to moderate hyponatremia are nonspecific: generalized weakness, lethargy, nausea, vomiting, and muscle cramps are common.
- Depending on the chronicity of the hyponatremia, some patients may be asymptomatic.

Critical Presentation

- Profound hyponatremia (< 120–125 mEq/L), or rapid drops in serum sodium level, may present with headache, encephalopathy, seizure, or respiratory arrest.

Diagnosis and Evaluation

History

- Medication culprits: diuretics, antidepressants, anticonvulsants, antipsychotics.
- Inquire about **volume loss** such as diarrhea, emesis, fever, diaphoresis, polyuria, or extreme exercise.
- Inquire about substance abuse, including **alcohol use** or illicit substances such as MDMA.
- Inquire about **volume gain** such as edema, ascites, oliguria.
- Look for systemic symptoms of hypothyroidism or adrenal insufficiency.

Physical Examination

- Perform a physical exam with special attention to: vital signs, orthostatics, jugular venous pressure, mucous membranes, skin turgor, capillary refill, peripheral edema, and other signs of volume status.
- Perform a bedside cardiac ultrasound looking for inferior vena cava diameter and degree of inspiratory collapse to help estimate intravascular volume status.

Diagnostic Evaluation

- Laboratory workup may include: basic metabolic panel, serum osmolality, urine sodium, urine osmolality, TSH, and morning cortisol.
- Urine labs must be obtained simultaneously with serum labs and, ideally, before any fluid resuscitation or diuresis is initiated.
- Note that conventional algorithms traditionally use volume status as a major branch point for assessment of hyponatremia; however, this is a challenging question, especially in the ED environment. It is also fraught with poor interrater reliability; as such, volume status may best be deferred until the final step of the algorithm.
- STEP ONE: Obtain a measured serum osmolality (normal = 280–295 mOsm/kg) to assess validity of hyponatremia.
  - Serum osmolality can help differentiate between hypertonic, isotonic, and hypotonic hyponatremia.
  - True hyponatremic patients are hypotonic.
  - If the patient is hypotonic, go to step 2.

- ○ If the patient is iso- or hypertonic, evaluate for the etiology of additional osmoles (e.g., hyperglycemia, hyperlipidemia, mannitol infusion, perioperative absorption of irrigation fluids).
- STEP TWO: Measure the urine osmolality to assess **ADH secretion.**
  - a. Urine osmolality < 100 mOsm/kg suggests ADH tone is LOW (e.g., indicates primary polydipsia, beer potomania syndrome, or reset osmostat).
  - b. Urine osmolality > 100 mOsm/kg suggests ADH tone is HIGH (i.e., an inappropriate ADH secretion status, to include SIADH (see below), hypothyroidism and adrenal insufficiency).
- STEP THREE: Measure the urine sodium concentration to assess **RAAS activation.**
  - ○ Urine sodium < 25 mEq/L suggests RAAS is active and is associated with a **low effective arterial blood volume compared to venous volume**, which can reflect hypovolemia, or, despite clinical hypervolemia, low cardiac output or peripheral vasodilation
    - i. In this case, volume status assessment is necessary to differentiate causes.
    - ii. Hypovolemia/volume depletion is common.
    - iii. Hypervolemic causes include:
      - a. Liver failure
      - b. Heart failure
      - c. Renal failure (if prerenal injury)
  - ○ Urine sodium > 25 mEq/L suggests RAAS is inactive and is associated with myriad distinct etiologies:
    - ○ SIADH
    - ○ Thyroid insufficiency
    - ○ Adrenal insufficiency
    - ○ Renal failure (if intrarenal injury)
    - ○ Diuretics (especially thiazides)

Possible Etiologies

Syndrome of Inappropriate Antidiuretic Hormone (SIADH)

- Antidiuretic hormone (ADH) secretion results in increased water absorption in the kidneys.

Table 35.1 Etiologies of syndrome of inappropriate antidiuretic hormone (SIADH)

CNS disturbances	Stroke, intracranial pathology, infection, trauma, psychosis
Malignancies	Small cell carcinoma, extrapulmonary small cell carcinomas, head and neck tumors
Drugs	Antidepressants (SSRIs, TCAs), anticonvulsants (e.g., carbamazepine), antipsychotics, anti-cancer drugs, anti-diabetic drugs, vasopressin analogues, opiates, NSAIDs, nicotine, amiodarone, proton pump inhibitors, MDMA (ecstasy)
Pulmonary disease	Pneumonias (viral, bacterial, tuberculous), obstructive lung disease (asthma, COPD)
Hormone deficiency	Hypopituitarism, hypothyroidism
Hormone administration	Vasopressin, desmopressin, oxytocin

- Normally, in euvolemic patients with adequate effective circulating volume, excess water intake decreases the serum tonicity and therefore suppresses ADH secretion, allowing for free water excretion.
- In SIADH, the ingestion of excess water does not suppress ADH, leading to an excess of water retention (and not a deficiency of sodium).
- The following conditions must be met to make a SIADH diagnosis:
  ○ Hypotonic hyponatremia
  ○ Urine osmolality > 100 mOsm/kg
  ○ Urine Na > 20 mEq/L
  ○ No evidence of diuretics, hypothyroidism, or adrenal insufficiency
- Treatment usually involves fluid restriction and treatment of the underlying cause.

Psychogenic or Primary Polydipsia

- Observed in patients with psychiatric disorders, or patients who have a CNS lesion that affects the thirst center.
- Patients drink excess large volumes of water that result in lower serum tonicity.

Critical Management

Critical Management Checklist

☑ **Airway management**: non-invasive ventilation or intubation as needed for symptomatic volume overload or alterations in mental status.

☑ Hemodynamic management to maintain **MAP > 65 mmHg.**

☑ Give intravenous fluid bolus if clinically hypovolemic.

☑ **Determine the degree, chronicity, and severity of symptoms of the hyponatremia.**

☑ **If severe symptoms (e.g., seizure/coma), give 100 mL bolus of 3% saline.**

☑ Consider adrenal insufficiency as a cause of hypotonic hyponatremia in patients with a suggestive history or those in shock.

☑ For critically ill patients or those with severe hyponatremia, consider ICU admission for serial sodium monitoring to avoid rapid overcorrection.

Critical management is based on the severity and duration of symptoms.

- **Duration: acute versus chronic**
  - Acute – developing in a period of < 48 hours
  - Chronic – developing in a period ≥ 48 hours
  - If unable to determine timing, **assume the hyponatremia is chronic**.
- **Degree of hyponatremia**
  - Mild: Na 130–134 mEq/L
  - Moderate: Na 120–129 mEq/L
  - Profound: Na < 120 mEq/L
- **Severity of symptoms**
  - Symptoms are on a spectrum from asymptomatic or mild to severe.
  - Severe symptoms such as seizures, altered mental status, coma, and death can be seen in patients with profound hyponatremia, and are more common with acute hyponatremia.
- Avoid overcorrection to reduce risk of osmotic demyelination syndrome; **care should be taken to raise the serum sodium level by no more than 0.5 mEq/hour or a total of 8–10 mEq/day.**

Acute Hyponatremia: Initial Management

- **Symptomatic** patients with Na < 130 mEq/L are treated with a 100 mL bolus of 3% saline, followed by additional 100 mL boluses if symptoms persist.

- Goal of therapy is to quickly increase the serum sodium by 4 to 6 mEq/L over a few hours.
- Desmopressin administration can help with rate of sodium correction in a more predictable fashion if there is concern for overcorrection.
- Consider 1–2 mcg of desmopressin every 6–8 hours IV or SQ in a 24- to 48-hour time period with hypertonic saline until the serum sodium is at least 125 mEq/L.
- For severe hyponatremia < 120 mEq/L, initiate a 3% saline infusion at a beginning rate of 0.25 mL/kg/hr.
- It is safe to initiate this through a peripheral IV line.
- **Asymptomatic** patients with Na < 130 mEq/L should be orally fluid restricted and receive treatment for the underlying etiology (e.g., diuresis or volume resuscitation as appropriate).
  - Watch for brisk urine output, suggesting a decrease in ADH tone and thus a risk for autocorrection; if this occurs, recheck serum sodium and urine ADH; if sodium is rapidly rising and ADH is dropping, clamp with desmopressin (see above).
  - Trend serum sodium concentration level every 1 to 2 hours.

Chronic Hyponatremia: Initial Management

- Similar to acute hyponatremia, **symptomatic** patients with Na < 130 mEq/L are treated with a 100 mL bolus of 3% saline, followed by additional 100 mL boluses if symptoms persist, with the goal of rapid correction of the Na level by 4–6 mEq/L over the next several hours.
- **Asymptomatic** patients with chronic hyponatremia are typically treated based on the severity and etiology of their condition.

Hyponatremia: Ongoing Treatment

- **Hypovolemic hypotonic hyponatremia:** Further management is focused on the use of sodium-containing fluids to replace intravascular volume, replenish serum sodium, and eliminate the stimulus for ADH. If the patient is hypotensive, normal saline boluses should be given as with any patient. Hold further resuscitation and consider desmopressin clamp (as above) if there is brisk urine output AND rapid sodium correction. To ensure an appropriate replacement, calculate the following:

- Total body water (TBW) in liters = 0.6 (male) or 0.5 (female) × weight (kg).
- Target serum sodium level (based on 0.5 mEq/hour or 8 mEq/day).
- Sodium deficit (mEq of sodium needed to reach target) = TBW × (Na target − Na serum).
- Total replacement fluid needed to provide sodium deficit = Na deficit (mEq)/Na replacement fluid (mEq/L).
- Hourly infusion rate: Amount of fluid/total replacement time.
- Replacement fluid options include normal saline (154 mEq/L), 2% saline (342 mEq/L), or 3% saline (513 mEq/L); 3% saline may require central venous access at various hospitals but is not required.
- Note: These examples assume a constant urine osmolality. In practice, Uosm will typically decrease as intravascular volume is replaced, the stimulus for ADH is removed, and free water is once again excreted. As this occurs, there can be an unintended increase in the rate of sodium correction.

- **Euvolemic hypotonic hyponatremia**: Restrict free water and treat underlying cause. In cases where Uosm is high, be careful not to give isotonic fluids (e.g., normal saline) unless the patient is hypotensive, as this can result in a net gain of free water and an unintended worsening of the hyponatremia. Recheck serum sodium levels frequently.
- **Hypervolemic hypotonic hyponatremia**: Restrict free water and treat underlying cause. Recheck serum sodium levels frequently.

Acute Decompensation

- For all patients who are moderately to severely hyponatremic (< 130 mEq/L) and are symptomatic, which includes any change in mental status, assess for airway management and hemodynamic status.
- Then, administer 100 mL bolus of 3% saline with 1– 2 mcg of desmopressin every 6 to 8 hours in the first 24 hours.
- Do not use mannitol, as it can lower sodium levels.
- As patients with mild hyponatremia (130–134 mEq/L) typically do not have severe symptoms, an alternate cause of deterioration should be suspected in this patient population.

Hypernatremia

Presentation

Classic Presentation

- As with hyponatremia, signs and symptoms of moderate hypernatremia are nonspecific, but generalized weakness and nausea are common.

Critical Presentation

- Severe hypernatremia, or rapid increases in serum sodium level, may present with confusion and seizure.

Diagnosis and Evaluation

History

- Elderly, impaired mental status and limited fluid intake, hospitalized patients requiring nasogastric suctioning.
- Inquire about sources of insensible losses (fever, tachypnea), diuretic use, osmotic diuresis (glycosuria), osmotic diarrhea (malabsorption, lactulose), and emesis.

Physical Examination

- Perform a physical examination assessing volume status, with an additional focus on mental status and mobility.

Diagnostic Tests

- Chemistry panel, urine osmolality, and urine sodium.
- Urine osmolality is a useful diagnostic test in the work-up of hypernatremia, as an appropriate response to a relative increase in serum sodium is to concentrate the urine and retain free water.
- Urine sodium is useful in *hypovolemic hypernatremia* as an indicator of the body's efforts to restore intravascular volume. Total body volume status assessment coupled with urine sodium and urine osmolality will help narrow the diagnosis.

Possible Etiologies

Hypovolemic Hypernatremia (Most Common)

- Urine will be concentrated, with Uosm > 600 mOsm/kg.
- A urine sodium < 20 suggests extrarenal losses, such as diarrhea, emesis, or dehydration.
- A urine sodium > 20 suggests renal losses, such as diuretic use or osmotic diuresis.

Euvolemic Hypernatremia

- Euvolemic hypernatremia results from increased insensible losses (diaphoresis) or loss of free water due to diabetes insipidus (DI).
- In patients with hypernatremia, the urine should be concentrated. In DI, a condition caused by either a deficiency of or insensitivity to ADH, the urine osmolality (Uosm) will be inappropriately low, often < 300 mOsm/kg.
- The diagnosis of DI is confirmed by testing the response to fluid restriction (urine osmolality should increase by > 30 mOsm/kg with this challenge). Once the diagnosis of DI is confirmed, distinguishing between central and nephrogenic DI requires administration of desmopressin (synthetic ADH) and rechecking urine osmolality. In central DI, desmopressin will make the urine more concentrated.

Hypervolemic Hypernatremia (Rare)

- Can be due to hypertonic saline administration.
- Also seen with mineralocorticoid excess, which causes suppression of ADH secretion.

Critical Management

Critical Management Checklist

- ☑ **Airway management**: intubation as needed for alterations in mental status.
- ☑ Hemodynamic management to maintain **MAP > 65 mmHg.**
- ☑ **Determine volume status** and begin to replace free water deficit.
- ☑ **Consider ICU admission** for critically ill patients or those requiring frequent sodium checks.
- ☑ Emergency treatment of diabetes insipidus (DI) centers on replacement of free water deficit. Definitive treatment of DI requires treatment of underlying cause and use of desmopressin.

- Management centers on replacement of the free water deficit.
- To ensure an appropriate rate of replacement, calculate the following:
  - Total body water (TBW) in liters = 0.6 (male) or 0.5 (female) × weight in kg.
  - Hourly infusion rate: amount of fluid/total replacement time.
  - Target serum sodium level (based on 0.5 mEq/hour or 8 mEq/day).
  - Liters of water required to reach target (water deficit) = TBW × [(Na serum/ Na target) − 1].
- **Care should be taken to lower the serum sodium level by no more than 0.5 mEq/hour, or by no more than 12 mEq/day.**

Sudden Deterioration

- Overly rapid correction of hypernatremia may lead to **cerebral edema** and seizure. However, this risk is less pronounced in older adults. Similar to hyponatremia, to ensure a safe and accurate replacement rate, sodium levels should be trended, though these patients almost never necessitate ICU level of care for sodium derangements alone.

Disorders of Potassium Regulation

Introduction

- Disorders of potassium, especially hyperkalemia, are the most feared electrolyte disorders due to their ability to cause life-threatening cardiac arrhythmia.
- Hypokalemia is defined as a serum potassium level of < 3.5 mEq/L.
- Hyperkalemia is defined as a serum potassium level of > 5.5 mEq/L.

Hypokalemia

Presentation

Classic Presentation

- Mild hypokalemia is usually asymptomatic, and symptoms may not manifest until the serum potassium falls below 3.0 mEq/L.

Table 35.2 Etiologies of hypokalemia

Renal losses: diuretics, primary mineralocorticoid excess, hypomagnesemia, renal tubular acidosis Type 1 or Type 2, diabetic ketoacidosis, salt wasting nephropathies, dialysis

Gastrointestinal losses: diarrhea, emesis, gastric suction, laxative abuse, malabsorption

Transcellular shift: metabolic or respiratory alkalosis, insulin use, inhaled beta-agonists/bronchodilators, hypothermia, catecholamines, hypokalemia or thyrotoxic periodic paralysis

Decreased potassium intake

Plasmapheresis

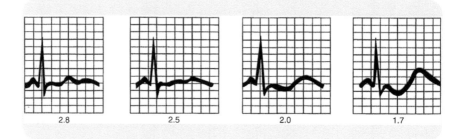

Figure 35.1 ECG changes associated with hypokalemia.

- Acute development of hypokalemia tends to be more symptomatic than chronic hypokalemia.
- Table 35.2 lists possible causes of hypokalemia.

Critical Presentation

- Severe hypokalemia (< 2.5 mEq/L) can present as severe muscle weakness or rhabdomyolysis, cardiac arrhythmias, or respiratory failure, as well as renal, GI, and neuromuscular aberrations.
- **Cardiovascular**: classic ECG changes follow a distinct pattern: flattened T waves > ST depression > U waves > QT interval prolongation > ventricular arrhythmia (Figure 35.1).
- **Renal**: impaired concentrating ability, increased ammonia production, or significant hypertension.
- **Gastrointestinal**: nausea, vomiting, ileus.
- **Neuromuscular**: weakness, muscle cramps, paralysis.

Diagnosis and Evaluation

- For many patients with hypokalemia, the cause is apparent from the history.
- Most common causes of hypokalemia are vomiting and diarrhea and use of diuretics.
- Urine potassium loss > 20mEq in a 24-hour period, spot urine potassium > 20 mEq/L or a spot urine potassium creatinine ratio > 20 mEq/g suggests renal losses.
- Urine potassium loss < 20mEq in a 24-hour period suggests transcellular shift, decreased oral intake, or extrarenal potassium losses.
  - In cases where the etiology is not clear, assessment of acid base disorder may be helpful, as some causes of hypokalemia are associated with metabolic alkalosis or acidosis.

Metabolic Etiologies

- Metabolic acidosis with severe hypokalemia is seen in diabetic ketoacidosis, type 1 (distal) or type 2 (proximal) renal tubular acidosis.
- Metabolic alkalosis with mild hypokalemia suggests diuretic use, vomiting, or laxative use.
- Metabolic alkalosis with severe hypokalemia and hypertension suggests primary mineralocorticoid excess or renovascular disease.

Critical Management

Critical Management Checklist

- ☑ **Airway management**: intubation as needed for depression in respiratory function or airway protection.
- ☑ **Place central line** for more expedient replacement in unstable or severely hypokalemic patients.
- ☑ **For severe hypokalemia, IV potassium chloride is indicated**.
- ☑ Continuous cardiac monitoring to assess for arrythmias.
- ☑ Obtain an **EKG** for assessment of cardiac involvement.
- ☑ Concomitantly correct serum magnesium.
- ☑ Treat severe acidosis or alkalosis if present.
- ☑ Be aware of rebound hyperkalemia in certain patients.
- ☑ Monitor potassium levels every 2 to 4 hours during repletion for critically ill patients.

- Treat underlying conditions that may worsen ongoing potassium losses in certain clinical settings (e.g., diarrhea, vomiting)
- Provide potassium supplementation with potassium chloride (KCl; preferred) or potassium bicarbonate.
- Generally, a dose of 10 mEq of KCl should raise the serum potassium by 0.1 mEq/L.
- Concomitantly correct serum magnesium. (Hypokalemia is difficult to correct in the setting of hypomagnesemia.)
- **Hypokalemic periodic paralysis** is a rare genetic or acquired disorder characterized by acute muscle flaccidness from an acute intracellular potassium shift. The familial form is often precipitated by exercise or high carb meals, whereas the acquired form occurs with thyrotoxicosis (most typically seen in male patients of Asian or Hispanic descent).

Sudden Deterioration

- Cardiac instability: 10–20 mEq/hr of KCl IV over 5–20 minutes, preferably through a central venous catheter.
- Potassium bicarbonate is preferred for patients with severe metabolic acidosis. Potassium chloride is preferred in almost all other circumstances.
- IV potassium replacement should be administered in saline instead of dextrose-containing fluids, as dextrose can stimulate insulin production, which can perpetuate hypokalemia.

Special Circumstances

- In patients with hyperglycemia or diabetic ketoacidosis, measured potassium levels may be falsely normal or even elevated despite a total body volume deficit of potassium, and administration of insulin may worsen hypokalemia; serum potassium should be closely followed during insulin therapy.
- Prior to insulin administration, potassium supplementation should occur for potassium levels less than 4.0 mEq/L, and potassium levels should be maintained between 4–4.5 mEq/L during treatment.

Hyperkalemia

Presentation

Classic Presentation

- Mild hyperkalemia is usually asymptomatic.
- Table 35.3 lists causes of hyperkalemia.

Critical Presentation

- Severe hyperkalemia can present with cardiac and neuromuscular abnormalities.
- **Cardiovascular**: classic ECG changes follow a distinct pattern: peaked T waves → shortening of QT interval arrows PR becomes prolonged arrows AV conduction blocks → sine waves arrows ventricular fibrillation and or asystole (Figure 35.2).
- **Neuromuscular**: paresthesia and weakness of the extremities, flaccid paralysis.

Table 35.3 Etiologies of hyperkalemia

Impaired excretion: renal insufficiency, potassium sparing diuretics, ACE-inhibitors

Transcellular shift: acidemia, lack of insulin, burns, tumor lysis, digoxin toxicity, beta-blockers, trauma, rhabdomyolysis, succinylcholine during anesthesia procedures

Hypoaldosteronism (type 4 RTA)

Excess intake

Pseudohyperkalemia: hemolysis of blood sample, elevated WBC or platelet count

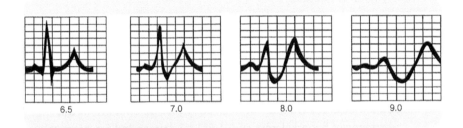

| 6.5 | 7.0 | 8.0 | 9.0 |

Figure 35.2 ECG changes associated with hyperkalemia.

Diagnosis and Evaluation

- In general, hyperkalemia is due to increased potassium release from cells, decreased urinary excretion or both.
- Exclude pseudohyperkalemia, usually due to cell lysis during phlebotomy or specimen processing; if suspected, repeat potassium in heparinized tubes or via blood gas.
- Measurement of 24-hour urinary potassium excretion is often of limited utility.

Critical Management

Critical Management Checklist

☑ **Airway management**: intubation as needed for depression in respiratory function or airway protection.
☑ Continuous cardiac monitoring to assess for arrythmias.
☑ Obtain **EKG** to assess for cardiac involvement.
☑ Stabilize cardiac cell membrane with calcium administration.
☑ Additional treatment to include insulin, albuterol, loop diuretics or potassium binders.
☑ **Place hemodialysis line** for emergent dialysis in conjunction with nephrology consultants.
☑ Be aware of rebound hyperkalemia in certain patients.

- **Stabilize cardiac myocardium:** for hyperkalemia with EKG changes, or any K > 7.0 mEq/L, give calcium chloride 1 g (ideally through a central venous catheter or large-bore peripheral IV); alternatively, calcium gluconate 3 g IV if access is limited to peripheral IVs; re-dose calcium every hour as needed.
- Drive potassium intracellularly
  - Administer insulin 10 units IV with 1 ampule of D50
  - Can consider addition of inhaled albuterol 10–20 mg
    - ○ Careful note: this is a higher dose than the standard adult dose and may cause tachycardia.
  - Sodium bicarbonate has not been shown to be effective in the treatment of hyperkalemia and is not recommended for patients without concomitant severe metabolic acidosis.

- Decrease total body potassium:
  - Loop diuretics (furosemide) 40 mg IV for patients without renal dysfunction.
  - May administer 1 mg/kg loop diuretic dose if concurrently overloaded.
  - Novel gastrointestinal cation exchangers patiromer (Veltassa) or zirconium cyclosilicate (Lokelma) are preferred over sodium polystyrene sulfonate (Kayexalate), due to its safety profile.
  - Hemodialysis for refractory hyperkalemia or unstable patients.

Sudden Deterioration

- Cardiac instability: IV calcium chloride 1 g (ideally via central line, but otherwise via the most patent available peripheral IV)
- Emergent hemodialysis.

Disorders of Calcium Regulation

Introduction

- Release of calcium stores into the circulation is regulated by extracellular calcium concentration, parathyroid hormone (PTH), vitamin D metabolites, and calcitonin.
- 40% of serum calcium is bound to protein, primarily albumin. 45% is physiologically free (not bound to albumin) and is measured as ionized calcium (iCa), which is the metabolically active form. 15% is bound to other anions.
  - Normal serum calcium measures 8.5–10.5 mg/dL and reflects total calcium (bound and unbound). Normal ionized calcium measures 4.5–5.6 mg/dL (1.05–1.37 mmol/L).
  - Decreases in albumin lower total serum calcium without affecting ionized calcium. Corrected calcium (mg/dL) = measured calcium + [0.8 × (4 − albumin)].
  - As iCa is the only biologically active fraction, it is always best to measure it directly in patients with low serum albumin.
    - Acidosis reduces albumin-calcium binding, while alkalosis enhances it.
    - Directly measure iCa in patients with acidosis or alkalosis for accuracy.

Hypocalcemia

Presentation

Classic Presentation

- Mild hypocalcemia is usually asymptomatic.
- Table 35.4 lists causes of hypocalcemia.

Critical Presentation

- Severe hypocalcemia (ionized calcium < 2 mg/dL or < 0.5 mmol/L) can manifest as tetany, seizures, cardiovascular complications, papilledema and psychiatric manifestations.

Table 35.4 Etiologies of hypocalcemia

Hypocalcemia with low parathyroid hormone (hypoparathyroidism)

- Primary: due to radiation therapy, surgery, infiltrative diseases, or genetic disorders
- Secondary (pseudohypoparathyroidism): end-organ resistance to parathyroid hormone (PTH)

Hypocalcemia with high PTH

- Vitamin D deficiency or resistance
- Renal disease
- Hepatic disease
- Decreased intake/malabsorption
- Hypomagnesemia (decreased sensitivity to PTH)

Calcium sequestration/precipitation

- Massive blood transfusion (calcium binds to citrate anticoagulant)
- Hyperphosphatemia
- Osteoblastic metastasis
- Pancreatitis
- Sepsis
- Post-surgical

- **Seizures**: generalized tonic clinic, generalized absence, or focal seizures.
- **Neuromuscular symptoms**: paresthesias (classically fingertips and perioral), muscle spasms, and tetany.
- **Circumoral and acral paresthesias**
- **Carpal-pedal spasm**
- **Cardiovascular**: prolonged QTc interval, ventricular arrythmias, hypotension, heart failure.
- **Papilledema**
- **Laryngospasm**

Diagnosis and Evaluation

- **Diagnostic tests**
  - Serum and ionized calcium, serum albumin, parathyroid hormone (PTH), phosphate (PO$_4$), magnesium, vitamin D, and renal function studies.
  - Order an EKG to evaluate for QTc interval prolongation.
  - Table 35.4 reviews different categories of causes of hypocalcemia, while Table 35.5 gives an overview of the diagnostic evaluation of hypocalcemia.

Table 35.5 Laboratory assessment of hypocalcemia

Etiology	Corrected calcium	PTH	PO$_4$	Mg	25 (OH) D	Cr
Hypo-parathyroidism	↓	↓	↑	Normal	Normal	Normal
Vitamin D deficiency	Normal or ↓	↑	Normal or ↓	Normal	↓	Normal
Chronic kidney disease	↓	↑	↑	Normal or ↓	Normal or ↓	↑
Hypo-magnesemia	↓	Normal or ↓	Normal	↓	Normal	Normal

Critical Management

Critical Management Checklist

☑ **Airway management**: intubation as needed for depression in respiratory function or airway protection.

☑ Continuous cardiac monitoring to assess for arrythmias.

☑ Obtain **EKG** to assess for QTc interval prolongation.

☑ **Verify** hypoglycemia by checking ionized calcium and correcting for albumin.

☑ IV calcium administration for patients with severe hypocalcemia or those with severe symptoms

- Treat patients with severe hypocalcemia and/or those with symptoms with IV calcium gluconate or calcium chloride.
  - Either 10% calcium gluconate or 10% calcium chloride may be used for initial replacement.
  - 1 to 2 grams of IV calcium gluconate is preferred as the initial strategy for patients with peripheral access.
  - Calcium should be infused over 20 minutes to reduce the risk of arrythmias and other cardiac side effects.
- The treatment effect above will be transient; a slow infusion of calcium should be given for patients with refractory or severe hypocalcemia.
- Check ionized calcium at regular intervals.
- Mild to moderate chronic hypocalcemia may be treated with oral calcium and vitamin D supplementation.
- Replete magnesium if low, as hypocalcemia will be difficult to normalize with low magnesium levels.
- Long term management of hypocalcemia involves diagnosis and treatment of the underlying etiology.
  - Many patients, including those with chronic kidney disease and hypoparathyroidism, will need concomitant supplementation of Vitamin D.

Sudden Deterioration

- Hypotension, ventricular arrhythmias, or seizures: cardiac monitoring and rapid correction with IV calcium chloride (ideally requires central venous access, but is not mandatory in an emergent situation).

Hypercalcemia

Presentation

Classic Presentation

- Mild to moderate cases are usually asymptomatic.
- Hypercalcemia has myriad causes (Table 35.6).

Critical Presentation

- Severe hypercalcemia (serum calcium level greater than 14 mg/dL) can produce acute neuropsychiatric, gastrointestinal, cardiovascular, renal, and skeletal symptoms (*"stones, bones, abdominal groans, and psychic overtones"*).
  - **Neuropsychiatric symptoms**: confusion, delirium, psychosis, weakness, and coma.
  - **Gastrointestinal symptoms**: abdominal pain, nausea, emesis, constipation, or ileus.

Table 35.6 Etiologies of hypercalcemia

Hyperparathyroidism (excessive release of PTH)
- Typically, due to a single adenoma; occasionally hyperplasia
- MEN syndromes

Malignancy
- Osteolysis: multiple myeloma, breast and bone cancer/metastasis
- Malignancy-associated PTH-related peptide

Familial hypocalciuric hypercalcemia (FHH)
- Genetic mutation in Ca-detecting receptor in parathyroid and kidney

Vitamin D excess
- Granulomatous disorders (tuberculosis, sarcoidosis, Wegener's syndrome)
- Vitamin D intoxication

Other
- Immobilization, thiazide diuretics, calcium antacids, milk-alkali syndrome

---

- **Cardiovascular symptoms**: hypertension, bradycardia, shortened QT interval.
- **Renal symptoms**: polyuria (with associated hypovolemia) and nephrolithiasis.
- **Skeletal**: osteopenia and associated fractures.

Diagnosis and Evaluation

- Favor **primary hyperparathyroidism** in post-menopausal female, asymptomatic patient with chronic hypercalcemia.
- Patients with **malignancy** present with higher calcium levels with more rapid increases and are more symptomatic (most common cause of hypercalcemia in a hospitalized patient).
- Check **serum and ionized calcium**, parathyroid hormone (**PTH**), **albumin** and **phosphate.**
  - Primary hyperparathyroidism: PTH is elevated, phosphorous is low.
  - Malignancy hypercalcemia: PTH is suppressed, phosphorous is low normal.
  - Multiple myeloma: PTH is suppressed, phosphorous is elevated. Measure SPEP, UPEP, serum free light chains.
- Check **Vitamin D** levels.
  - High calcium, high 1-25 hydroxyvitamin D: lymphoma or granulomatous disease (sarcoidosis, tuberculosis).
  - High calcium, high 25-hydroxyvitamin D: Vitamin D intoxication.
- Measure PTH-related protein: if elevated, likely related to malignancy.
- Other causes include Vitamin A intoxication, hyperthyroidism.

Critical Management

Critical Management Checklist

☐ **Airway management**: intubation as needed for depression in respiratory function or airway protection.

☐ Continuous cardiac monitoring to assess for arrythmias.

☐ Obtain **EKG** to assess for cardiac involvement.

☐ **Verify** hypercalcemia by checking ionized calcium and correcting for albumin.

☐ For symptomatic patients or significantly increased calcium levels, start fluid administration immediately.

☐ Consider administration of calcium-lowering agents as soon as possible.

☐ Initiate hemodialysis for patients with serum calcium levels > 18 mg/dL or severe symptoms.

- Mild to moderate elevations may not require immediate treatment.
- **Treat serum calcium level greater than 14 mg/dL, regardless of symptoms**.
- Mild hypercalcemia ($<$ 12mg/dL): address underlying cause (thiazide diuretics, lithium, volume depletion, prolonged bed rest) and hydrate appropriately.
- Moderate hypercalcemia (12 to 14 mg/dL): follow same precautions as above; any acute rise in serum levels can cause mental status changes which would then necessitate more aggressive therapy.
- Severe hypercalcemia ($>$ 14mg/dL)
  - Volume expansion with isotonic saline (200–300 mL/hour) to maintain a urine output of 100–150 mL/hour. (Note: Unless there is concomitant renal or heart failure, loop diuretics to increase calcium excretion are not recommended because of potential complications).
  - Administer calcitonin 4 IU/kg every 12 hours IV or SQ up to 48 hours (up to four doses) and obtain repeat serum calcium; a longer duration of administering the drug increases risk of tachyphylaxis
  - Consider co-administration one-time doses of zoledronic acid (4 mg IV over 15 minutes) – contraindicated in renal disease or CrCl $<$ 35 mL/min
  - Volume expansion with calcitonin should reduce calcium concentrations within 12–48 hours. Subsequently, the bisphosphonate will take effect, therefore maintaining control of the calcium level.
- Emergent or urgent hemodialysis should be considered in patients with Ca $>$ 18–20 mg/dL and with altered mental status, or in those with severe hypercalcemia with renal failure.
- In these cases (particularly if hypercalcemia is from malignancy or a toxic etiology), one can also administer denosumab with calcitonin

Sudden Deterioration

- Sudden change in mental status or hemodynamics: rapid volume expansion, emergent hemodialysis.

Disorders of Magnesium Regulation

Introduction

- **Magnesium** is one of the most abundant cations in the body and plays a large role in cardiac contractility as well as nerve conduction.
- The majority of magnesium is stored in the bone, with about 1% stored in the extracellular fluid compartment.
- Consequentially, it is important to note that plasma magnesium levels may not provide an accurate assessment of total body magnesium content.

Hypomagnesemia

Presentation

Classic Presentation

- Mild hypomagnesemia is usually asymptomatic, but failure to correct low serum magnesium may contribute to refractory hypokalemia and hypocalcemia.
- Table 35.7 lists causes of hypomagnesemia.

Table 35.7 Etiologies of hypomagnesemia

Gastrointestinal losses
Acute pancreatitis
Medications (PPIs)
Diarrhea, malabsorption, small bowel syndrome
Renal losses
Loop and thiazide diuretics, alcohol-induced
Medications (antibiotics, cisplatin)
Diabetes
Hypercalcemia

Critical Presentation

- Severe hypomagnesemia (serum levels less than 1 mg/dL) may affect the cardiovascular and neurological systems.
  - **Cardiovascular**: prolonged QT, QRS widening, atrial and ventricular tachyarrhythmias.
  - **Neurological**: neuromuscular hyperexcitability (e.g., tremor, tetany, convulsions), muscle weakness, delirium, coma.

Diagnosis and Evaluation

- Typically, the source of hypomagnesemia is apparent. If the etiology is unclear, GI and renal losses can be differentiated by measuring a 24-hour urine magnesium excretion.
  - 24-hour urine Mg is elevated in renal losses.
  - 24-hour urine Mg is low in GI losses.
- Obtain serum electrolytes with magnesium and calcium.
  - Hypomagnesemia and hypokalemia can suggest urine potassium wasting.
  - Hypomagnesemia with hypocalcemia suggests low PTH secretion.
- For mild hypomagnesemia, begin repletion with 2 g magnesium sulfate ($MgSO_4$) IV over 2 hours.
- Risks of rapid magnesium sulfate repletion include diaphoresis, flushing, hypotension, and possible bradycardia.

Sudden Deterioration

- Seizure: 4 g IV $MgSO_4$ as needed.
- Ventricular arrhythmias: 1–2 g $MgSO_4$ IV over several minutes.
  - This dose can be repeated up to 4 mg in a patient with ventricular tachycardia and prolonged QTc, or up to 6 mg for ventricular fibrillation or pulseless ventricular tachycardia.
- In renal impairment, reduce IV replacement doses by 50% and monitor serial plasma magnesium daily.

Special Circumstances

- Preeclampsia or pregnancy induced hypertension (PIH): 4–6 g $MgSO_4$ in 100 mL IV over 30 minutes as a loading dose, followed by 2–3 g of Mg SO_4 maintenance per hour while monitoring reflexes, mental status, and respiratory status.

Critical Management

Critical Management Checklist

☑ **Airway management**: intubation as needed for respiratory depression or airway protection.
☑ Continuous cardiac monitoring to assess for arrythmias.
☑ Obtain **EKG** to assess for cardiac involvement.
☑ Symptomatic patients should receive immediate IV replacement.
☑ Magnesium replacement should be performed judiciously in patients with renal failure.

Hypermagnesemia

Presentation

Classic Presentation

- Most cases are asymptomatic.
- Table 35.8 lists causes of hypermagnesemia.

Critical Presentation

- Severe hypermagnesemia (serum levels > 4.0 mg/dL) may affect the cardiovascular and neurological systems.
- **Neurological**: absent deep tendon reflex, lethargy, encephalopathy, flaccid paralysis, apnea.
- **Cardiovascular**: bradyarrhythmia, slowing of atrioventricular conduction, pulmonary edema, hemodynamic collapse.

Table 35.8 Etiologies of hypermagnesemia

Renal insufficiency
Excessive ingestion or administration (e.g., magnesium enemas, magnesium infusions for preeclampsia, oral supplementation)

Diagnosis and Evaluation

- A detailed history regarding medications such as oral supplementation, antacids, laxatives and discontinuing the use of these.
- Obtain serum electrolytes with magnesium and calcium.

Sudden Deterioration

- For patients receiving magnesium supplementation, indications to stop administering magnesium include: loss of deep tendon reflexes, urine output less than 30 mL per hour, or decreased respiratory effort.
- If the patient becomes hemodynamically unstable, administer calcium gluconate 1 g IV over 2–3 minutes in addition to beginning IV fluids and loop diuretics.
- If the patient is in renal failure, hemodialysis may be required

Critical Management

Critical Management Checklist

☑ **Airway management**: intubation as needed for respiratory depression or airway protection.

☑ **Stop all magnesium sources.**

☑ Administer **calcium gluconate 1g IV** over 2–3 minutes.

☑ Continuous cardiac monitoring to assess for arrythmias.

☑ Obtain **EKG** to assess for cardiac involvement.

BIBLIOGRAPHY

al-Ghamdi SM, Cameron EC, Sutton RA. Magnesium deficiency: pathophysiologic and clinical overview. *Am J Kidney Dis* 1994;24(5):737–52. https://doi.org/10.1016/s0272-6386(12)80667-6

Braun M, Barstow C, Pyzocha N, et al. Diagnosis and management of sodium disorders: hyponatremia and hypernatremia. AAFP Guidelines, 2015.

Bullard Z, Dattero J, Zimmerman LH, et al. In-hospital hypocalcemia. *Crit Care Med* 2019;47:126. https://doi.org/10.1097/01.ccm.0000551044.21178.02

Grams ME, Hoenig MP, Hoorn EJ. Evaluation of hypokalemia. *JAMA* 2021;325 (12):1216–1217. https://doi.org/10.1001/jama.2020.17672

Levis JT. ECG diagnosis: hypokalemia. *Perm J* 2012;16(2):57.

Pepe J, Colangelo L, Biamonte F, et al. Diagnosis and management of hypocalcemia. *Endocrine* 2020;69(3):485–495. https://doi.org/10.1007/s12020-020-02324-2

Shepshelovich D, Leibovitch C, Klein A, et al. The syndrome of inappropriate antidiuretic hormone secretion: distribution and characterization according to etiologies. *Eur J Int Med* 2015;26(10):819–824. https://doi.org/10.1016/j.ejim.2015.10.020

Shepshelovich D, Schechter A, Calvarysky B, et al. Medication-induced SIADH: distribution and characterization according to medication class. *Br J Clin Pharmacol* 2017;83(8):1801–1807. https://doi.org/10.1111/bcp.13256

Sood L, Sterns RH, Hix JK, et al. Hypertonic saline and desmopressin: a simple strategy for safe correction of severe hyponatremia. *Am J Kidney Dis* 2013;61(4):571–578; https://doi.org/10.1053/j.ajkd.2012.11.032

Spasovski G, Vanholder R, Allolio B, et al. Hyponatraemia Guideline Development Group. Clinical practice guideline on diagnosis and treatment of hyponatraemia. *Eur J Endocrinol* 2014;170(3):G1–G47.

36

Acute Kidney Injury and Emergent Dialysis

ADAM L. GOTTULA AND FERAS H. KHAN

Chapter 36:
AKI

KDIGO Definition:

+ Increase in serum creatinine by ≥ 0.3 mg/dL within 48 hours, or

+ Increase in serum creatinine to ≥ 1.5 times baseline within the prior 7 days, or

+ Urine volume < 0.5 mL/kg/hour for 6 hours.

Most common etiologies: pre-renal azotemia and acute tubular necrosis.

 Presentation

Classic: Vague symptoms, may include lethargy, nausea, decreased urine output, dark or turbid urine, pulmonary/peripheral edema.

Critical Presentation: AMS, seizures, arrhythmia, and/or pulmonary edema resulting in respiratory failure.

Often with history of physiological insult or other precipitating factor (e.g., medications).

 Diagnosis and Evaluation

Thorough history in attempt to understand etiology.

Bloodwork: CMP, calcium, phosphorus, creatinine, BUN, relevant drug levels.

Urine: UA, microscopy, creatinine, osmolality, urine electrolytes.

Catheter insertion to monitor urine output.

Echocardiography, ECG.
✿ *Assess for arrythmia and uremic pericarditis/tamponade.*

Bladder/Renal US.

Chapter 36:
AKI

 ## Management

Airway management and
hemodynamic monitoring.
✿ *Goal MAP > 65 mmHg*

Stop nephrotoxic drugs and
dose-adjust renally excreted drugs.

Consider urgent RRT.

Sudden deterioration: Assess for
electrolyte derangements.

Address underlying etiology.

Monitor ECG for arrythmia.
✿ *If evidence of hyperkalemia,
administer calcium.*

Consider sodium bicarbonate drip
in severe acidosis.

◉ Consider Urgent Hemodialysis in:

✿ Severe acidosis
and hypotension.

✿ Hyperkalemia.

✿ Volume overload.

✿ Specific toxins.

✿ Uremia (relative
indication).

Introduction

- Acute kidney injury (AKI) is defined as a fall in glomerular filtration rate (GFR) leading to the accumulation of nitrogenous wastes.
- There are many competing criteria for diagnosing AKI. The **Kidney Disease Improving Global Outcomes (KDIGO)** group defines AKI as:
  - Increase in serum creatinine by $\geq$ 0.3 mg/dL within 48 hours, or
  - Increase in serum creatinine to $\geq$ 1.5 times baseline within the prior 7 days, or
  - Urine volume < 0.5 mL/kg/hour for 6 hours.
- There are three **classes of AKI**:
  - **Prerenal:** inadequate perfusion of the kidney (most common).
  - **Intrinsic (Renal):** diseases intrinsic to the kidney.
  - **Postrenal:** obstruction distal to the kidney.

Etiology

- There are many etiologies of AKI (see Table 36.1).
- Two major causes, prerenal azotemia and acute tubular necrosis (ATN), account for nearly 75% of AKI.

Table 36.1 Etiologies of acute kidney injury

Prerenal	Intrinsic (renal)	Postrenal
• **Shock*** • **Hepatorenal syndrome** • **Cardiorenal syndrome** • **Drugs** (angiotensin-converting enzyme inhibitor, NSAIDs, etc.)	• **Acute interstitial nephritis (AIN):** beta-lactam, sulfa-based drugs, NSAIDs • **Renal ischemia** (including ATN) • **Antimicrobials:** aminoglycosides, amphotericin B • **Intravascular hemolysis:** HUS, TTP • **Rhabdomyolysis** • **Direct nephrotoxic agents**	• **Papillary necrosis** • **Prostatic hypertrophy** • **Retroperitoneal mass** • **Obstruction:** urethral stricture, occluded urinary catheter, etc.

HUS: hemolytic uremic syndrome; TTP: thrombotic thrombocytopenic purpura; *of all etiologies: hypovolemia, distributive, cardiogenic, obstructive.

- Prerenal azotemia is the result of decreased renal perfusion without ischemic injury.
- Untreated prerenal azotemia can progress to ischemic ATN.
- ATN, an intrinsic renal disease commonly caused by hypotension or nephrotoxic drugs, is the result of acute tubular cell injury.
- ATN, unlike prerenal azotemia, is unresponsive to fluids and treated with supportive care.

Presentation

Classic Presentation

- Findings on initial examination are vague, but include:
  - Decreased urine output.
  - Lethargy, fatigability, anorexia, nausea, and vomiting.
  - Dark or turbid urine.
  - Pulmonary and peripheral edema.

Critical Presentation

- Altered mental status and seizure.
- Hyperkalemia with associated arrhythmias.
- Pulmonary edema causing respiratory failure.

Diagnosis and Evaluation

- **History and physical examination**
  - A patient's history will frequently reveal etiology of renal failure (e.g., medications or gastrointestinal illness).
- **Diagnostic tests**
  - **Blood studies:** standard electrolytes, calcium, phosphorus, creatinine, BUN, and relevant drug levels (vancomycin, aminoglycosides, etc.).
  - **Urine studies**: urinalysis, microscopy, creatinine, osmolality, and urine electrolytes (Table 36.2).
  - **Bladder catheter:** enables monitoring of urine output and treats postrenal obstruction.

Table 36.2 Urine microscopy/sediment findings: probable etiology

- Hyaline casts: prerenal (hypovolemia)
- Muddy brown casts: ATN
- White blood cells casts and eosinophils: AIN
- Pigmented casts: myoglobinuria

- ○ **Renal ultrasound:** demonstrates signs of urinary obstruction including hydronephrosis and evaluates kidney size to determine acuity of injury.
- **Calculations**
  - ○ **Fractional excretion of sodium (FENa) = (U Na/P Na)/(U Cr/P Cr)**
    - FENa < 1% suggests prerenal condition with oliguria.
    - A single FENa and urine sodium level should play a limited role in determining the etiology of AKI. Patients on diuretics, with chronic kidney disease, or congestive heart failure have an unreliable FENa and urine sodium.
    - The absence of FENa < 1% should not be used to exclude prerenal AKI.
  - ○ **Fractional excretion of urea (FEUrea) = (Serum$_{Cr}$ * U$_{Urea}$)/ (Serum$_{Urea}$ x U$_{Cr}$) %**
    - Should be considered instead of FENa for patients on diuretics.
    - FEUrea is not effective when proximal tubule effected (acetazolamide, mannitol, etc.)
    - FEUrea > 50%: Intrinsic renal disease
    - FEUrea < 35%: Prerenal cause
  - ○ **Creatinine clearance (CrCl)** may be calculated to assess general kidney function: CrCl = (140 − age [years]) × weight (kg)/72 × Cr (mg/dL) × 0.85 (in women)
  - ○ **Acute kidney injury may be classified as prerenal, intrinsic, or postrenal based on serum and urine laboratory findings (Table 36.3)**
- **KDIGO AKI Severity Score** is used to define the degree of kidney injury.
  - ○ **Stage 1:** 1.5–1.9 times baseline, *or* ≥ 0.3 mg/dL increase in the serum creatinine, *or* urine output < 0.5 mL/kg/hour for 6–12 hours.
  - ○ **Stage 2:** 2.0–2.9 times baseline increase in the serum creatinine, *or* urine output < 0.5 mL/kg/hour for 6–12 hours.
  - ○ **Stage 3:** > 3 times baseline increase in the serum creatinine, *or* increase in serum creatinine to ≥ 4.0 mg/dL, *or* urine output of < 0.3 mL/kg/hour for > 24 hours, *or* anuria for ≥ 12 hours, *or* the initiation of renal replacement therapy, *or*, in patients < 18 years old, decrease in estimated GFR to < 35 mL/minute per 1.73 m^2.

Table 36.3 Classifications of acute kidney injury

Type	U_{OSM}	U_{na}	Fe_{Na}	BUN/Cr	Fe_{UREA}
Prerenal	> 500	< 10	< 1%	> 20	< 35%
Intrinsic	< 350	> 20	> 2%	< 10–15	> 50%
Postrenal	< 350	> 40	> 4%	> 20	Not applicable

- The clinical utility of AKI scoring systems is uncertain, but they help predict mortality.

Critical Management

Critical Management Checklist

☑ **Airway management**: noninvasive positive-pressure ventilation or intubation for symptomatic volume overload.

☑ Hemodynamic management to maintain **MAP > 65 mmHg.**

   ☑ Consider **fluid bolus** if hypovolemic.

   ☑ Consider **vasopressors** if fluid unresponsive or clinically volume overloaded.

   ☑ Consider **inotropes** if evidence of cardiogenic shock.

☑ **Treat identifiable cause.**

☑ Evaluate for **indications for emergent dialysis.**

☑ **Stop** all **nephrotoxic drugs** and **potassium** supplements.

   ☑ Dose-adjust all other renally excreted drugs.

☑ Complete bladder and renal **ultrasound.**

☑ Complete echocardiography.

☑ Complete EKG.

☑ Administer calcium if evidence of hyperkalemia on EKG.

☑ If severely acidotic, consider a sodium bicarbonate drip.

- **Airway management**:
  - Volume overload due to AKI can lead to pulmonary edema, which may require respiratory support including noninvasive positive-pressure ventilation and/or intubation.
- **Hemodynamic management:**
  - The shock state should be treated. Correcting hemodynamic instability, while targeting euvolemia, is critical to preserve renal function.

- ○ Patients with prerenal failure, clinical hypovolemia, and hypotension require resuscitation with intravenous fluids and vasopressors to normalize blood pressure (mean arterial pressure > 65 mmHg).
- ○ Intravenous fluid resuscitation should be used with caution in patients with oliguric AKI who are not clinically hypovolemic.
- ○ Inotropes should be considered if there is evidence of cardiogenic shock.
- ○ Bolus doses of furosemide or other diuretics to promote urinary output have not been shown to be useful. In patients who are adequately resuscitated with persistent oliguria, diuretics may provide prognostic information and symptomatic improvement in patients who are volume overloaded.
- A careful patient history, physical exam, and appropriate laboratory testing should reveal the cause and class of AKI.
  - ○ **Treat any identifiable cause.**
- Once AKI is diagnosed, **all drugs that cause renal injury and potassium supplementation orders should be discontinued**.
- Dose-adjust all renally cleared drugs.
- A complete **bladder and renal ultrasound** should be completed and **foley catheter** placement should be considered.
- **Renal replacement therapy (RRT):**
  - ○ Indications for emergent dialysis include:
    - ▪ Volume overload
    - ▪ Metabolic acidosis
    - ▪ Uremia (encephalopathy, pericarditis)
    - ▪ Hyperkalemia
    - ▪ Toxins (small, non-protein bound; see Table 36.4)
  - ○ Vascular access: a large-bore venous catheter, with multiple lumens, is placed in either the internal jugular, subclavian or femoral vein.
- Types of renal replacement therapy (RRT): the type of therapy that a patient will receive varies based on institution, familiarity with each technique, hemodynamics and indications.
  - ○ *Hemodialysis (HD):* Blood flows alongside dialysate across a semipermeable membrane in opposite directions (countercurrent mechanism). Solutes are removed by diffusion.
    - ▪ Disadvantages: critically ill patients with hypotension may not tolerate HD due to the high-flow rates required to achieve diffusive clearance.
    - ▪ Advantages: solutes are cleared rapidly, so it requires less time to complete.

Table 36.4 Common dialyzable drugs/toxins

- INH
- Isopropyl alcohol
- Salicylates
- Theophylline
- Methanol
- Barbiturates
- Lithium
- Ethylene glycol
- Dabigatran (Pradaxa)
- Divalproex (Depakote)

- ○ *Hemofiltration/continuous veno-venous hemofiltration (CVVH)*
  - Uses convection to remove solutes.
  - Fluid balance is controlled closely through continuous changing of the amount of fluid given back to the patient.
  - Causes less hypotension as lower flow rates result in less dramatic fluid shifts.
  - Advantages: hemodynamic stability, slower fluid shifts, volume control.
  - Disadvantages: requires continuous monitoring; patient must remain immobile during therapy; hypothermia.
- ○ *Sustained low-efficiency dialysis (SLED)*
  - Like HD except that this modality uses slower blood-pump speeds and low dialysate flow rates for 6–12 hours daily.
  - Advantages: high solute clearance, requires less time than CVVH, uses the same machines as HD.
  - Disadvantages: longer time requirement than HD.

Sudden Deterioration

- Patients with AKI who suddenly decompensate should be rapidly evaluated for electrolyte imbalances. Hyperkalemia, which can cause cardiac arrhythmias, is the most concerning. Empiric calcium administration should be considered in unstable patients.
- AKI resulting in metabolic acidosis can cause hypotension. Temporary treatment includes volume resuscitation and vasopressors.

A sodium bicarbonate infusion can be considered while preparing for dialysis.

- Any patient with uremia and hypotension should be evaluated with echocardiography for pericardial tamponade from uremic pericarditis.

Special Circumstances

- **Acute interstitial nephritis:** an inflammatory reaction that impairs kidney function, typically caused by a medication hypersensitivity reaction.
  - Common causes include antibiotics (aminoglycosides, cephalosporins, penicillins), NSAIDs, and diuretics.
  - Fever, rash, and eosinophilia may be seen but are not always present.
  - WBC casts and eosinophils may be seen on urinalysis.
  - Renal biopsy can be used to make a definitive diagnosis.
  - Treat by stopping offending agent and consider steroids.
- **Contrast-induced nephropathy (CIN):** an acute injury to the renal tubular epithelial cells caused by iodinated radiocontrast agents used in radiological procedures.
  - Previously prevalent with hyper-osmolar contrast. When using iso- and low-osmolar contrast agents, CIN is not observed.
  - Risk factors include renal transplant, underlying renal disease, advanced age, diabetes, dehydration, and congestive heart failure.
  - Given limitations of the evidence, in patients with **serum creatinine ≥ 4.0 mg/dL or renal transplant,** consider withholding contrast. Otherwise, imaging with contrast should not be limited because of concern for AKI.
  - The American College of Radiology/National Kidney Foundation recommends:
    - Prophylaxis with intravenous normal saline for patients without contraindication who have an AKI or an estimated glomerular filtration rate less than 30 mL/min/1.73 m^2 who are not undergoing maintenance dialysis.
    - Prophylaxis with intravenous normal saline may be considered in individual high-risk circumstances with an eGFR of 30–44 mL/min/1.73 m^2 at the discretion of the ordering clinician.
    - The presence of a solitary kidney should not independently influence decision making regarding the risk of contrast-induced AKI.

- **Rhabdomyolysis** occurs when myoglobin released by injured muscle damages the renal tubular epithelial cells.
- Diagnosis is confirmed by testing for CK and urine myoglobin.
- Aggressive volume administration with isotonic fluids is the standard of care.
- Severe cases may require hemodialysis.

BIBLIOGRAPHY

Davenport MS, Perazella M, Yee J, et al. Use of intravenous iodinated contrast media in patients with kidney disease: consensus statements from the American College of Radiology and the National Kidney Foundation. *Radiology* 2020;294(3):660–668. https://doi.org/10.1148/radiol.2019192094

Gauthier PM, & Szerlip HM. Metabolic acidosis in the intensive care unit. *Crit Care Clin* 2002;18:289–308.

Ho KM, & Sheridan DJ. Meta-analysis of furosemide to prevent or treat acute renal failure. *BMJ* 2006;333:420.

Kidney Disease: Improving Global Outcomes (KDIGO) Acute Kidney Injury Work Group. KDIGO Clinical Practice Guideline for Acute Kidney Injury. *Kidney Int Suppl* 2012;2:1–138.

Koyner J, Davison D, Brasha-Mitchell E, et al. Furosemide stress test and biomarkers for the prediction of AKI severity. *J Am Soc Nephrol* 2015;26(8):2023–2031.

Matsuura R, Komaru Y, Miyamoto Y, et al. Response to different furosemide doses predicts AKI progression in ICU patients with elevated plasma NGAL levels. *Ann Intensive Care* 2018;8(1):8.

Mehran R, & Nikolsky E. Contrast-induced nephropathy: definition, epidemiology, and patients at risk. *Kidney Int Suppl* 2006:S11–15.

Legrand M, Le C, Perbet S, et al. Urine sodium concentration to predict fluid responsiveness in oliguric ICU patients: a prospective multicenter observational study. *Crit Care* 2016;20(1):165.

Ostermann M, & Joannidis M. Acute kidney injury 2016: diagnosis and diagnostic workup. *Crit Care* 2016;20(1):299.

Stevens MA, McCullough PA, Tobin KJ, et al. A prospective randomized trial of prevention measures in patients at high risk for contrast nephropathy: results of the P.R.I.N.C.E. Study. Prevention of Radiocontrast Induced Nephropathy Clinical Evaluation. *J Am Coll Cardiol* 1999;33:403–411.

SECTION 8

Hematology–Oncology Emergencies

JASON BLOCK

37

Reversal of Anticoagulation

CALVIN E. HWANG

Chapter 37:
Anticoagulant Reversal

 Presentation

History of anticoagulation therapy.

Bleeding (i.e. trauma-related, gastrointestinal, epistaxis).
May present in hemorrhagic shock.

Maintain high index of suspicion for intracranial hemorrhage.
May present with neurological findings.

 Diagnosis and Evaluation

Obtain non-contrast head CT to rule out intracranial hemorrhage in anticoagulated pts with encephalopathy or head trauma.

Labwork: CBC, BMP, type and screen, and coagulation studies including PT/INR and aPTT.
- *TT in patients taking dabigatran.*
- *Chromogenic anti-Xa activity assay in patients taking factor Xa inhibitors (rivaroxaban, apixaban, edoxaban) or enoxaparin.*

 Management

Establish patent airway and hemodynamic monitoring.

Reverse anticoagulation.

Establish large-bore IV access for transfusions as needed.

Sudden deterioration often requires aggressive resuscitation with blood products and surgical/neurosurgical /interventional radiology involvement to control bleeding.

Introduction

- The use of direct oral anticoagulants (e.g., dabigatran, rivaroxaban, apixaban, edoxaban) over more traditional agents like warfarin has significantly increased over the past decade.
- These patients require prompt reversal of their bleeding diathesis during resuscitation.
- Common anticoagulants and their mechanism of action are presented in Table 37.1.

Presentation

Classic Presentation

- Common sources of bleeding in patients on anticoagulation include gastrointestinal, intracranial, epistaxis and trauma-associated.
- Maintain a high level of suspicion for ICH in patients on anticoagulation, even in the absence of trauma, and particularly in those patients with a supratherapeutic INR.

Table 37.1 Mechanism of action of common anticoagulants

Warfarin	Inhibits the synthesis of vitamin K-dependent coagulation factors (II, VII, IX, X) and proteins C and S
Heparin	Activates antithrombin III, leading to inactivation of thrombin and other coagulation factors
Enoxaparin	Similar to heparin, activates antithrombin III, but preferentially inhibits factor Xa
Dabigatran	Direct thrombin inhibitor
Rivaroxaban/ Apixaban/Edoxaban	Direct inhibitor of factor Xa
Aspirin	Inhibits cyclooxygenase-1 and -2 enzymes, leading to inhibition of platelet aggregation
Clopidogrel	Inhibits platelet ADP receptors, preventing platelet aggregation

Critical Presentation

- Patients may present in hemorrhagic shock from gastrointestinal hemorrhage, traumatic hemorrhage, or epistaxis.
- Patients with more significant ICH may present acutely with encephalopathy or with focal neurological findings such as hemiplegia, cranial nerve deficits, or seizures.

Diagnosis and Evaluation

- **Imaging**
  - In anticoagulated patients with encephalopathy or possible head trauma, an emergent non-contrast computed tomography (CT) of the head is integral to identify ICH.
- **Laboratory tests**
  - All patients with serious bleeding should receive a complete blood count, basic metabolic panel, coagulation studies, and type and cross-match.
  - For patients on warfarin, PT/INR is crucial to assess the degree of coagulopathy.
  - Thrombin time should be obtained in all patients on dabigatran. A normal thrombin time rules out any clinically significant level of dabigatran in the system. If a thrombin time is not available, a normal aPTT value typically excludes clinically significant levels of dabigatran.
  - Levels of factor Xa inhibitors (rivaroxaban, apixaban, edoxaban) can be measured using a chromogenic anti-Xa activity assay, if available. A negative result excludes clinically significant levels of factor Xa inhibitor in the patient's system.
  - Patients treated with heparin can be monitored using the aPTT or heparin activity level.
  - The aPTT test is not reliable for patients on enoxaparin and an anti-Xa activity level should be obtained instead.
  - In some populations (e.g., ECMO), thromboelastography R-time and aPTT have been similarly used to manage anticoagulation status.

Critical Management

Critical Management Checklist

☑ Airway management as needed
☑ Large-bore IV access
☑ Maintain hemodynamic stability
☑ Reversal of anticoagulation
☑ Specialist consultation as indicated for specific location of hemorrhage
☑ Blood transfusion as necessary

- Airway management with endotracheal intubation should be performed for those not protecting their airway.
- Perform a hemodynamically neutral intubation in patients with ICH to avoid cerebral hypoperfusion or expansion of the hemorrhage.
- Obtain intravascular access with two large-bore intravenous lines for possible massive transfusion of blood products.
- **Patients on warfarin**
  - All patients with serious or life-threatening bleeding should receive vitamin K 10 mg IV for sustained reversal of warfarin-induced anticoagulation.
  - If available, four-factor prothrombin complex concentrates (4F-PCCs, dose generally weight-based and variable per pretreatment INR) have been shown to result in faster correction of INR and require less total volume of infusion than fresh frozen plasma (FFP).
  - In institutions where 4F-PCC is not available, these patients should receive FFP, initially dosed at 10–15 mL/kg. This may be difficult in patients with medical comorbidities such as heart failure.
- **Patients on dabigatran**
  - Those with life-threatening bleeding or requiring urgent/emergent surgery can be reversed with idarucizumab, a monoclonal antibody that binds to dabigatran. The dose of idarucizumab is 5 g, administered in two 2.5 g vials, either as a bolus or consecutive infusions.
  - If idarucizumab is not available, activated prothrombin complex concentrate (aPCC, FEIBA®) 50 units/kg IV should be given.
  - If aPCC is not available, 4F-PCC 50 units/kg can be given.
  - If available and clinically feasible, dialysis can remove approximately 60% of dabigatran at 2 hours.

Table 37.2 Dosing recommendations for andexanet alfa

Drug	Last dose	Last drug dose < 8 hours prior/ unknown	Last drug dose ≥ 8 hours prior
Rivaroxaban	≤ 10 mg	low dose	low dose
Rivaroxaban	> 10 mg / unknown	high dose	low dose
Apixaban	≤ 5 mg	low dose	low dose
Apixaban	> 5 mg / unknown	high dose	low dose
Edoxaban	≤ 30 mg	low dose	low dose
Edoxaban	> 30 mg	high dose	low dose
Enoxaparin	≤ 40 mg	low dose	low dose
Enoxaparin	> 40 mg	high dose	low dose

- **Patients on Factor Xa inhibitors (apixaban, rivaroxaban, edoxaban)**
  - ○ 4F-PCC, aPCC or andexanet alfa can be used for the reversal of anticoagulation in patients on Factor Xa inhibitors. To date, studies have not shown superiority of one product over another in this setting.
  - ○ 4F-PCC or aPCC should be administered 50 units/kg IV x 1.
  - ○ The dose of andexanet alfa is dependent on the patient's factor Xa dosage and timing of last dose (Table 37.2).
- Low dose: 400 mg over 15 minutes IV bolus followed by infusion of 480 mg over 2 hours.
- High dose: 800 mg over 30 minutes IV bolus followed by infusion of 960 mg over 2 hours.
  - ○ **Patients on heparin**
    - ▪ Heparin can be reversed emergently in patients with severe bleeding through the use of protamine sulfate at a ratio of 1 mg protamine sulfate/ 100 units heparin.
    - ▪ This may need to be titrated further in patients on subcutaneous heparin as its absorption will be slower.
  - ○ **Patients on enoxaparin**
    - ▪ Although protamine sulfate does not reverse the anti-Xa activity of enoxaparin, its administration at a ratio of 1 mg/mg of enoxaparin may reduce clinical bleeding.
    - ▪ Andexanet alfa can also be used for reversal of enoxaparin (Table 37.2).

- **Patients on antiplatelet medications**
    - For severe bleeding, platelet transfusion may be beneficial, as some antiplatelet medications irreversibly inactivate platelets.
    - Desmopressin (DDAVP) dosed at 0.3 mcg/kg can be used in patients with platelet dysfunction to enhance platelet adhesion to the vessel walls and increase factor VIII and von Willebrand factor.

Sudden Deterioration

- Deterioration usually occurs because of hemorrhagic shock or worsening ICH.
    - Patients with ongoing hemorrhage should have a balanced blood product resuscitation in concert with anticoagulant reversal. Surgical or interventional radiology consultation may be necessary to help control the source of bleeding.
    - For patients with suspected or confirmed ICH, a neurosurgical consult should be obtained immediately for consideration of operative management.

Vasopressor of choice: Patients on anticoagulants presenting in shock will need to be aggressively resuscitated with blood products. Infusion of crystalloids and use of vasopressors such as norepinephrine may be initiated as a temporizing measure, keeping in mind patients with hemorrhagic shock should be managed with permissive hypotension.

BIBLIOGRAPHY

Baugh CW, Levine M, Cornutt D, et al. Anticoagulant reversal strategies in the emergency department setting: recommendations of a multidisciplinary expert panel. *Ann Emerg Med* 2020;76(4):470–485.

Bliden KP, Chaudhary R, Mohammed N, et al. Determination of non-Vitamin K oral anticoagulant (NOAC) effects using a new-generation thrombelastography TEG 6s system. *J Thromb Thrombolysis* 2017;43(4):437–445.

Connolly SJ, Crowther M, Eikelboom JW, et al. Full study report of andexanet alfa for bleeding associated with Factor Xa inhibitors. *N Engl J Med* 2019;380 (14):1326–1335.

Pollack CV, Reilly PA, van Ryn J, et al. Idarucizumab for dabigatran reversal — full cohort analysis. *N Engl J Med* 2017;377(5):431–441.

Schulman S, Ritchie B, Nahirniak S, et al. Reversal of dabigatran-associated major bleeding with activated prothrombin concentrate: a prospective cohort study. *Thromb Res* 2017;152:44–48.

Tomaselli GF, Mahaffey KW, Cuker A, et al. 2017 ACC expert consensus decision pathway on management of bleeding in patients on oral anticoagulants: a report of the American College of Cardiology Task Force on Expert Consensus Decision Pathways. *J Am Coll Cardiol* 2017;70(24):3042–3067.

38

Thrombotic Thrombocytopenic Purpura/ Hemolytic Uremic Syndrome and Disseminated Intravascular Coagulation

JAI MADHOK

Chapter 38:
DIC

 ## Presentation

History of recent physiological insult.

Petechiae, purpura, bleeding from mucous membranes, and oozing from surgical/IV sites.

 ## Diagnosis and Evaluation

Prolonged PT/INR/PTT.

Anemia, low fibrinogen, increased D-dimer, thrombocytopenia.

 ## Management

Correct underlying disorder.

Transfuse blood in cases of active bleeding.

Platelet administration in bleeding patient if platelet count below 50 x 10^6/mL.

Prophylactic platelet administration in non-bleeding patient if platelet count below 10 x 10^6/mL.

If INR >2 or two-fold prolongation of aPTT: administer FFP 10–15 mL/kg.

Administer cryoprecipitate with FFP in bleeding patients where fibrinogen < 100 mg/dL.

Hematologist consultation.

In sudden deterioration, assess for hemorrhage or ischemia: Head CT, CXR, ECG, echocardiogram, GI bleed workup.

Chapter 38:
TTP/HUS

Presentation

Often with three or more of the following: Fever, neurological signs, anemia, thrombocytopenia, and renal dysfunction.

TTP is more common in adults.

HUS is more common in children, often after infection with enterohemorrhagic E. Coli infection.

Neurological dysfunction is more common in TTP, renal dysfunction is more common in HUS.

Diagnosis and Evaluation

Thrombocytopenia, normal or increased D-dimer and fibrinogen.

Increased LDH, increased indirect bilirubin, and decreased haptoglobin can indicate presence/degree of hemolysis.

Schistocytes on blood smear.

BMP to determine degree of renal dysfunction, especially in HUS.

Measurement of ADAMTS13 activity: Activity of less than 10% supports diagnosis of TTP.

Management

Consult hematology

Avoid platelet transfusion.

TTP: Plasmapheresis and plasma exchange with FFP.

HUS in adults: more likely to require blood products, plasmapheresis, plasma exchange.

HUS in children: supportive care, severe cases may require dialysis.

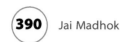

Introduction

- Thrombotic microangiopathies (TMA) are a group of conditions characterized by excessive platelet activation resulting in microvascular thrombi and platelet consumption (thrombocytopenia). The thrombosed microvasculature shears red blood cells (RBCs) causing microangiopathic hemolytic anemia.
- Primary TMAs include thrombotic thrombocytopenic purpura (TTP) and hemolytic uremic syndrome (HUS) while secondary TMAs result from infection, pregnancy, malignancy, drugs and toxins among other causes (Table 38.1).
- TMAs do not directly involve the coagulation cascade, and therefore do not prolong coagulation studies. Microthrombi may result in ischemic complications in any organ system.
- Disseminated intravascular coagulation (DIC) refers to the consumptive coagulopathy triggered by exposure of the blood to foreign antigens, resulting in a vicious cycle of coagulation and fibrinolysis.

Table 38.1 Conditions associated with disseminated intravascular coagulation

Severe infection/sepsis
Trauma (including neurotrauma)
Solid and myeloproliferative malignancies Transfusion reactions
Rheumatological conditions (adult-onset Still's disease, systemic lupus erythematosus) Obstetric complications (amniotic fluid embolism, abruptio placentae, HELLP syndrome (hemolysis, elevated liver enzymes, low platelets), (pre) eclampsia)
Vascular abnormalities (Kasabach–Merritt syndrome, large vascular aneurysms)
Liver failure Envenomation Hyperthermia/heatstroke
Hemorrhagic skin necrosis (purpura fulminans) Transplant rejection

Presentation

Classic Presentation of Disseminated Intravascular Coagulation

- DIC usually develops 6–48 hours after a physiological insult. Most patients that develop DIC are already hospitalized.
- Patients will have petechiae, purpura, bleeding from mucous membranes, and diffuse oozing from intravenous or surgical sites.
- Prolonged coagulation studies: due to consumption of coagulation factors.
- Hypofibrinogenemia and increased D-dimer: from fibrin deposition and fibrinolysis (increased fibrin-degradation products) though fibrinogen's role as acute phase reactant may result in normal fibrinogen levels.
- Thrombocytopenia: due to platelet activation.
- Anemia (consumptive and destructive): secondary to microvascular thrombosis.
- Microhemorrhage (petechiae, purpura, mucous membrane bleeding, oozing at intravenous sites) from decreased procoagulant reserves and impaired hemostasis.

Critical Presentation of Disseminated Intravascular Coagulation

- Patients with DIC may present with a variety of life-threatening conditions associated with severe coagulopathy or hypercoagulable stress.

Classic Presentation of Thrombotic Thrombocytopenic Purpura/Hemolytic Uremic Syndrome

- The classic presentation of TTP involves a **pentad** of symptoms that include fever, neurological signs, anemia, thrombocytopenia, and renal dysfunction.

Table 38.2 Symptoms associated with thrombotic thrombocytopenic purpura

Finding	Mechanism
Fever	Acute-phase reaction
Altered mental status	Cerebral microvascular thrombosis
Anemia	Microangiopathic hemolytic anemia
Thrombocytopenia	Direct platelet activation and consumption
Renal dysfunction	Renal microvascular thrombosis

- This constellation of symptoms is only seen in 20–30% of cases and it is strongly recommended to suspect the condition and manage it as such if a patient exhibits three or more of these features (Table 38.2).
- While TTP is more common in adults, HUS is most commonly seen in children and often follows an infectious illness, usually diarrhea (classically associated with *E. coli* O157:H7).
- While neurologic dysfunction predominates TTP, renal dysfunction is more common in HUS.
- Atypical HUS (complement-mediated HUS) is a genetic disorder that results in uncontrolled complement activation. Atypical HUS accounts for 10% of HUS cases but carries much higher mortality (25%).
- Despite the aforementioned differences, these two entities are often referred to as TTP/HUS given similarities in their pathophysiology.

Critical Presentation of Thrombotic Thrombocytopenic Purpura/Hemolytic Uremic Syndrome

- Morbidity and mortality with TTP/HUS are usually attributed to thrombosis rather than anemia and bleeding.
- Patients with TTP can present with neurological symptoms that can be life-threatening themselves or complicated by a life-threatening event such as stroke, seizure, myocardial infarction, arrhythmias, etc.
- Patients (usually children) presenting with HUS may have significant renal dysfunction that may require renal replacement therapy.

Table 38.3 Laboratory parameters in disseminated intravascular coagulation versus thrombotic thrombocytopenic purpura/hemolytic uremic syndrome

Parameter	Smear	Platelets	PT/INR	aPTT	Fibrinogen	D-Dimer
DIC	schistocytes ↓	↑	↑	↓/-		↑
TTP/HUS	schistocytes ↓	-	-	-/↑		-/↑

Diagnosis and Evaluation

- DIC is suspected when a patient who has suffered a physiological insult is showing overt signs of bleeding, but most commonly DIC presents with coagulopathic oozing from intravenous or surgical sites or mucus membranes.
- No single laboratory test is sensitive or specific to diagnose DIC but general findings are listed in Table 38.3.
- The diagnosis of TTP/HUS should be suspected in patients presenting with three or more of the classic pentad of symptoms (Table 38.2).
- The laboratory hallmark of TTP is **ADAMTS13 deficiency** which is either autoimmune or acquired (majority of cases) versus congenital.
  - ○ The measurement of ADMATS13 activity, ADAMTS13 inhibitor, and ADAMTS13 antibody can support the diagnosis of TTP and help distinguish it from other TMAs such as HUS, immune thrombocytopenic purpura, etc.
  - ○ ADAMTS13 activity < 10% supports a diagnosis of TTP, while levels > 10% suggest other causes of TMA.
- Other laboratory investigations can help strengthen the diagnosis of TTP/HUS and assess for possible complications. The laboratory hematologic abnormalities most commonly seen are as shown in Table 38.3. In addition, basic metabolic panel will help stratify the severity of renal dysfunction (more severe in HUS versus TTP), and lactate dehydrogenase (↑), haptoglobin (↓), and indirect bilirubin (↑) can help determine the presence and degree of hemolysis.

Critical Management

Disseminated Intravascular Coagulation

- Initial management of DIC should be directed at the underlying disorder.
- Administration of blood products should be guided by clinical necessity such as active bleeding or the need to perform an invasive procedure.
  - Routine administration of platelets and coagulation factors is not indicated in the stable non-bleeding patient.
  - Platelet administration should be considered in the bleeding patient if the platelet count falls below 50×10^6/mL.
  - Prophylactic platelet transfusions should be considered in the nonbleeding patient if the count falls below 10×10^6/mL.
  - Bleeding patients with an elevated INR (> 2) or a two-fold prolongation of aPTT should receive fresh frozen plasma (FFP) at a starting dose of 10–15 mL/kg.
  - Cryoprecipitate should be administered as an adjunct to FFP in bleeding patients with fibrinogen <100 mg/dL.
  - Prothrombin concentrates (PCCs) allow for administration of select factors for DIC but do not contain all the factors lost in the consumptive coagulopathy.
  - Low-dose heparin (5–10 units/kg/hour) without a bolus may be considered for DIC if there is purpura fulminans, ongoing ischemia, skin infarction, extremity thrombus (arterial or venous), or other thromboembolic events. The decision to initiate anticoagulation in these patients should be made in consultation with a hematologist.

Thrombotic Thrombocytopenic Purpura

- Since mortality from TTP can decrease from 90% to 10% with appropriate management, treatment should be initiated as soon as possible after consultation with a hematologist in patients exhibiting three or more criteria listed in Table 38.3.
- The therapy of choice for TTP is plasmapheresis and plasma exchange with FFP which removes any circulating antibodies and replenishes functional ADAMSTS13.

- Patients may be effectively temporized by FFP transfusions until plasmapheresis is available.
- Immunosuppressive agents such as glucocorticoids and rituximab are often administered to patients with TTP at the direction of a hematologist.

Hemolytic Uremic Syndrome

- The mainstay of treatment for HUS (Shiga-toxin associated) is supportive care.
- In children, HUS can often be managed without blood product transfusion, plasmapheresis, or plasma exchange. This is not usually the case with adult patients presenting with HUS.
- Antibiotic use for typical HUS is controversial, with theoretical concern for increasing Shiga-toxin release and exacerbating the disease process.
- Patients with HUS may require dialysis if the renal dysfunction is severe.
- Adults with atypical HUS may be treated with eculizumab as directed by the hematologist.

General Principles for Thrombotic Thrombocytopenic Purpura/Hemolytic Uremic Syndrome

- Platelet transfusion should be avoided in patients suspected of having TTP/HUS as transfusion can provide further substrate for intravascular thrombosis. Platelet transfusion may be considered for life-threatening bleeding, but the decision to transfuse should be made in consultation with a hematologist.

Sudden Deterioration

Consider both thrombotic and/or hemorrhagic complications

- **Acute change in mental status**
  - Obtain a CT head to rule out ICH or stroke.
- **Hemorrhage in DIC**

○ Patients with life-threatening hemorrhage should be managed with balanced blood product transfusion to replace clotting factors, fibrinogen, and platelets.

- **Life- or limb-threatening thromboembolism**
  ○ Consider heparin infusion without bolus at 5–10 units/kg/hour in consultation with a hematologist.
  ○ For large vessel thrombi, consider consulting an interventional radiologist or a vascular surgeon for catheter-directed thrombolysis or thrombectomy.
- **Respiratory failure**
  ○ Obtain a chest radiograph to rule out pulmonary hemorrhage.
  ○ PE should remain high on the differential for these patients.
- **Hypotension**
  ○ An ECG should be performed to rule out myocardial ischemia due to microvascular thrombosis.
  ○ Perform a bedside echocardiogram to rule out cardiac tamponade and evaluate for wall motion abnormalities.
  ○ Consider workup for gastrointestinal bleed.

Vasopressor of choice: the hypotensive patient in DIC may need resuscitation with blood products. In a patient with normal cardiac function, vasopressors such as norepinephrine or vasopressin can be initiated along with crystalloids to temporize these patients until blood products are available.

BIBLIOGRAPHY

Levi M. Disseminated intravascular coagulation. *Crit Care Med* 2007;35:2191–2195.

Levi M, & Ten Cate H. Disseminated intravascular coagulation. *N Engl J Med* 1999;341:586–592.

Levi M, Toh CH, Thachil J, et al. Guidelines for the diagnosis and management of disseminated intravascular coagulation. *Br J Haematol* 2009;145:24–33.

Masias C, Cataland SR. The role of ADAMTS13 testing in the diagnosis and management of thrombotic microangiopathies and thrombosis. *Blood* 2018;132 (9):903–910.

Noris M, Remuzzi G. Atypical hemolytic-uremic syndrome. *N Engl J Med* 2009;361 (17):1676–1687.

Scott SB. Emergency department management of hematologic and oncologic complications in the patient infected with HIV. *Emerg Med Clin North Am* 2010;28:325–333.

39

Sickle Cell Emergencies

CHARLES LEI

Chapter 39:
Sickle Cell Emergencies

Routinely draw CBC, reticulocyte count, and type and screen

| Vaso-occlusive crisis | Priapism | Infection |

Presentation

Ischemic pain, often back, abdomen, and/or extremities.

Sustained penile erection in the absence of sexual desire.

Always rule out infection in the presence of fever.

Diagnosis and Evaluation

Diagnosis of exlcusion: rule out other etiologies (i.e. cellulitis, septic arthritis, ostemyelitis).

Cavernosal blood gas.

CBC, blood cultures, UA and culture, CXR, consider LP/ arthrocentesis.

Management

Pain management, judicious IV fluids, antibiotics, O2 for saturation under 92%, transfusion not shown to be effective.

IV fluids, analgesics, aspiration/irrigation of corpus cavernosa, intracavernosal phenylephrine.

Prompt broad -spectrum antibiotics, fluids and vaso pressors as needed.

Chapter 39:
Sickle Cell Emergencies

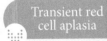 Transient red cell aplasia

 Hemolytic Crisis

 Splenic Sequestration (critical!)

Presentation

 Acute anemia: dyspnea, fatigue, pallor.

Commonly associated with Parvovirus B19.

Acute anemia: dyspnea, fatigue, pallor.

Fatigue, abdominal pain and fullness (esp. LUQ), tachycardia, may progress to hemorrhagic shock.

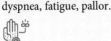 Diagnosis and Evaluation

 Decreased reticulocyte count.

 High indirect bilirubin, high LDH, low haptoglobin, **increased** reticulocyte count, conider iron studies.

 Sudden splenic enlargement and acute decrease in hemoglobin > 2 g/dL, **increased** reticulocyte count.

Management

 Simple transfusion for symptomatic anemia.

 Simple transfusion for symptomatic anemia.

 Immediate transfusion of packed RBCs, serial hemoglobin monitoring.

Chapter 39:
Sickle Cell Emergencies

| Acute Chest Syndrome (critical!) | Stroke | Eye Trauma |

 ## Presentation

Fever, cough, dyspnea, chest pain, hypoxemia, tachypnea, abnormal breath sounds.

Ischemic: typically focal neurologic deficits, possible seizures, encephalopathy.

Pain and decreased visual acuity in affected eye.

Caused by vaso-occlusion of the pulmonary vasculature.

Hemorrhagic: headache, vomiting, encephalopathy, neurologic deficits.

May present even after minor trauma.

 ## Diagnosis and Evaluation

New infiltrate on CXR.

Emergent Head CT.

Hyphema and elevated IOP.

 ## Management

Prompt broad-spectrum antibiotics, analgesics, IV fluid, O2 (for saturation < 92%), exchange transfusion (goal HbS < 30%), bronchodilators as necessary.

Exchange transfusion (goal HbS < 30%, Hgb approx. 10 g/dL).

Consult ophthamology.

Topical IOP-lowering medications.

Thrombolytics contraindicated in children, may consider in adults but must not delay exchange transfusion.

Head of bed to 30°.

Serial IOP measurements.

Introduction

- Sickle cell disease (SCD) is caused by an autosomal recessive mutation in the β-globin chain of hemoglobin A (HbA) causing the mutated hemoglobin S (HbS).
- A vaso-occlusive crisis (VOC) occurs when sickled RBCs increase the viscosity of blood and cause microvascular occlusion contributing to hypoxemia, acidosis, and further sickling.
- **The clinical manifestations of SCD are diverse, and are related to chronic hemolysis with periodic episodes of vascular occlusion that can affect nearly every organ system.**

Presentation

Classic Presentations

Vaso-Occlusive Crisis

- Vaso-occlusive crisis causes ischemic pain, most commonly affecting the back and extremities.
- **VOC is a diagnosis of exclusion.** Warmth, swelling, erythema, or fever are more suggestive of an infection such as cellulitis or osteomyelitis. Limited range of motion of a joint should raise suspicion for septic arthritis.
- The abdomen is the second most common site of ischemic pain in VOC.
- Triggers include infection, dehydration, change in weather or altitude, and stress, but there may be no identifiable precipitant.
- Young children may present with dactylitis, characterized by painful swelling of the hands and feet caused by obstruction of the arteries of the metacarpals and metatarsals.

Transient Red Cell Aplasia

- Aplastic crisis is characterized by a rapid decline in RBC production with associated acute anemia, fatigue, dyspnea and pallor.
- It is most commonly caused by an acute infection with parvovirus B19.

Priapism

- Priapism is a sustained penile erection in the absence of sexual desire.

- Patients with SCD typically develop low-flow priapism as a result of venous stasis, hypoxemia, and ischemia.
- Recurrent episodes can lead to fibrosis and impotence.

Infection

- **Patients with SCD are functionally asplenic and therefore immunocompromised after early childhood, placing them at increased risk of infection from encapsulated organisms.**
- Infections associated with SCD include pneumonia, bacteremia, meningitis, septic arthritis, and osteomyelitis.

Critical Presentations

Acute Chest Syndrome

- **Acute chest syndrome (ACS) is the leading cause of death in patients with SCD.**
- ACS is caused by vaso-occlusion in the pulmonary vasculature, which leads to pulmonary ischemia and infarction. The resultant hypoxemia and acidosis further aggravate the vaso-occlusion.
- **ACS is defined as a new infiltrate on chest radiography plus at least one new sign or symptom**: fever, cough, dyspnea, chest pain, hypoxemia, tachypnea, rales, wheezing, or retractions.
- Potential etiologies of ACS are listed in Table 39.1.

Table 39.1 Causes of acute chest syndrome

Pulmonary infection
Thromboembolism
Fat embolism
Rib infarction
Pulmonary sequestration
Iatrogenic (e.g., excessive hydration, excessive opioid use)

Splenic Sequestration

- Splenic sequestration, or intrasplenic trapping of RBCs, is a major cause of morbidity and mortality in SCD. It is most common in children who have not yet developed splenic auto-infarction.
- **It is characterized by a sudden enlargement of the spleen accompanied by an acute decrease in the hemoglobin level (> 2 g/dL below baseline).**
- Symptoms may include fatigue, abdominal fullness, and left upper quadrant abdominal pain.
- Physical examination may reveal tachycardia, pallor, and splenomegaly.
- A large volume of blood can quickly become sequestered within the spleen, leading to hypovolemic shock. The condition can be fatal within hours.

Stroke

- Patients with ischemic stroke typically present with focal neurologic deficits, but may present with seizure or encephalopathy. Vague or resolving symptoms consistent with a transient ischemic attack (TIA) may herald an ischemic stroke.
- Patients with hemorrhagic stroke may exhibit headache, vomiting, or encephalopathy.
- Approximately 10% of patients experience a clinically apparent stroke before the age of 20 years.

Eye Trauma

- Even minor trauma to the eye can cause hemorrhage (hyphema) into the anterior chamber in patients with SCD. Patients with sickle cell trait are also at increased risk for hyphema and its complications.
- When hyphema develops, sickled RBCs may obstruct the trabecular meshwork resulting in acute glaucoma.
- Symptoms include pain and decreased visual acuity in the affected eye.
- Physical examination may reveal hyphema and elevated intraocular pressure (IOP).
- Patients with SCD are also more susceptible to rebleeding and delayed complications such as optic nerve atrophy and central retinal artery occlusion.

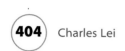

Diagnosis and Evaluation

- **The reticulocyte count can help to differentiate between splenic sequestration and transient red cell aplasia** (Table 39.2).
- High indirect bilirubin, high lactate dehydrogenase, and low haptoglobin are indicative of hemolysis.
- Perform complete blood count, blood type and screen.
- Patients with a fever should be evaluated for infection (Table 39.3).
- Many patients with SCD have a baseline leukocytosis. A white blood cell count > 20,000/mcL with an increased number of bands should raise suspicion for an infection.
- Chest radiography can identify the presence of a new infiltrate. The lower lobes are most commonly involved, but any lobe can be affected.
- Emergent head computed tomography (CT) should be performed in patients with suspected acute stroke.

Table 39.2 Differentiating common causes of acute anemia in sickle cell disease

Etiology	Anemia	Markers of hemolysis	Reticulocyte count
Hemolysis	Severe	Present	Increased
Splenic sequestration	Severe	Absent	Increased
Transient red cell aplasia	Severe	Absent	Decreased

Table 39.3 Diagnostic tests for patients with sickle cell disease and fever

Complete blood count
Blood cultures
Urinalysis and culture

Chest radiography

Lumbar puncture (for toxic-appearing children)
Arthrocentesis (for acute arthritis)

Critical Management

Critical Management Checklist

- ☑ Pain management with IV opioids
- ☑ Hydration with IV crystalloids
- ☑ Simple transfusion (symptomatic anemia, transient red cell aplasia, splenic sequestration)
- ☑ Exchange transfusion (acute chest syndrome, ischemic stroke)
- ☑ Antibiotics (infection, acute chest syndrome)

Vaso-Occlusive Crisis

- **Initial management includes aggressive pain management and rehydration.**
- Treatment of pain usually requires opioids.
- In the absence of intravenous (IV) access, oral administration of medications is preferred over the intramuscular route due to unpredictable muscle absorption and concerns for hematoma formation.
- Non-steroidal anti-inflammatory drugs should be used cautiously as patients with SCD have some degree of renal dysfunction from microinfarction.
- Fluid rehydration should be performed judiciously. Use boluses of IV crystalloids if there is overt hypovolemia (e.g., sepsis, vomiting, diarrhea). While no clear consensus exists, hypotonic solutions such as 5% dextrose in half-normal saline are thought to favorably affect RBC membrane stiffness.
- IV fluid therapy should not exceed 1.5 times maintenance to avoid pulmonary edema, which may lead to ACS.
- **Transfusion has not been shown to be effective for VOC and should be reserved for other complications of SCD.**
- Supplemental oxygen is recommended only if the patient's oxygen saturation falls below 92%.

Transient Red Cell Aplasia

- Patients should be transfused only if they develop symptomatic anemia.
- Because parvovirus B19 is highly communicable, patients with aplastic crisis should be isolated from pregnant or immunocompromised individuals.

Priapism

- Treatment of low-flow priapism includes IV fluids, analgesics, aspiration and irrigation of the corpus cavernosa, and intracavernosal injection of phenylephrine.
- There is insufficient evidence to support the use of simple or exchange transfusion in treating SCD-associated priapism.

Infection

- **Patients who are systemically ill should be treated promptly with broad-spectrum IV antibiotics.** Once a causative organism is identified, therapy can be tailored according to its antibiotic sensitivity.
- Septic patients should be treated with IV fluids and vasopressors as per evidence-based guidelines.

Acute Chest Syndrome

- Treatment of ACS parallels that of VOC, including use of analgesics, IV fluids, and supplemental oxygen.
- **Patients with ACS should receive antibiotics to cover both typical and atypical organisms**. A full course of antibiotics is recommended regardless of culture results.
- **Transfusion therapy may be lifesaving in ACS.** Exchange transfusion is preferred over simple transfusion in patients with deteriorating conditions, particularly in those with relatively high hemoglobin (> 9 g/dL). The goal for exchange transfusion therapy is to decrease the HbS concentration to < 30%.

- Bronchospasm may accompany ACS. Administer bronchodilators to patients with wheezing and continue the treatment if a response is elicited.
- Steroids are not recommended in ACS unless there is evidence of concurrent reactive airway disease.

Splenic Sequestration

- **All patients with acute splenic sequestration should immediately be transfused with packed RBCs.**
- Serial hemoglobin measurements should be performed to evaluate the adequacy of transfusion.

Stroke

- **Patients with acute ischemic stroke or TIA should be treated with simple or exchange transfusion, with a goal to decrease the HbS concentration to < 30% and increase the total hemoglobin level to 10 g/dL. Exchange transfusion is the preferred therapy, if available.**
- Thrombolysis is contraindicated in children with acute ischemic stroke. In adults, thrombolytics may be considered but should not replace or delay transfusion therapy.

Eye Trauma

- Patients who sustain eye trauma with or without hyphema require emergent ophthalmologic evaluation to identify and treat elevated IOP.
- Treatment of hyphema includes head-of-bed elevation to 30° and topical medications for lowering IOP (e.g., beta-blockers, alpha-2 agonists).
- Mannitol and carbonic anhydrase inhibitors should be avoided because of their potential to promote sickling.
- Patients with SCD or sickle cell trait presenting with hyphema should be admitted for medical therapy and serial IOP measurements. The threshold for surgical hyphema evacuation is lower in these patients than in the general population.

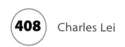

Sudden Deterioration

Respiratory Distress

- Causes of acute respiratory distress include pneumonia, pulmonary edema, pulmonary embolism, and fat embolism.
- Chest radiography should be obtained to help determine the etiology of the patient's respiratory compromise.
- Noninvasive positive-pressure ventilation may improve oxygenation and ventilation in patients with pulmonary edema and decrease the need for intubation.
- Patients with impending respiratory failure should be emergently intubated.

Hypotension

- Splenic sequestration, pulmonary embolism, and septic shock can all cause a precipitous drop in blood pressure.
- Measures to monitor and support the blood pressure should be initiated. This may include invasive hemodynamic monitoring, bedside ultrasonography, central venous access, IV fluid resuscitation, packed RBC transfusion, or vasopressor support.

Altered Mental Status

- Patients with focal neurological deficits or encephalopathy should undergo emergent head CT to evaluate for ischemic or hemorrhagic stroke.
- **Encephalopathy may be an ominous sign in patients with splenic sequestration. Emergent RBC transfusion is imperative.**
- Patients with VOC may develop a depressed level of consciousness as a result of excessive opiate use. Naloxone may be used to reverse the respiratory depression. Patients with persistent respiratory compromise may require endotracheal intubation.

Vasopressor of choice: Patients presenting with septic physiology should receive norepinephrine as the first-line vasopressor.

BIBLIOGRAPHY

Simon E, Long B, Koyfman A. Emergency medicine management of sickle cell disease complications: an evidence-based update. *J Emerg Med* 2016;51:370–381.

Ware RE, de Montalembert M, Tshilolo L, et al. Sickle cell disease. *Lancet* 2017;390:311–323.

SECTION 9

Endocrine Emergencies

BRANDON GODBOUT

40

Diabetic Ketoacidosis and Hyperglycemic Hyperosmolar State

BENJAMIN ZABAR

Chapter 40:
DKA

 Presentation

Polyuria, polydipsia, polyphagia, dizziness, weakness.

Abdominal pain, nausea, vomiting.

AMS

Kussmaul respirations, fruity breath odor.

Critical: hypotension, coma, acidemia.

 Diagnosis and Evaluation

POCT glucose.
🔴 *> 250 mg/dL.*

CMP

Serum acetone or beta-hydroxybutyrate, blood gas, CXR, lipase, UA, ECG.
🔴 *Absence of urine ketones does not exclude DKA.*

 Management

Airway management and hemodynamic support.

IV Fluid replacement, potassium repletion, electrolyte correction.

After potassium repletion, initiate insulin drip.

Consider sodium bicarbonate for pH < 7.0.

Serial chemistry/ glucose monitoring.

Chapter 40:
HHS

 ## Presentation

AMS in an elderly person with multiple comorbidities.

Polyuria, polydipsia.

Critical: severely obtunded, comatose, hypotension.

 ## Diagnosis and Evaluation

POCT glucose.

- *Often too high for glucometer to register.*

CMP

- *Significant osmolal gap.*
- *HHS in isolation does not cause high anion gap metabolic acidosis, although precipitating factor may.*

Blood gas, lactate, UA.

Consider precipitating cause (injury, infection, stroke).

 ## Management

Airway management and hemodynamic support.

IV fluid replacement, potassium repletion, electrolyte correction.

After significant fluid replacement and potassium repletion, initiate insulin (usually via a drip).

Serial chemistry/glucose monitoring.

Diabetic Ketoacidosis

Introduction

- **Diabetic ketoacidosis (DKA)** is a critical state of hyperglycemia that results in both hyperketonemia and acidosis.
- Despite elevated serum glucose in DKA, the cells are "starving" due to the lack of insulin to facilitate glucose uptake. Therefore, fatty acids are utilized which produce ketones and an anion gap ketoacidosis.
- Hyperglycemia causes glucose to spill into the urine, resulting in an osmotic diuresis that leads to dehydration and electrolyte derangements.
- The acidosis causes K^+ to shift out of cells, leading to serum hyperkalemia. K^+ and bicarbonate are lost in the urine, depleting whole body potassium. The loss of bicarbonate further exacerbates the acidosis.

Presentation

Classic Presentation

- Classic symptoms of hyperglycemia including polyuria, polydipsia, polyphagia, dizziness, and weakness.
- Abdominal pain, nausea, and vomiting.
- Altered mental status.
- Deep breathing (Kussmaul respiration) with fruity odor.
- Table 40.1 lists the differential diagnoses of patients in DKA.

Table 40.1 Differential diagnosis of diabetic ketoacidosis

Ketoacidosis

- Alcoholic ketoacidosis

Anion-gap acidosis

- Salicylate toxicity
- Toxic alcohols (methanol, ethylene glycol, propylene glycol)
- Uremia
- Lactic acidosis (sepsis, shock)

Hypoglycemia
Trauma

Critical Presentation

- Profound hypotension due to severe dehydration.
- Coma, requiring airway protection.
- Acidemia with the corresponding compensatory mechanisms

Diagnosis and Evaluation

Diagnostic Tests

- **Glucometry** – point of care glucose level is typically greater than 250 mg/dL (13.89 mmol/L) (may read "high").
- **Chemistry** is critical for obtaining glucose and electrolyte levels and calculating anion gap (anion gap = sodium – [chloride + bicarbonate]).
  - Serum potassium is often elevated and will correct with insulin therapy, fluid replacement, and correction of acidosis. **Remember: DKA patients are often depleted in total body potassium**.
  - Other electrolytes such as magnesium, phosphate, and calcium may also be depleted during DKA and monitoring them is important.
  - Consider checking serum lipase to exclude pancreatitis as a precipitating factor for the hyperglycemia. But keep in mind that hyperglycemia can cause pancreatitis as well.
  - Serial chemistry monitoring every 1–2 hours is recommended during insulin infusion because of rapid fluid and electrolyte shifting.
  - Sodium should be adjusted for elevated glucose – profound hyperglycemia will show corresponding sodium levels lower than they actually are. Na^+ artificially decreases approximately 1.6 mEq/L for every 100 mg/dL the glucose is above normal. Additionally, with glucose levels above 400 mg/dL, a correction factor of 2.4 mEq/L appears to be more accurate than 1.6 mEq/L.
- **Serum acetone or beta-hydroxybutyrate** measurement indicates presence of ketonemia and may correlate with the degree of dehydration and breakdown of fatty acids that occur in DKA.
- **Blood gas** measurement is important for determining the resultant acidemia. Venous blood gas has been demonstrated to be as reliable as arterial blood gas for pH monitoring.
- **Chest radiography** to exclude pneumonia as a precipitating cause of DKA.
- **Urinalysis** evaluates the presence of ketonuria (commonly acetoacetate) and/or presence of urinary tract infection.

- *Critical pitfall: Negative urine ketone testing does not exclude the presence of DKA.*
- **ECG** evaluates the presence of ischemia or STEMI (ST-segment elevation myocardial infarction) and may indicate significant electrolyte abnormalities.

Critical Management

Critical Management Checklist

- ☑ ABCs
- ☑ Aggressive fluid replacement
- ☑ Insulin (0.1 units/kg/hour IV infusion)
- ☑ Potassium and other electrolyte repletion
- ☑ Treat underlying cause (e.g., infection, AMI, stroke)
- ☑ Consider sodium bicarbonate for pH < 7.0

Manage Airway, Breathing, and Circulation

- Rapid sequence intubation may be necessary for airway protection in obtunded patients or those that are severely hypoxic. Remember to match the ventilatory rate with the patient's respiratory rate pre-intubation; typically, tachypnea is a compensation for metabolic acidosis.
- Establish **two large-bore IVs.**

Aggressive Fluid Replacement

- Patients are **often depleted 4–8 liters of total body volume**.
- For adults begin with 2–4 liters of balanced crystalloid solution; avoid normal saline as resuscitative fluid given potential to exacerbate acidosis/acidemia with concomitant hyperchloremic non-anion gap acidosis.
- Titrate further fluid replacement (boluses or infusion) to the clinical status of the patient and the acid/base physiology.

Insulin Therapy

- Insulin therapy decreases serum glucose by shifting it into cells and signals cells to stop fatty acid breakdown and begin metabolizing existing ketones. Reversal of ketoacidosis is the goal of the insulin drip, not the correction of the serum glucose.

- Regular insulin has a short half-life of 3–5 minutes. It will reach a steady state in five half-lives (15–25 minutes); therefore, it is generally unnecessary to give a bolus dose when starting an insulin drip. Also, data show potential harm when giving a bolus of insulin in DKA patients.
- Begin an IV drip at 0.1 units/kg/hour, titrating up to 5–10 units/hour (depending on the weight of the patient), with a goal of reducing glucose 50–100 mg/ dL/hour (2.77–5.55 mmol/L/hour).
- Check blood glucose by glucometer every 30–60 minutes to prevent hypoglycemia.
- Once serum glucose reaches 250 mg/dL (13.89 mmol/L), add dextrose to the IV fluids at a rate that allows a normal steady serum glucose level while continuing IV insulin therapy (typically D5–½NS or D5–1/2LR at 100–150 mL/hour). Insulin will still be required to remove ketones despite normalization of glucose at a dose typically half the starting dose.
- Continue the insulin drip until normalization of the anion gap ("gap closure").
- One hour prior to termination of the insulin drip, administer long-acting insulin to prevent rebound hyperglycemia (i.e., insulin glargine 10–20 units subcutaneously).
- Note: Some institutions and recent research have investigated the utility of a q2h insulin dosing (using subcutaneous lispro at 0.2U/kg) and blood glucose check schedule with some success in the uncomplicated DKA population to avoid ICU admission.

Potassium Repletion

- **Remember that DKA patients are often depleted in total body potassium** (Table 40.2).
- Potassium will shift into the cells during insulin treatment and should be repleted even if slightly elevated.
- Check potassium before starting insulin drip.
- Resist the temptation to give further potassium-lowering agents such as Kayexalate unless the patient is exhibiting dysrhythmias as a result of hyperkalemia. Always ensure that the patient can produce urine prior to giving potassium.

Table 40.2 Potassium repletion in diabetic ketoacidosis

Measured potassium (mEq/L)	mEq of K⁺ to give per hour
< 3	40
3–4	30
4–5	20
5–6	10
> 6	0

Other Electrolyte Repletion

- Repletion of magnesium, calcium, and phosphate are often necessary, especially after the first day of treatment.

Sodium Bicarbonate

- Some authors advocate administering sodium bicarbonate if pH < 7.0. The utility of bicarbonate in patients with renal dysfunction has an evolving literature basis with some signal for benefit in select populations.

Hyperglycemic Hyperosmolar State

Introduction

- **Hyperglycemic hyperosmolar state (HHS)** (formerly hyperglycemic hyperosmolar nonketotic coma) is a critical state of hyperglycemia, hyperosmolarity, and dehydration similar to DKA but without development of ketoacidosis. As with DKA, HHS is sometimes the result of a precipitating stressor like infection, myocardial infarction, or stroke.
- In HHS it is believed that the body produces enough insulin to prevent ketoacidosis; however, the state of severe hyperglycemia continues to result in osmotic diuresis, hyperosmolar state, and electrolyte abnormalities.
- HHS occurs most frequently in elderly, confused, and bed-bound persons with underlying renal insufficiency who are unable to access enough fluids to match losses or obtain needed medications.

- The diagnosis is associated with a high mortality, up to 50% even with treatment. Note that this is much greater than in patients with DKA.
- The average fluid deficit is 9 liters.

Presentation

Classic Presentation

- Altered mental status in an elderly person with multiple comorbidities.
- Polyuria, polydipsia.

Critical Presentation

- Severely obtunded, comatose, lack of airway protection.
- Hypotensive.

Diagnosis and Evaluation

Same as DKA with the following differences:

- **Glucometry** – The value is too "high" to register and presents with a glucose significantly more elevated than in DKA, at times in excess of 800–1000 mg/dL (44.40–55.50 mmol/L).
- **Chemistry** – HHS does not primarily cause high anion gap acidosis as in DKA (there is not a primary excess of ketones); however, precipitating illnesses may lead to anion gap acidosis (i.e., renal failure, lactic acidosis). A significant osmolal gap will be present with plasma osmolality > 320 mOsm/L.
- **Blood gas** – While HHS patients are usually less acidotic than with DKA, a low pH should prompt consideration of metabolic disturbances other than HHS.
- **Lactate** – A high lactate may indicate inadequate tissue perfusion, from dehydration or sepsis.
- **Urinalysis** is less likely to show ketones than in DKA. Urinalysis helps evaluate the presence of urinary tract infection.
- A diagnosis of HHS must prompt the question why the patient was unable to maintain hydration. New causes of incapacity such as stroke, infection, or injury should be considered.

Critical Management

Same as for DKA with following differences:

- **ABCs** – Due to profound mental status changes, patients with HHS more often lack airway protection than patients with DKA.
- **Insulin therapy** – Patients with HHS need IV fluids for profound dehydration. Although severe hyperglycemia causes osmotic diuresis, HHS occurs in individuals capable of making insulin with some degree of effectiveness. Thus, in contrast to DKA, insulin is not an urgent component of treatment. Once significant replacement of fluids occurs, electrolyte abnormalities are corrected, and adequate urine output is ensured, patients with HHS may benefit from IV insulin 0.1 U/kg/hour to slow continuing osmotic diuresis.

Sudden Deterioration in Diabetic Ketoacidosis and Hyperglycemic Hyperosmolar State

Acute Change in Mental Status

- Hypoglycemia can occur as a result of "overcorrection" of hyperglycemia with insulin drip. Immediately check bedside glucometry and if necessary, stop insulin therapy and give D50W.
- Cerebral edema may occur as a result of rapid fluid shifts, particularly in the pediatric population. If it occurs, stop fluid replacement and consider rapid sequence intubation, hyperventilation, and administration of IV mannitol.

Acute Muscle Weakness

- This is most often a result of an electrolyte abnormality occurring during therapy, most notably hypophosphatemia. Hold insulin and fluids and immediately obtain an ECG, chemistry panel (including calcium, magnesium, and phosphate), and whole-blood potassium. Replete the abnormal electrolyte, monitor closely, and resume therapy after improvement of weakness.

Acute Respiratory Distress

- Consider pulmonary vascular congestion as a result of aggressive fluid replacement. Provide additional oxygen and immediately obtain a portable chest radiograph. Avoid diuretics if the chest radiograph shows congestion as this will worsen intravascular fluid depletion and may cause a further drop in potassium. Slowing/stopping IV fluids is usually sufficient; in certain instances noninvasive positive-pressure ventilation or rapid sequence intubation are necessary.

BIBLIOGRAPHY

Cydulka RK, & Gerald ME. Diabetes mellitus and disorders of glucose homeostasis. In: Marx JA, Hockberger RS, Walls RM, et al., eds. *Rosen's Emergency Medicine: Concepts and Clinical Practice*, 7th ed. Philadelphia, PA: Mosby Elsevier, 2010.

Graber MN. Diabetes and hyperglycemia. In: Adams, JG, ed. *Emergency Medicine*. Philadelphia, PA: Elsevier Saunders, 2008.

Marino PL. *The ICU Book*, 3rd ed. Philadelphia, PA: Lippincott Williams & Wilkins, 2007.

41

Thyroid Storm

YVES DUROSEAU

Chapter 41:
Thyroid Storm

 ## Presentation

Classic: Marked tachycardia (often 140 +), fever, diaphoresis, abdominal pain, agitation.

History of thyroid disorder.

Critical: A-fib with rapid ventricular repsonse, severely altered mental status.

Presence of precipitating factor (infection, surgery, other physiological insult).

 ## Diagnosis and Evaluation

Labwork: TSH, T3, T4, free T4, CBC, BMP, lactate, lipase, LFTs, cardiac markers, BNP, and cultures. *Normal TSH virtually excludes thyroid storm.*

ECG: assess for arrhythmia.

Imaging: CXR/Head CT to rule alternate etiology, echocardiography to establish baseline function.

 ## Management

Airway managment.

Fluid resuscitation.

Hemodynamic monitoring.

Aggressive cooling (ice packs, fans, acetominophen).

Control agitation (benzodiazepines).

Medical Therapy
In this order: IV Esmolol/IV Propranolol, PTU/methimazole, Dexamethasone, SSKI.

Introduction

- Thyrotoxicosis is a clinical state of hyperdynamic metabolism as a result of excessive circulating thyroid hormone.
- The most notable causes of thyrotoxicosis are Graves' disease, Hashimoto thyroiditis, subacute (De Quervain) thyroiditis, and TSH/thyroid hormone-secreting tumors.
- **Excessive circulating thyroid hormone can have critical effects on many organ systems.**
  - *Cardiovascular system:*
    - Direct positive chronotropic and inotropic effects on the heart.
    - Indirectly increases cardiac output secondary to increased peripheral tissue oxygen consumption and thermogenesis.
    - Indirectly increases cardiac output due to decreased peripheral vascular resistance and increased dilatation of arterioles.
  - *Pulmonary system:*
    - Hyperventilation secondary to increased CO_2 production resulting from elevated tissue metabolism.
    - Respiratory muscle fatigue.
  - *Renal system:*
    - Increase in blood volume and preload due to increased production of erythropoietin.
- **Thyroid storm** is a life-threatening decompensation of thyrotoxicosis (thought to be due to acute increase in catecholamine binding sites), which occurs in approximately 1–2% of persons with thyrotoxicosis and carries an 8–25% mortality.
- Since many disease processes can increase circulating catecholamines, precipitation of thyroid storm is not simply a sudden increase in the levels of thyroid hormones but rather an exaggerated response to internal/external stressors.
- Infection is the most common precipitating factor in thyroid storm (Table 41.1).

Presentation

- The broad clinical picture is one suggestive of a hypermetabolic state with increased beta-adrenergic activity.
- Often more than one disease process may be occurring at once, which makes rapid identification of thyroid storm very difficult. The key is to have a high index of suspicion.

Table 41.1 Common precipitants of thyroid storm

Infection/sepsis

Surgery

Acute coronary syndrome/myocardial infarction

Cerebral vascular accident

Trauma (especially neck trauma)

Medication noncompliance

Thyroid hormone ingestion

Iodine contrast

Classic Presentation

- Marked tachycardia, often with ventricular rates exceeding 140 bpm.
- Fever, temperatures sometimes exceeding 41°C (106°F).
- Diaphoresis.
- GI symptoms, such as abdominal pain, nausea, vomiting, diarrhea.
- CNS dysfunction, agitation, confusion, delirium.

Critical Presentation

- High-output cardiac failure and shock.
- Atrial fibrillation with rapid ventricular response.
- Severely obtunded state, coma, seizure.

Diagnosis and Evaluation

- The diagnosis of thyroid storm is made based on clinical findings and laboratory analysis.
- **Burch and Wartofsky scoring system**
  - Given the spectrum of illness, Burch and Wartofsky developed a scoring system to help clinically distinguish uncomplicated thyrotoxicosis from impending thyroid storm and true thyroid storm (Table 41.2).
  - A score of 45 or more is highly suggestive of thyroid storm, a score of 25–44 is suggestive of impending thyroid storm, and a score below 25 makes the diagnosis of thyroid storm unlikely.

Table 41.2 Burch and Wartofsky scoring system for thyroid storm

Thermoregulatory dysfunction (°F)	
99–99.9	5
100–100.9	10
101–101.9	15
102–102.9	20
103–103.9	25
≥ 104	30
Tachycardia (beats/minute)	
90–109	5
110–119	10
120–129	15
130–139	20
≥ 140	25
CNS effects	
Mild agitation	10
Delirium/psychosis/lethargy	20
Seizure/coma	30
Heart failure	
Pedal edema	5
Bibasilar rales	10
Atrial fibrillation	10
Pulmonary edema	15
Gastrointestinal-hepatic dysfunction	
Diarrhea/nausea/vomiting/abdominal pain	10
Unexplained jaundice	20
Precipitant history	
Positive	10

- **Laboratory testing**
  - Laboratory evaluation is primarily directed at assessing the severity of the disease and searching for potential precipitants.
  - TSH, T_3, T_4, free T_4
  - CBC, basic metabolic profile, lactate, hepatic function panel, lipase.
  - Cardiac markers, brain natriuretic peptide (BNP).
  - Blood, urine and possibly CNS cultures/analysis.
  - **A normal TSH virtually excludes the diagnosis of thyroid storm**.
- **ECG**
  - Evaluate for the presence of atrial fibrillation, other cardiac arrhythmias, or evidence of acute myocardial ischemia.
  - The most common cardiac rhythm is sinus tachycardia.
- **Echocardiography**
  - Will help establish baseline cardiac function if patient further decompensates.
  - Can help distinguish between high output cardiac failure versus hypokinesis.
- **Imaging**
  - Chest radiography to rule out pneumonia and to evaluate for evidence of congestive heart failure (CHF).
  - Consider CT of the head to assess for other potential etiologies of altered mental status.

Critical Management

Critical Management Checklist

- ☑ ABC
- ☑ Fluid resuscitation
- ☑ Control agitation
- ☑ Aggressive cooling
- ☑ Treat precipitating/concomitant illness
- ☑ Inhibit toxic peripheral effects of excess thyroid hormone (beta-blockade)
- ☑ Inhibit further thyroid hormone synthesis (propylthiouracil [PTU]/methimazole)
- ☑ Prevent peripheral conversion $T_4 \rightarrow T_3$ (dexamethasone)
- ☑ Inhibit thyroid hormone release (iodine)

- **Management of ABCs and general supportive measures**
  - Insert IV line, provide supplemental O_2, and place on continuous monitoring.
  - Sit the patient upright to reduce symptomatic pulmonary congestion.
  - Consider rapid sequence intubation for respiratory distress/failure.
  - A low threshold for broad-spectrum antibiotics should be considered as SIRS criteria is often present and a source of infection may not be apparent.
  - Steroids should be considered in life-threatening thyroid storm to address associated adrenal insufficiency and prevent peripheral T4->T3 conversion.
  - *Fluid resuscitation:*
    - Thyroid storm is a hypermetabolic state, which means patients are often severely dehydrated with depleted glycogen stores.
    - Vigorous crystalloid administration is indicated unless signs of CHF are present.
    - Addition of glucose-containing isotonic fluid is often necessary.
  - *Control hyperthermia:*
    - Antipyretics – Acetaminophen is preferred; be cautious with aspirin as it is thought to increase free T_3 and T_4 levels by affecting protein binding.
    - Consider cooling blankets, ice packs, fans, and other methods of active/passive cooling.
  - *Control agitation:*
    - Benzodiazepines to control agitation and decrease sympathomimetic state.
    - Avoid agents that increase sympathomimetic tone – ketamine, amiodarone, albuterol, etc.
- **Specific therapy for thyroid storm**
  - *The order of treatment is important in thyroid storm.* Following the ABCs, treat the life-threatening hypermetabolic state with beta-blockade first. Wait at least 1 hour after the time PTU/methimazole administration prior to giving iodine (see #4 below).
  - *#1: Inhibit toxic adrenergic effects of thyroid hormone:*
    - A short-acting IV agent such as esmolol is preferred in severe disease as it allows for rapid titration.
      - 250–500 micrograms/kg loading dose, followed by an infusion at 50–100 micrograms/kg/minute.
    - Alternatively, IV propranolol (non-cardiac specific) can be selected. Although more difficult to titrate, it has the physiological advantage of blocking peripheral conversion of T_4 to T_3.

- 0.5–1 mg IV slow push, repeat every 15 minutes to effect.
  - ○ *#2: Inhibit thyroid hormone synthesis:*
    - Propylthiouracil ([PTU] generally less favored due to liver toxicity [but used in pregnancy]) and methimazole are thionamides that block synthesis of thyroid hormone in the thyroid gland.
    - PTU is preferred for its additional advantage of blocking peripheral conversion of T_4 to T_3.
    - PTU: 600–1000 mg PO loading dose, 200–250 mg PO every 4 hours.
  - ○ *#3: Prevent peripheral conversion of $T_4 {\rightarrow} T_3$:*
    - Dexamethasone.
      - 2–4 mg IV every 6 hours.
  - ○ *#4: Inhibit thyroid hormone release options (administer at least 1 hour after thionamide):*
    - Large doses of iodine paradoxically suppress thyroid hormone release.
    - Saturated solution of potassium iodide – five drops PO/NG/PR every 6 hours.
    - Lugol solution – 8 drops PO/NG/PR every 8 hours.
    - Sodium iodide – 500 mg IV every 12 hours.
    - If there is iodine allergy, lithium carbonate 300 mg PO/NG every 6 hours.

Sudden Deterioration

- **High-output cardiac failure** can be a devastating complication in thyroid storm. It is the result of excessive tachycardia and may result in pulmonary edema despite volume depletion. This can be complicated by the development of atrial fibrillation with rapid ventricular response, further worsening hemodynamics.
- The goal is to decrease fever and heart rate and to judiciously increase intravascular volume while decreasing excessive circulating thyroid hormone.
- Avoid the use of diuretics.
- Use a titratable beta-blockade to decrease the heart rate and increase cardiac filling time, but caution if inotropy is acutely needed.
- Consider noninvasive positive-pressure ventilation to reduce the work of breathing.

BIBLIOGRAPHY

Hackstadt D, & Korley F. Thyroid disorders. In: Adams JG, ed. *Emergency Medicine*. Philadelphia, PA: Elsevier Saunders, 2008.

Mills L, & Lim S. Identifying and treating thyroid storm and myxedema coma in the emergency department. *Emerg Med Pract*. EBMedicine.net, August 2009. Available at www.ebmedicine.net/topics/endocrine/thyroid-storm-myxedema-coma Zull D. Thyroid and adrenal disorders. In: Marx JA, Hockberger RS, Walls RM, et al, eds. *Rosen's Emergency Medicine: Concepts and Clinical Practice*, 7th ed. Philadelphia, PA: Mosby Elsevier, 2010.

42

Adrenal Crisis

RAYMOND HOU AND DANIEL ROLSTON

Chapter 42:
Adrenal Crisis

Presentation

Often non-specific symptoms like fatigue, weakness, abdominal pain, fever, depression.

Often with history of precipitating factor, like surgery, HIV, steroid use, infection, pituitary damage.

Critical Presentation: Persistent hypotension despite fluids and vasopressors.

Diagnosis and Evaluation

Vital signs are main identifier of illness as symptoms are non-specific.

✿ *Hypotension and lack of reflexive tachycardia (*note negative chronotropic medications may also blunt reflex tachycardia).*

AM Cortisol Levels: <3 mcg/dL is diagnostic, while >15 mcg/dL excludes the diagnosis.

Thorough history, physical exam, and dermatologial evaulation may help identify underlying cause.

Labwork: Hyponatremia, hyperkalemia, and hypoglycemia.

Management

Airway management and hemodynamic monitoring.

Rule out sepsis or other acute illness.

Crystalloid bolus, inotropes/vasopressors as needed.

After sending serum cortisol and ACTH, administer hydrocortisone.

Consider underlying cause.

Introduction

- Adrenal insufficiency can either be primary, resulting from destruction of the adrenal gland; or secondary, resulting from a deficiency of ACTH (adrenocorticotropic hormone, corticotropin).
- Tables 42.1 and 42.2 list the causes of chronic and acute adrenal insufficiency, respectively.
- **Adrenal crisis** is either the acute development of severe adrenal insufficiency or a rapid deterioration from baseline chronic adrenal insufficiency (which is often insidious) brought on by a stressor.
- **Pathophysiology**
  - The adrenal gland (made up of cortex and medulla) produces three categories of steroids: glucocorticoids (cortisol), mineralocorticoids (aldosterone) and gonadocorticoids (sex hormones).
  - Aldosterone levels change in response to volume status and sodium intake. It maintains sodium and potassium concentration, and regulates water balance.
  - Primary adrenal insufficiency (Addison disease) occurs when the adrenal gland loses approximately 90% of its function and can no longer produce cortisol or aldosterone.

Table 42.1 Common causes of chronic adrenal insufficiency

Chronic steroid use
HIV/AIDS
Tuberculosis
Autoimmune adrenalitis
Congenital (congenital adrenal hyperplasia, adrenoleukodystrophy)
Infiltrative (sarcoidosis, hemochromatosis, amyloidosis)
Cancer
Surgery/irradiation
Hepatic failure Pancreatitis

Table 42.2 Etiologies of acute adrenal insufficiency

Drugs (steroids, etomidate, ketoconazole) Systemic infection/sepsis
Adrenal hemorrhage (meningococcemia/Waterhouse–Friderichsen, anticoagulation, antiphospholipid antibody syndrome)
Pituitary hemorrhage (pituitary apoplexy) Postpartum pituitary necrosis (Sheehan syndrome) Trauma
Hepatic failure Pancreatitis

- ○ Secondary adrenal insufficiency occurs because of decreased production of ACTH by the pituitary gland, and therefore decreased cortisol production. The most common etiology includes hypoaldosteronism caused by prolonged glucocorticoid use.
- ○ ACTH is released by the pituitary gland and stimulates the adrenal gland to produce and release cortisol.

Presentation

Classic Presentation

- Patients with adrenal insufficiency usually present with nonspecific symptoms including weakness/fatigue, weight loss, anorexia, abdominal pain, fever, and depression.
- The classic finding in adrenal crisis is refractory hypotension.
- These patients can frequently appear to be in septic shock, and they may in fact be septic, but their body is not able to respond appropriately because of a lack of cortisol.
- A thorough history including steroid use/drug use, surgeries, history of HIV, and precipitating symptoms should be elicited.
- Consider this diagnosis in symptomatic patients who have received doses of prednisone > 7.5 mg per day or equivalent for longer than 3 weeks. Patients receiving topical, intranasal, inhalation or PR route steroids are typically at less risk for hypothalamus-pituitary-adrenal axis suppression.

Critical Presentation

- Consider adrenal crisis in the patient who is persistently hypotensive despite multiple liters of fluid boluses and high doses of multiple vasopressors.
- Acute adrenal insufficiency can appear to be a severe gastroenteritis with fever, vomiting, and dehydration, but this can quickly progress to vascular collapse and death.

Diagnosis and Evaluation

- *The diagnosis of adrenal insufficiency is difficult to make because the most common symptoms are nonspecific, including fatigue, weight loss, GI symptoms, and depression, so a broad differential must be considered.*
- **Vital signs** are the main identifier of illness since the symptoms are non-specific.
  - **Refractory hypotension** is the hallmark of adrenal crisis as discussed above.
  - The **lack of reflexive tachycardia** in a hypotensive state should increase concern for adrenal crisis since cortisol deficiency blunts the physiological vasoconstriction and catecholamine synthesis. However, many patients are on beta-blockers, calcium channel blockers or other antiarrhythmic drugs that can cause this discrepancy.
  - Consider adrenal crisis or neurogenic shock in a hypotensive patient with a normal heart rate not taking negative chronotrope medications.
- **Physical examination** is frequently unimpressive, but a thorough examination can help determine the underlying cause.
  - First assess for signs of infection, which can precipitate a crisis:
    - Focal lung findings: crackles or rhonchi or wheezes
    - Altered mental status
    - Abdominal tenderness
    - Rashes
    - Joint swelling and erythema.

- ○ Dermatological examination can be especially helpful if adrenal crisis is suspected:
  - Hyperpigmentation of sun-exposed areas, axilla, palmar creases, and mucous membranes (Addison disease). The increased ACTH secreted by the pituitary stimulates melanin production.
  - Petechial rash (meningococcemia).
  - Vitiligo (white patches of amelanotic skin) can be seen in polyglandular autoimmune (PGA) syndrome type I.
- **Diagnostic tests**
  - ○ *Laboratory tests:*
    - Hyponatremia is seen in primary adrenal insufficiency because of the aldosterone deficiency. Additionally, the lack of cortisol leads to increased antidiuretic hormone (ADH) secretion, increased free water absorption, and worsening hyponatremia.
    - The lack of aldosterone also causes hyperkalemia, with an accompanying mild hyperchloremic metabolic acidosis.
    - Hypoglycemia can be seen in both primary and secondary adrenal insufficiency because of a lack of cortisol and decreased appetite. Additionally, in secondary adrenal insufficiency, growth hormone and ACTH deficiency contribute further to hypoglycemia.
  - ○ *Serum cortisol level (exact cutoffs vary by guidelines):*
    - Should be elevated with acute illness because of physiological stress on the body. Naturally, cortisol is generally higher (10–20 mcg/dL) in the AM and lower in the afternoon (3–10 mcg/dL).
    - Generally accepted cutoffs for AM levels: cortisol level < 3 mcg/dL is diagnostic of adrenal crisis; levels 3–15 mcg/dL is indeterminate; levels > 15 mcg/dL exclude the diagnosis.
    - Meta-analysis has shown no difference between low dose (1–2 micrograms) and high dose (250 micrograms) ACTH stimulation tests. The high dose (250 micrograms) ACTH (cosyntropin) stimulation test with results of less than a 9 micrograms/dL increase in serum cortisol is often diagnostically used to classify those who may benefit from stress corticosteroids (200 mg/day hydrocortisone or equivalent). There is no evidence that testing improves mortality outcomes in the septic population. Dexamethasone does not alter the cortisol assay and can be used instead of hydrocortisone if treatment is emergent and a stimulation test will be performed later.
    - Keep in mind that laboratories currently measure total cortisol only and the majority of cortisol is protein bound. As such, cortisol values might not reflect the true active cortisol level in the patient (Figure 42.1) .

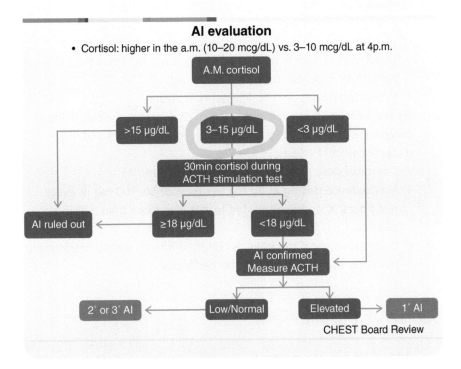

AI evaluation
- Cortisol: higher in the a.m. (10–20 mcg/dL) vs. 3–10 mcg/dL at 4p.m.

A.M. cortisol

>15 µg/dL | 3–15 µg/dL | <3 µg/dL

30min cortisol during ACTH stimulation test

AI ruled out ← ≥18 µg/dL | <18 µg/dL

AI confirmed Measure ACTH

2° or 3° AI ← Low/Normal | Elevated → 1° AI

CHEST Board Review

Figure 42.1 AI evaluation for cortisol levels.

Critical Management

Critical Management Checklist

- ☑ ABCs
- ☑ Give normal saline bolus for hypotension
- ☑ Rule out sepsis/other acute illness
- ☑ Consider antibiotic coverage
- ☑ Start inotropes/vasopressors as needed
- ☑ Consider adrenal crisis in patients with hypotension refractory to vasopressors
- ☑ Send serum cortisol and ACTH levels prior to steroids
- ☑ Give hydrocortisone

- ○ **Manage ABCs**
  - ▪ Airway and breathing.
  - ▪ Place patients on cardiac monitor and pulse oximeter.
  - ▪ Hypotensive patients require 2–3 liters of normal saline fluid boluses (with D5W if the patient is hypoglycemic).
  - ▪ Vasopressors/inotropes to maintain circulation.
- ○ **Hydrocortisone** is the initial therapy of choice once the possibility of adrenal crisis is recognized because of its glucocorticoid and mineralocorticoid effects.
  - ▪ The initial dose of hydrocortisone is 50–100 mg IV.
  - ▪ Maintenance dosing at 20 mg per hour or 50–100 mg IV every 6–8 hours. It is recommended to not give more than 300 mg per day.
  - ▪ Dexamethasone 4 mg bolus is preferred if rapid adrenocorticotropic hormone stimulation test will be performed.

Sudden Deterioration

- Administer mineralocorticoid
- Vasopressors
  - ▪ If the patient with suspected adrenal insufficiency experiences sudden cardiovascular collapse, adrenal hemorrhage must be considered. Hydrocortisone 100 mg IV should be started and central venous access obtained to give fluids and vasopressors for resuscitation. If the BP does not improve, fludrocortisone can be added. If the patient continues to deteriorate, another cause should be suspected.

Special Circumstances

- **Steroids and sepsis**
  - ○ The most recent meta-analysis evaluating acute management with corticosteroids for sepsis demonstrated an improvement in mortality. Currently, this topic is very controversial. Current guidelines recommend giving steroids in septic patients with hypotension not responsive to vasopressors.

- **Chronic adrenal insufficiency and sepsis**
  - ○ Patients with known adrenal insufficiency or chronic corticosteroid use should receive hydrocortisone to generate an appropriate stress response to sepsis. If the BP is stable, 50 mg of hydrocortisone is probably appropriate.
- **Chronic adrenal insufficiency and procedures**
  - ○ Patients with chronic adrenal insufficiency who need to have moderate sedation or a significant procedure in the emergency department should also receive 50–100 mg of hydrocortisone prior to the procedure.
  - ○ Etomidate is a first-line agent used in rapid sequence intubation, which may decrease available cortisol. The clinical relevance of this adrenal suppression is still under debate. Some studies show no difference in outcome, while some smaller studies have linked etomidate to a higher risk of pneumonia in trauma patients (56% versus 26%).
- **HIV and AIDS**
  - ○ Adrenal insufficiency has been seen in 5–20% of tested patients with HIV. This may be from HIV-related infection or associated therapeutic agents (megestrol, rifampin, ketoconazole). Autopsies of AIDS patients reveals adrenal injury in > 50% of cases.
- **Pregnancy**
  - ○ Most women with primary adrenal insufficiency are able to undergo healthy pregnancy, labor and delivery. They may require adjustment of glucocorticoid doses, especially during labor.
  - ○ During labor, adequate saline hydration and 25 mg hydrocortisone should be administered intravenously q6 hours. During delivery, 100 mg q6 or a continuous infusion can be given. After delivery, the dose can be rapidly tapered to maintenance within 3 days.

Vasopressor of choice: norepinephrine.

BIBLIOGRAPHY

Annane BE. Corticosteroids in the treatment of severe sepsis and septic shock in adults: a systematic review. *JAMA* 2009;301:2362–2375.

Fang F, Zhang Y, Tang J, et al. Association of corticosteroid treatment with outcomes in adult patients with sepsis: a systematic review and meta-analysis. *JAMA Intern Med* 2019;179(2):213–223. https://doi.org/10.1001/jamainternmed.2018.5849

Salvatori R. Adrenal insufficiency. *JAMA* 2005;294:2481–2488.

Torrey SP. Recognition and management of adrenal emergencies. *Emerg Med Clin North Am* 2005;23:687–702, viii.

Zull D. Thyroid and adrenal disorders. In: Marx JA, Hockberger RS, Walls RM, et al., eds. *Rosen's Emergency Medicine: Concepts and Clinical Practice*, 7th ed. Philadelphia, PA: Mosby Elsevier, 2010.

SECTION 10

Environmental Emergencies

CHRISTIAN RENNE

43

. . . .

Anaphylaxis

DAVID CONVISSAR

Chapter 43:
Anaphylaxis

 ## Presentation

Warmth, tingling, urticaria, abdominal pain, nausea, chest tightness, respiratory distress, facial swelling, light-headedness.

Critical: Advancing to stridor, hypersalivation, hypotension, loss of consciousness.

Known allergy/recent history of allergen exposure.

 ## Diagnosis and Evaluation

Clinical diagnosis.

CBC, BMP, ECG, CXR, and serial blood gasses may be used to assess severity/guide treatment.

 ## Management

Airway Management.

Bronchodilators.

Antihistamines.

 Pharmacological Interventions.

- *Epinephrine IM or IV (Most Important!)*
  - *IM 0.3–0.5 mg 1:1000 concentration.*
  - *IV continuous infusion to maintain a MAP > 65 mmHg, 1–10 mcg/min, titrate for response.*

***DO NOT ADMINISTER CARDIAC ARREST DOSE (1 mg of 1:10,000 IV).

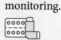 Fluid resuscitation and hemodynamic monitoring.

 Corticosteroids–slower onset of action, but can use to mitigate persistent reactions.

 ## Consider This

- Patients on beta blockers may be refractory to epi and require glucagon administration. Always give with antiemetic.

Introduction

- Anaphylaxis is a life-threatening allergic syndrome characterized by multi-organ involvement and rapid onset which can lead to life-threatening airway compromise and cardiovascular collapse.
- Anaphylaxis is an IgE-mediated (type I or immediate) hypersensitivity reaction, resulting in mast cell degranulation and release of mediators including histamine and cytokines. The release of these chemical mediators results in a constellation of symptoms within 30 minutes of exposure.
- The term *anaphylactoid reaction* describes a similar clinical syndrome that is not mediated by IgE. However, the clinical presentation and treatment are identical.
- There are approximately 100,000 cases of anaphylaxis each year in the United States where the mortality is approximately 1%.
- Foods and medications are among the most common causative agents (Table 43.1); however, the offending agent is not identified in up to 1/3 of cases.
- Other etiologies may mimic the presentation of anaphylaxis (Table 43.2), although they usually lack the multi-system involvement seen in anaphylaxis.

Table 43.1 Etiologies of anaphylaxis

Foods: nuts, shellfish, eggs, cow's milk, soy, wheat, fruits

Antibiotics: penicillin, cephalosporins, sulfonamides, nitrofurantoin, tetracycline
Other therapeutics: methylparaben, rabies vaccine, egg-based vaccines

Insect stings
Latex

Heterologous and human sera
Local anesthetics (ester family)

Direct mast cell degranulation: radiocontrast media, opiates, curare, protamine
Immune complex-mediated: whole blood, immunoglobulins

Arachidonic acid metabolism: aspirin, NSAIDs, benzoates
Physical factors: exercise, temperature

Idiopathic

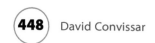

Table 43.2 Differential diagnoses

Flush syndromes: alcohol-induced, scombroidosis, carcinoid syndrome
Stridor: epiglottitis, retropharyngeal or peritonsillar abscess, laryngeal spasm, foreign body
Dyspnea: acute asthma exacerbation, COPD exacerbation, mucus plug, pneumothorax, pulmonary embolism
Syncope: vasovagal, seizure, hypoglycemia, cardiac dysrhythmia, stroke, acute coronary syndrome
Shock: sepsis, spinal shock, cardiogenic, hypovolemic

Presentation

Classic Presentation

- The severity of the presentation may vary depending on a number of factors including the degree of hyper-sensitivity, the quantity and route of exposure, and the sensitivity and responsiveness of the target organs.
- Rapid onset of symptoms (5–30 minutes) after exposure.
  - Generalized warmth and tingling of the face, mouth, chest, hands, and areas of exposure.
  - Pruritis
  - Flushing
  - Urticarial rash (hives)
  - Nasal congestion, sneezing, tearing.
  - Crampy abdominal pain, nausea, vomiting, diarrhea, tenesmus.
  - Cough, chest tightness, dyspnea, and wheezing.
  - Lightheadedness or syncope.

Critical Presentation

True anaphylaxis entails an allergic response with evidence of end-organ dysfunction: e.g., airway, breathing, circulatory, neurologic compromise. To that end, presentation may include:

- **Airway:** Hoarseness, stridor, and hypersalivation secondary to oropharyngeal/laryngeal edema and swelling.

- **Breathing:** Coughing, wheezing, decreased air entry secondary to diffuse bronchoconstriction.
- **Circulatory:** Refractory hypotension and tachycardia secondary to circulatory collapse from diffuse vasodilation, and increased vascular permeability; dysrhythmias may also occur.
- **Neurologic:** Altered mental status, loss of consciousness, or seizure may occur secondary to decreased cerebral perfusion in the setting of shock.
- **Hematologic:** Fibrinolysis and disseminated intravascular coagulation, manifesting as abnormal bleeding or bruising, may develop as the reaction continues.

Diagnosis and Evaluation

- Anaphylaxis is a clinical diagnosis. However, some laboratory tests may be helpful in evaluating the severity of the reaction, guide treatment, and rule out concurrent emergencies.
- Laboratory studies: complete blood count (CBC), complete metabolic panel (CMP).
- Electrocardiogram (ECG) to rule out dysrhythmias.
- Chest radiograph.
- Depending on the clinical situation: cardiac enzymes, serial blood gases, cultures, computed tomography (CT) of the head, neck soft tissue radiographs, indirect or direct laryngoscopy.
- Serum tryptase if there is diagnostic uncertainty (although this is most useful for outpatient follow-up as the results do not come back in in real-time).

Critical Management

- Most fatalities occur within 30 minutes of antigen exposure.
- The rapidity of symptom onset after exposure is usually indicative of the severity of the reaction.

Critical Management Checklist

☑ Epinephrine IM or IV
☑ Airway management

☑ Volume resuscitation
☑ Epinephrine IV to maintain **MAP > 65 mmHg**
☑ Bronchodilators for wheezing
☑ Systemic corticosteroids (delay to effect ~ 4 hours)

- **Initial steps**
  - Secure the airway via endotracheal intubation if indicated based on evidence of stridor, or angioedema.
    - It is critical to have backup airway tools available including a video laryngoscope and surgical airway equipment as oral and laryngeal swelling may result in inability to successfully place the endotracheal tube from the mouth.
  - Remove the offending agent if still present.
  - Obtain adequate intravenous (IV) access and begin crystalloid administration.
  - Cardiac monitoring, pulse oximetry.
- **Interventions**
  - Epinephrine is the primary treatment of anaphylaxis and is indicated in all cases with suspected airway, breathing, or circulatory compromise.
    - The route of epinephrine administration depends on the severity of the clinical presentation.
    - For most cases of anaphylaxis, epinephrine should be administered intramuscularly (IM); the adult dose is **0.3–0.5 mL** of **1:1,000** concentration.
    - Indications for **IV epinephrine** include severe upper airway obstruction, acute respiratory failure, or systolic BP < 80 mmHg. Patients receiving epinephrine should be placed on cardiac monitors.
    - IV epinephrine is most safely and efficaciously administered as a **continuous infusion.**
    - For patients with imminent cardiovascular collapse, provide a loading dose with the infusion at 20 mcg/min for 2 minutes and then rapidly down-titrate (to < 10 mcg/min) as able.
    - For less-severe patients, the infusion can be titrated to improvement of symptoms from 1 to 10 mcg/min.
    - Much confusion exists over proper epinephrine dosing: **extreme care must be taken not to mistakenly administer the cardiac arrest dose (1 mg of 1:10,000 concentration) in anaphylaxis, as it may lead to potentially lethal cardiac and hypertensive complications.**

- If an IV epinephrine infusion cannot be initiated quickly or there is provider unfamiliarity with this method, give epinephrine IM without delay.
- **Antihistamines** such as diphenhydramine should also be administered.
  - H2 antagonists such as famotidine and rantidine have been shown to potentiate the effect of H1 antagonists and can be used as well.
- **Inhaled beta-agonists** may be used for bronchospasm refractory to epinephrine. In cases of severe bronchospasm, inhaled medications may be less efficacious due to inability to penetrate to the lower obstructed airway. Nonetheless, epinephrine is always the mainstay of therapy.
- **Systemic corticosteroids** are of limited benefit in the acute treatment of anaphylaxis as the onset of action is approximately 4–6 hours; however, they may be useful for persistent bronchospasm and to prevent delayed reactions.
- Patients on beta-blockers may be refractory to epinephrine. In these cases, **glucagon** may be used to counteract the beta-blockade (1–5 mg IV over 5 minutes, followed by 5–15 micrograms/minute by continuous infusion). Due to glucagon's common side effect of vomiting, consider pre-treating with an antiemetic such as ondansetron.
- **Airway considerations:** In the setting of critical anaphylaxis, the airway may be compromised due to hypersalivation as well as oropharyngeal and laryngeal edema. Video laryngoscopy or, depending on the degree of stridor, fiberoptic intubation may be employed. Preparations should always be made for cricothyrotomy as a backup plan in these high-risk airways.
- **Disposition**
  - Most patients with mild to moderate anaphylaxis who respond appropriately to initial treatment may be discharged home.
  - Due to the potential for rebound reaction, patients should be observed for 2–6 hours prior to discharge, depending on the severity of the reaction.
  - Patients should be provided with oral antihistamines and corticosteroid therapy for 7–10 days.
  - Indications for admission include any persistent/recurrent hypotension, upper airway involvement or prolonged bronchospasm.
  - Prior to discharge, every patient with anaphylaxis should be prescribed a **home epinephrine auto injector.**

Sudden Deterioration

- **Hypotension**
  - Additional crystalloid should be considered; colloid solutions such as 5% albumin may also be considered given the increased vascular permeability involved in anaphylaxis, though there are no data to support this.
  - If hypotension persists, vasopressor should be added.
  - Epinephrine infusion is the vasopressor of choice.
- **Airway compromise**
  - Airway swelling refractory to IV epinephrine necessitates emergent airway management, which may be attempted fiberoptically (oral or nasal) but should ALWAYS occur in tandem with a double setup for potential surgical airway.

BIBLIOGRAPHY

Anchor J, & Settipane RA. Appropriate use of epinephrine in anaphylaxis. *Am J Emerg Med* 2004;22:488–490.

Gavalas M, Sadana A, & Metcalf A. Guidelines for the management of anaphylaxis in the emergency department. *J Accid Emerg Med* 1998;15:96–98.

Kanwar M, Irvin CB, Frank JJ, et al. Confusion about epinephrine dosing leading to iatrogenic overdose: a life-threatening problem with a potential solution. *Ann Emerg Med* 2010;55:341–344.

Marx JA, Hockberger RS, Walls RM, et al, eds. *Rosen's Emergency Medicine: Concepts and Clinical Practice*, 7th ed. Philadelphia, PA: Mosby Elsevier, 2010.

Hyperthermia

AMY CAGGIULA AND DANIEL HERBERT-COHEN

Introduction

- Body temperature usually follows a diurnal fluctuation, going from a baseline of around 36°C in the morning, to 37.5°C in the late afternoon at rest.
- The human body has many physiological compensatory mechanisms such as shivering and sweating for maintaining a state of thermal homeostasis.
- Occasionally these mechanisms become overwhelmed resulting in a continuum of heat-related injuries and illnesses.
- Heat edema, syncope, cramps, and exhaustion comprise the milder manifestations of temperature illness. This chapter will focus on the more critical presentations of hyperthermia, including **heatstroke** and **toxicological hyperthermia**.

Heatstroke

Overview

- Two main pathophysiological mechanisms exist:
  1. *Classic heatstroke:* Occurs during heat waves and is most commonly observed in the elderly, debilitated patients, psychiatric patients, and young children. These patients may not have easy access to oral fluids or may be taking medications that impair their body's ability to respond appropriately to increases in temperature. Additionally, these populations can lack sufficient physiologic thermoregulatory responses to increased ambient temperature.
     - Medications predisposing to heat illnesses include neuroleptics, sympathomimetics, diuretics, anticholinergics, and antihypertensive agents that diminish the compensatory cardiovascular response to heat exposure.
  2. *Exertional heatstroke:* Generally seen in young, healthy patients and athletes such as distance runners and military personnel training in hot climates. These patients' heat-dispelling mechanisms are usually overwhelmed by endogenous heat production.
- Differential diagnosis for heatstroke
  - Sepsis
  - Meningitis/encephalitis
  - Malignant hyperthermia (MH)
  - Neuroleptic malignant syndrome (NMS)
  - Serotonin syndrome
  - Toxins/drugs
  - Thyroid storm
  - Pheochromocytoma
  - Intracranial hemorrhage

Presentation

Classic Presentation

- Elevated core temperature ($> 40.5°C$).
- Central nervous system (CNS) dysfunction such as confusion, delirium, agitation, psychosis, ataxia, coma, seizures, and posturing.
- Elevated transaminases

- Acid–base disturbances:
  - ○ Lactic acidosis is more frequently seen among victims of exertional heat-stroke due to the increase in aerobic glycolysis occurring during strenuous physical activity and associated adrenergic surge.
  - ○ Primary respiratory alkalosis with little or no metabolic acidosis is usually observed in sufferers of classic heatstroke.
- Impaired sweating leading to impaired evaporation contribute to the development and exacerbation of heatstroke. Medications that inhibit sweating such as anticholinergics intensify heat-related injury. However, the presence of sweating should not be used as exclusion criteria for the diagnosis of heatstroke, as anhidrosis is common but not universal in these patients.

Critical Presentation

- Elevated creatine phosphokinase (CPK), rhabdomyolysis, and acute renal failure are more commonly seen in exertional heatstroke.
- Hypotension from peripheral vasodilation and dehydration can occur as well.
- Coagulopathy and disseminated intravascular coagulation (DIC) presenting as gastrointestinal bleeding, genitourinary bleeding, petechiae, purpura, epistaxis, hemoptysis, or oozing from venipuncture sites.

Diagnosis and Evaluation

- A rectal temperature should be obtained on all patients with a concern for hyperthermia.
- Helpful laboratory tests include:
  - ○ Comprehensive metabolic panel to assess electrolyte abnormalities and renal function.
  - ○ CPK to assess for rhabdomyolysis.
  - ○ Liver function tests.
  - ○ Coagulation studies including fibrinogen if there is suspicion for DIC.
  - ○ pH from arterial or venous blood gas to help determine severity of illness.
- A head CT followed by lumbar puncture can be performed in patients presenting with any hyperthermia and neurological dysfunction in whom the diagnosis of heatstroke is less likely and when risk factors for heat-related illness are not present.

Critical Management

- The goal of treatment is **to rapidly decrease the core temperature** to less than 40°C. A urinary or rectal temperature probe should be placed for continuous monitoring of core body temperature.
- The rapidity of cooling cannot be stressed enough; the magnitude of organ dysfunction increases with time spent hyperthermic. As such, hyperthermia should be considered a truly time-sensitive emergency and cooling measures should be initiated **before** any investigations into the hyperthermia etiology.
  - Cooling can be initiated in the field by placing ice packs on the patient's neck, groin, and axillae until more effective cooling measures are available.
  - Various methods may be utilized but evaporative cooling and ice water immersion remain the mainstays of management.
  - **Evaporative cooling** is quick and effective. The patient is sprayed with room temperature water and positioned under large fans to simulate the body's own response to heat.
  - **Ice water immersion** is also common and the quickest method for lowering body temperature rapidly. Benzodiazepines can be administered to prevent shivering. If no ice water bath is available, the patient can be placed in a body bag filled with ice and cold water, leaving the head portion of the bag open.
  - Central cooling has been employed to some benefit. These methods include cold intravenous fluids, cardiopulmonary bypass, and peritoneal, gastric, and bladder lavage. These methods are invasive and labor intensive, however, and their efficacy when compared with standard measures is unknown. They are thus often used as adjuncts to evaporative or immersion cooling.
  - Cooling should be stopped when the body temperature decreases below 40°C in order to avoid a hypothermic overshoot.

- ○ Antipyretics such as acetaminophen and NSAIDs play no role in noninfectious hyperthermia and should be avoided.

Sudden Deterioration

- Airway management is the initial priority, and endotracheal intubation is often indicated in the altered or seizing patient. These patients are at high risk for aspiration, particularly if they present with persistent seizures or severe central nervous system (CNS) manifestations.
- Given the possibility of rhabdomyolysis and associated hyperkalemia in patients suffering from exertional heatstroke, a nondepolarizing muscle relaxant (e.g., rocuronium) should be used for rapid sequence intubation (RSI).
- Initiate fluid resuscitation with crystalloids if the patient is hypotensive or presents with signs of rhabdomyolysis. A urinary catheter should be placed to titrate fluid administration to a urine output of 1–1.5 mL/kg/hour.
- Persistent anuria, uremia, or hyperkalemia are indications for consideration of hemodialysis.

Malignant Hyperthermia

Overview

- Malignant hyperthermia (MH) is a disease state occasionally observed in patients undergoing **general anesthesia.**
- An inherited autosomal dominant disorder predisposes to excessive calcium release from the sarcoplasmic reticulum of skeletal muscles, resulting in hyper-metabolism and hyperthermia.
- While this condition is most often seen in the operating room because of its association with inhaled anesthetic gases such as halothane, it can also be precipitated by **succinylcholine** which is frequently used for airway management in the emergency department.

Presentation

Classic/Critical presentation

- Malignant hyperthermia presents during or shortly after exposure to inhaled anesthetic agents such as halothane, sevoflurane, and desflurane, or the depolarizing muscle relaxant succinylcholine.

- The **hypercatabolic state** results in rapid-onset, severe hyperthermia ($> 40.5°C$), tachycardia, and tachypnea.
- Muscular rigidity, metabolic acidosis, and rising end-tidal CO_2 are also classic early findings.
- Patients can also have altered mental status, autonomic instability (including arrhythmias), rhabdomyolysis, and DIC.

Diagnosis and Evaluation

- The diagnosis of MH should be suspected in the individual exposed to inhaled anesthetics or succinylcholine who develops the constellation of **hyperthermia, rising end-tidal CO_2** (due to chest wall rigidity), and **muscle rigidity.**
- Additional investigations can help diagnose any associated complications but play no role in the diagnosis of MH and should therefore not delay essential interventions.

Critical Management

Critical Management Checklist

☑ Discontinue offending agent
☑ Airway & ventilatory management as needed with **nondepolarizing** paralytics
☑ Cooling measures
☑ Supportive care with benzodiazepines
☑ Administer dantrolene 2.5 mg/kg IV q5 mins up to 10 mg/kg IV

- Discontinue the offending agent.
- Initiate cooling measures as described above.
- Provide sedation and muscle relaxation using **benzodiazepines**.
- Certain patients will need to be mechanically ventilated in order to assist ventilation and help overcome chest stiffness.
  - ○ N.B. Since malignant hyperthermia is due to an intrinsic problem with the muscle cells, neuromuscular blockade will provide no benefit in these patients.
  - ○ A nondepolarizing paralytic agent can be used to improve intubation conditions, although it is unlikely to result in complete muscle relaxation in these patients.
- Assess for rhabdomyolysis and manage electrolyte abnormalities.

- **Dantrolene 2.5 mg/kg intravenously (IV)** will decrease the amount of calcium released from the sarcoplasmic reticulum of muscle cells. This bolus can be repeated every 5 minutes until the signs of MH are reversed, or up to a cumulative dose of 10 mg/kg IV.

Neuroleptic Malignant Syndrome

Overview

- Neuroleptic malignant syndrome (NMS) is a pathological condition in which hyperthermia is encountered due to excessive blockage of dopaminergic receptors by some antipsychotics, as well as by withdrawal of dopaminergic drugs.

Presentation

Classic/Critical Presentation

- It most often presents within the first few weeks of starting antipsychotic medications but can present earlier (after as little as one dose) or after years of consistent treatment.
- NMS is classically seen with "typical" neuroleptics such as haloperidol or fluphenazine but can also be seen with "atypical" neuroleptics such as clozapine or risperidone.
- Typical features:
  - Fever with altered mentation (e.g., agitation, delirium, catatonia).
  - Neuromuscular abnormalities often described as **"lead pipe rigidity"** due to increased muscle tone.
  - Autonomic instability:
    - Life-threatening hyperthermia
    - Hypertension or hypotension
  - Rhabdomyolysis
- Other abnormalities:
  - Arrhythmias, cardiomyopathy or myocardial infarction
  - Electrolyte abnormalities
  - Acute renal/hepatic failure
  - Hypercarbic respiratory failure from chest wall rigidity
  - Coagulopathies and DIC

Diagnosis and Evaluation

- NMS is a clinical diagnosis. Remember the **FEVER** mnemonic: **F**ever, **E**ncephalopathy, **V**ital sign instability, **E**levated enzymes (CPK), **R**igidity.
- Medication history is crucial to make the diagnosis.
- Appropriate workup for sepsis, encephalitis, or meningitis should be considered.
- Computed tomography (CT) of the brain is indicated as well as lumbar puncture if the diagnosis is not certain.

Critical Management

Critical Management Checklist

- ☑ Discontinue offending agent
- ☑ Airway & ventilatory management as needed with **nondepolarizing paralytics**
- ☑ Cooling measures
- ☑ Supportive care with benzodiazepines
- ☑ Consider bromocriptine 2.5–5 mg PO q6–12 hours

- Discontinue the offending drug.
- Initiate cooling measures.
- Administer sedation and muscle relaxation using benzodiazepines.
- Neuromuscular blockade can be used for refractory hyperthermia or for airway management.
- Assess for rhabdomyolysis and manage electrolyte abnormalities.
- **Bromocriptine** has central dopaminergic agonist effects and can be used in patients with refractory symptoms. It is only available as an oral formulation and therefore a nasogastric tube will have to be placed for administration if the patient is intubated or at risk for aspiration. It is given in doses of 2.5–5 mg PO every 6–12 hours.

Serotonin Syndrome

Overview

- Serotonin syndrome is caused by excessive stimulation of serotonin receptors.
- It is usually precipitated by medication changes such as:
  - Addition of a new serotonergic agent
  - Increase in dosage of usual medications
  - Overdose

Presentation

Classic/Critical Presentation

- **Classic triad**
  - Cognitive effects: altered mental status, agitation, delirium, hallucinations.
  - Autonomic effects: hyperthermia, shivering, sweating, hypertension, tachycardia, nausea, vomiting, diarrhea.
  - Somatic effects: hyperreflexia, and clonus (more prominent in the lower extremities).
- **Other abnormalities**
  - Rhabdomyolysis
  - Acute renal failure
  - Seizures
  - Coagulopathies and DIC

Diagnosis and Evaluation

- The Hunter criteria (Table 44.1) can help make the diagnosis of serotonin syndrome. To meet the Hunter criteria, a patient must have recently taken a serotonergic agent and present with at least one symptom presented in the table below.

Table 44.1 Hunter criteria

Spontaneous clonus

Inducible clonus *plus* agitation or diaphoresis

Ocular clonus *plus* agitation or diaphoresis

Tremor *plus* hyperreflexia

Hypertonia *plus* temperature above 38°C *plus* ocular clonus or inducible clonus

Table 44.2 Serotonin syndrome (SS) versus neuroleptic malignant syndrome (NMS)

	SS	NMS
Onset	24 hours	Days to weeks
Precipitating medications	Serotonergic agents (e.g., SSRIs, MAOIs, meperidine, linezolid, psychoactive drugs of abuse)	Antipsychotics (e.g., phenothiazines, butyrophenones, thioxanthines)
Mechanism of action	Stimulation of serotonin receptors	Dopamine blockade
Neuromuscular abnormality	Clonus	Rigidity
Specific treatment	Cyproheptadine	Bromocriptine

Abbreviations: MAOI, monoamine oxidase inhibitor; SSRI, selective serotonin re-uptake inhibitor.

- Patients usually present with clonus that is more prominent in the lower extremities. This clinical finding as well as certain historical clues can help to differentiate serotonin syndrome from neuroleptic malignant syndrome (see Table 44.2).
- Sepsis, encephalitis, or meningitis should be in the differential diagnosis of all these patients, especially because rigors and myoclonus can often look similar. A sepsis workup should be initiated.
- Consider computed tomography of the brain as well as lumbar puncture.

Critical Management

Critical Management Checklist

☑ Discontinue offending agent
☑ Airway & ventilatory management as needed with **nondepolarizing** paralytics

☑ Cooling measures
☑ Fluid resuscitation
☑ Supportive care with benzodiazepines
☑ Consider cyproheptadine 12 mg PO and 2 mg q 2 hours to effect

- Discontinue the offending drug.
- Initiate cooling measures as described above.
- Patients should be supported with intravenous fluids aimed at treating dehydration and normalizing vital signs.
- Benzodiazepines should be administered to help decrease motor tone.
- Assess for rhabdomyolysis and managed electrolyte abnormalities.
- Neuromuscular blockade can be used for refractory hyperthermia or for airway management.
- Cyproheptadine has nonspecific serotonin antagonism effects and can be used in patients with refractory symptoms. While the classic antidote for serotonin syndrome, many toxicologists feel only supportive care with benzodiazepines is necessary. It is only available as an oral formulation and therefore a nasogastric tube will have to be placed for administration if the patient is intubated or at risk for aspiration. It is given as an initial dose of 12 mg PO (via NG) followed by 2 mg every 2 hours pending patient improvement.

Vasopressor of choice: Patients with hypotension associated with hyperthermia can exhibit either a hypodynamic state with low cardiac index, or a hyperdynamic state with decreased systemic vascular resistance. A clinical assessment of the patient complemented by an evaluation of the cardiac function by ultrasound will help determine whether the patient would benefit more from additional fluids, a vasopressor (i.e., norepinephrine), or an inotrope (i.e., epinephrine).

BIBLIOGRAPHY

Boyer EW, & Shannon M. The serotonin syndrome. *N Engl J Med* 2005;352:1112–1120.

Epstein Y, & Yanovich R. Heatstroke. *N Engl J Med* 2019;380(25):2449–2459.

Gaudio FG, & Grissom CK. Cooling methods in heat stroke. *J Emerg Med* 2016;50(4): 607–616.

Gauer R, Meyers BK. Heat-related illnesses. *Am Family Physician* 2019;99(8):482–489.

Litman RS, Smith VI, Larach MG, et al. Consensus Statement of the Malignant Hyperthermia Association of the United States on Unresolved Clinical Questions Concerning the Management of Patients with Malignant Hyperthermia. *Anesth Analg* 2019;128(4):652–659.

Sloan BK, Kraft EM, Clark D, et al. On-site treatment of exertional heat stroke. *Am J Sports Med* 2015;43(4):823–829.

Hypothermia

SHAN MODI

Introduction

- Hypothermia is defined as a **core temperature below 35°C (95°F).**
- **Primary hypothermia** occurs when the body is exposed to a cold environment that overwhelms the body's compensatory mechanisms to heat loss such as increased muscle tone, shivering, and vasoconstriction.
- **Secondary hypothermia** is due to the body being unable to maintain normothermia due to a medical condition such as hypothyroidism, adrenal insufficiency, or hypoglycemia.
- Secondary hypothermia is often refractory to rewarming techniques and requires treatment of the underlying medical condition.

Presentation

Classic Presentation

- Presentation can be classified using the Swiss staging system (Table 45.1).

Table 45.1 Swiss staging system for hypothermia

Stage	Body temperature	Presentation
I (Mild)	32–35°C	Alert and shivering
II (Moderate)	28–32°C	Altered ± shivering
III (Severe)	24–28°C	Unconscious
IV (Severe)	< 24°C	No vital signs

- **Mild Hypothermia** – from 32°C to 35°C:
  - Patient usually will be alert and oriented.
  - Can present with vague complaints including nausea, myalgias, and fatigue.
  - Shivering and increased muscle tone occur for thermogenesis.
  - Tachycardia, and tachypnea are often present.
  - Peripheral vasoconstriction can lead to hypertension and cold diuresis.

Critical Presentation

- **Moderate Hypothermia** – from 28°C to 32°C:
  - Patient will be lethargic or obtunded.
  - Hyporeflexia and unreactive pupils can occur from CNS depression.
  - **The likelihood of dysrhythmias increases** (most common is atrial fibrillation).
  - Bradycardia, bradypnea, and hypotension begin to occur.
- **Severe Hypothermia** – less than 28°C:
  - Patient will be unresponsive.
  - Increased susceptibility to junctional dysrhythmia (ventricular fibrillation).
  - Areflexia occurs with further CNS depression.
  - Progressive decrease in cardiac output with increased pulmonary congestion leads to cardiopulmonary collapse.

Diagnosis and Evaluation

- **Measure core temperature** using a rectal thermometer, a temperature-sensing Foley catheter, or esophageal thermometer.

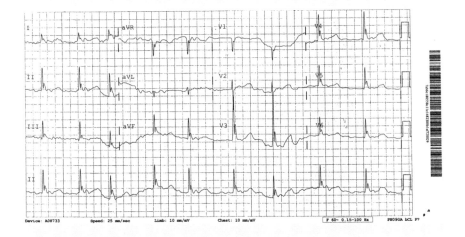

Figure 45.1 ECG of a patient with hypothermia and Osborn waves.

- Hypothermia is often a clinical diagnosis however it is important to ascertain the cause of why patient had prolonged exposure to a cold environment. For example, a patient could be obtunded from slipping on ice leading to an ICH with concomitant hypothermia.
- **Laboratory studies**: Finger stick glucose, complete blood count (CBC), basic metabolic panel, coagulation studies, thyroid function tests, cortisol levels, blood cultures.
  - Can assist in determining causes for secondary hypothermia.
  - **Serial basic metabolic panels should be performed during rewarming** due to severe electrolyte derangements in hypothermic patient (**hyperkalemia).**
  - Coagulation studies often falsely normal due to requirement to rewarm sample for analysis.
- **ECG:** Typically progresses from sinus bradycardia with Osborn (J) waves (Figure 45.1) to atrial fibrillation (with slow ventricular response) and then ventricular fibrillation.
- **Imaging Studies:**
  - Chest X-ray: may show pulmonary edema secondary to cardiorespiratory collapse.
  - Bedside ultrasound: Can be used as an adjunct to assess cardiac function in moderate to severe hypothermia.
  - CT Scan: Can be obtained in relation to clinical presentation (e.g., trauma).

Table 45.2 Rewarming modality with hypothermia severity

Stage	Rewarming modality
I (Mild)	Passive rewarming
II (Moderate)	Active external rewarming and minimally invasive rewarming
III (Severe)	Active internal rewarming
IV (Severe)	Active internal rewarming ± ACLS

Critical Management

See "Critical Management Checklist" and Table 45.2.

> ## Critical Management Checklist
> ☑ Airway and ventilatory support as needed
> ☑ Remove wet clothing
> ☑ For mild hypothermia, initiate passive rewarming
> ☑ For moderate hypothermia, actively rewarm trunk then extremities
> ☑ For severe hypothermia, consider early ECMO or CVVH

- **Initial approach**
  - Secure the airway if necessary.
  - Remove wet clothing.
  - Obtain intravenous (IV) access.
  - Start cardiac monitoring and temperature monitoring.
- **Passive rewarming**
  - Indicated for **mild hypothermia** (32–35°C).
  - Warm environment with warm clothing and blankets.
  - Encourage PO intake of warm sweet drinks to support metabolic demands.
- **Active external rewarming and minimally invasive rewarming**
  - Indicated for **moderate hypothermia** (28–32°C).
  - Apply forced air heating elements (e.g., Bair Hugger) or warming blankets.
  - Start warmed intravenous fluids (40°C D5NS preferred in undifferentiated hypothermia to prevent rebound hypoglycemia during rewarming).

- Heated high-flow nasal cannula can be used to increase temperature if the patient is not intubated. Warmed humidified air can be used if patient intubated.
- Heat should be applied initially to trunk before extremities to avoid **core temperature after drop.**
  - Thought to occur when cold blood from the extremities returns to central circulation as peripheral vessels dilate during the rewarming process leading to hypotension.
- **Avoid excessive movement of patient as it can lead to dysrhythmia.**
- **Active internal rewarming**
  - Indicated for **severe hypothermia** ($< 28°C$).
  - Secure airway if not already intubated.
  - Correct any unstable dysrhythmias.
    - Atrial fibrillation/atrial flutter will usually resolve with rewarming.
    - Ventricular fibrillation can occur and is usually refractory until patient is rewarmed, but defibrillation should be attempted.
  - Vasopressor support (norepinephrine) should be initiated as needed for hypotension.
  - **ECMO if available is preferred rewarming modality.**
  - If ECMO unavailable, CVVH or hemodialysis can be performed.
    - Femoral access preferred for temporary dialysis catheter to avoid irritation of myocardium leading to dysrhythmia.
  - If none of the above modalities are available, body cavity lavage via thoracic, GI tract, bladder, or peritoneum can be performed although limited in evidence.
    - Thoracic cavity lavage: Insertion of anterior chest tube with warm fluid infusion and drainage via posteriorly inserted chest tube connected to suction.

Sudden Deterioration

- Hypothermic patients that are deteriorating will need to have their airway managed. There is no contraindication to performing rapid sequence induction (RSI) with the usual drug regimen in these patients.
- Patients who develop pulseless arrhythmias secondary to shockable rhythms should be initially managed by advanced cardiac life support

guidelines. While CPR should be initiated promptly, epinephrine boluses should be avoided absent aystole, and defibrillation should be attempted only when the patient has been rewarmed to more than 30°C.

BIBLIOGRAPHY

Austin MA, Maynes EJ, O'Malley TJ, et al. Outcomes of extracorporeal life support use in accidental hypothermia: a systematic review. *Ann Thorac Surg* 2020;110 (6):1926–1932.

Brown DJA, Brugger H, Boyd J, et al. Accidental hypothermia. *New Engl J Med* 2012;367 (20):1930–1938.

Cline DM. *Tintinalli's Emergency Medicine Manual*, 7th ed. New York, NY: McGraw Hill, 2012.

Duong H, Patel G. Hypothermia. In: *StatPearls*. StatPearls Publishing; 2021. Available at: www.ncbi.nlm.nih.gov/books/NBK545239/

Marx JA, Hockberger RS, Walls RM, et al., eds. *Rosen's Emergency Medicine: Concepts and Clinical Practice*, 7th ed. Philadelphia, PA: Mosby Elsevier, 2010.

McCullough L, Arora S. Diagnosis and treatment of hypothermia. *Am Fam Physician* 2004;70:2325–2332.

Mulcahy A, & Watts M. Accidental hypothermia: an evidence-based approach. *Emerg Med Pract* 2009;11:1.

Sawamoto K, Tanno K, Takeyama Y, et al. Successful treatment of severe accidental hypothermia with cardiac arrest for a long time using cardiopulmonary bypass – report of a case. *Int J Emerg Med* 2012;5.

46

Overdoses

CHRISTOPHER SHAW AND DANIEL HERBERT-COHEN

Chapter 46:
Overdose

❖ Engage pharmacy early

❖ Always rule out coingestions and consult toxicology as needed!

Acetaminophen

Salicylates

 Presentation

24 hours after ingestion: asymptomatic or nausea/malaise.

24-72 hours after ingestion: RUQ pain, rising transaminases, possible hyoptension/ tachycardia.

72-96 hours after ingestion: Signs of liver failure, cerebral edema, AKI, metabolic acidosis, ARDS.

Classic: Tinnitus, vertigo, nausea, hyperventiliation.

Critical: Cerebral edema, noncardiogenic pulmonary edema, AKI, coagulopathy, severe acid-base disturbance.

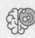

 Associated Lab Value

Serial serum APAP levels, urine pregnancy, CMP, LFTs, coagulation studies, ECG to evaluate for co-ingestion, CT if concern for cerebral edema.

Serial ASA levels, CMP, blood gas (anion-gap metabolic acidosis).

 Principles of Management

Activated charcoal if < 4 hrs since ingestion, N-acetylcysteine based on Rumack-Matthewnomogram and poison control recommendations.

Activated charcoal if < 4 hrs since ingestion and no evidence of GI hemhorrage, sodium bicarbonate, consider need for RRT, adjust ventilation to compensate for metabolic acidemia.

 Notes

Sudden Deterioration: Consider hypoglycemia, AKI/Electrolyte derangments, cerebral edema.

Considered high-risk intubation: administer bolus dextrose and sodium bicarbonate prior to intubation even in euglycemia, Be aware of risk for GI bleeding.

Chapter 46:
Overdose

Tricyclic Antidepressants | Digoxin

 Presentation

 Classic: Anti-cholinergic toxidrome, ECG changes.

 Critical: Seizures, arrhythmia, coma, shock.

 Classic: Headache, nausea, lethargy, visual disturbance, PVCs.

 Critical: Hyperkalemia, ventricular arrythmias, delirium, seizures.

 Associated Lab Value

 Blood gas, CMP, ECG may reveal: widened QRS, broad terminal R wave in avR, right axis deviation.

 Electrolytes, ECG (classic digitalis changes do not necessarily indicate toxicity), note drug levels drawn < 6 hrs post ingestion may be inaccurate and high drug levels alone are not diagnostic of toxicity.

 Principles of Management

 Activated charcoal if < 2 hrs since ingestion, fluids/vasopressors as needed, sodium bicarbonate, benzodiazepines as needed for seizures.

 Activated charcoal if < 2 hrs since ingestion.

 Correct hypokalemia (Target: 4.0-5.0 mmol/L) before adimistration of antidigoxin Fab.

Notes

✿ IV lipid emulsion in cardiac arrest/severe shock, physostigmine contraindicated despite anticholinergic syndrome,

✿ Avoid phenytoin, fosphenytoin, and Class IA/IC antiarrythmics.

✿ In cardiac arrest, administer ACLS for at least 30 minutes after 20 vials of antidigoxin Fab have been administered.

✿ Monitor for anaphylaxis and recurrence of toxicity 24-72 hours post-administration of antidigoxin Fab.

✿ *Digitalis toxicity is common given low TI, note presence of precipitating event (i.e. kidney failure, drug regimen change).*

Chapter 46:
Overdose

Calcium Channel Blockers	Beta-Blockers

 Presentation

 Classic: Hypotension with relatively clear mental status, hyperglycemia, early reflex tachycardia (dihydropyridines).

 Critical: Symptomatic bradycardia, hypotension, pulmonary edema, cardiogenic shock.

 May be asymptomatic in young healthy patient, or present as bradycardia, hypotension, respiratory depression, seizures, coma.

 Associated Lab Value

 ECG (intervals may be normal), CMP, POCT glucose.

 ECG (intervals may be normal), CMP, POCT glucose.

 Principles of Management

 Activated charcoal if < 2 hrs since ingestion, glucagon and atropine for symptomatic bradycardia, calcium chloride/gluconate, pressor as needed, **high dose insulin euglycemia therapy.**

 Activated charcoal if < 2 hrs since ingestion, glucagon and atropine for symptomatic bradycardia, calcium chloride/gluconate, pressor as needed, **high dose insulin euglycemia therapy.**

 Notes

- ✿ Administer IV lipid emulsion in cardiac arrest or hemodynamic instability.

- ✿ Closely monitor potassium and blood glucose during HIET.

- ✿ Consider ECMO, methylene blue, and/or plasma exchange in refractory instability.

- ✿ Administer IV lipid emulsion in cardiac arrest or hemodynamic instability.

- ✿ Closely monitor potassium and blood glucose during HIET.

- ✿ Consider ECMO in refractory instability.

Introduction

- Many common medications are toxic when taken at higher dosages.
- Ingestions can be accidental or a suicidal gesture.
- **Patients presenting with intentional ingestion are often unreliable historians; thus collateral information is essential. This may be obtained from family, friends, or emergency medical service personnel and include observed and reported behavior, medication history, or empty pill bottles found at the scene.**
- History and physical examination are crucial to establish a diagnosis and to guide treatment.
- Co-ingestions are common in intentional overdoses, specifically acetaminophen and salicylate, which are commonly available over the counter in multiple preparations.
- Urine toxicology screens do not detect drugs most commonly used in the setting of overdose, are notoriously inaccurate, and rarely contribute meaningfully to the workup of a poisoned patient.
- Patients may become critically ill if not promptly assessed and provided with the appropriate antidote.
- This chapter will cover a selection of common drug overdoses such as acetaminophen, salicylates, tricyclic antidepressants, beta-blockers, calcium channel blockers, and digoxin.

Acetaminophen

Overview

- Acetaminophen (APAP) is the most common medication overdose reported to poison control centers in the United States and is a leading cause of acute liver failure nationally.
- APAP is a common co-ingestant.
- It is rapidly absorbed enterically with peak plasma concentration usually occurring within 4 hours of ingestion, but large overdoses may delay absorption.
- In therapeutic dosing the majority of APAP is metabolized by the liver into harmless conjugates that are excreted in the urine.

- A small percentage is metabolized by cytochrome P450 into NAPQI (*N*-acetyl-*p*-benzoquinone imine), a highly toxic metabolite, which is then reduced to nontoxic conjugates by glutathione.
- In overdose, the normal metabolic pathways are saturated, and thus glutathione is depleted, and NAPQI accumulates, leading to hepatocellular destruction.

Presentation

Classic Presentation

- During phase 1 (0–24 hours after ingestion) patients can be asymptomatic or experience nausea, vomiting, anorexia, or general malaise.
- During phase 2 (24–72 hours after ingestion) patients usually develop right upper quadrant (RUQ) abdominal pain. Serum transaminase levels are continuously rising at this point, and tachycardia and hypotension can be present.

Critical Presentation

- **Critical symptoms generally appear during phase 3 (72–96 hours after ingestion).**
- Hepatic necrosis may produce signs of acute liver injury, including jaundice, coagulopathy, and hypoglycemia, and liver failure (encephalopathy).
- Multisystem organ failure may result, including acute kidney injury, metabolic acidosis, and acute respiratory distress syndrome (ARDS).
- Cerebral edema is an ominous and late finding reflecting severe hepatic encephalopathy.

Diagnosis and Evaluation

- A thorough history is imperative. The time of ingestion and amount of drug taken are both critically important in guiding management.
- Examination findings such as RUQ tenderness, jaundice, altered mental status, or hemodynamic instability suggest a late presentation.

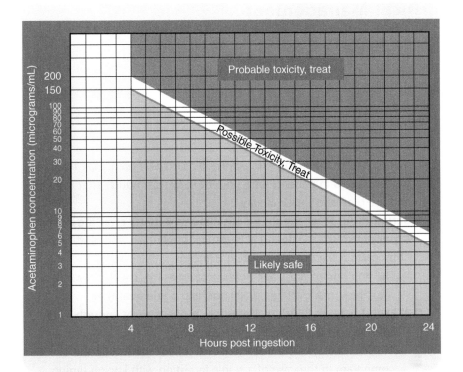

Figure 46.1 Rumack–Matthew nomogram.

(Courtesy of Graham Walker, MD.)

- **Serum APAP level should be plotted on the Rumack-Matthew nomogram in the case of single ingestion with a known time of ingestion** (Figure 46.1).
- 150 mg/kg, or 12 g, is considered a toxic dose of APAP.
- Liver enzymes (ALT, AST), bilirubin, prothrombin time (PT), and international normalized ratio (INR), may initially be normal but will rise over time as liver injury develops.
- Routine imaging has a limited role. If the patient is demonstrating signs of encephalopathy, consider a computed tomography (CT) of the head to evaluate for cerebral edema.
- The electrocardiogram (ECG) is expected to be normal but remains an important screening tool given the frequency of co-ingestion.
- Pregnancy status must be established as acetaminophen freely crosses the placenta.

Critical Management

Critical Management Checklist

- ☑ Airway and ventilatory support as needed
- ☑ Activated charcoal (1 g/kg max 100 g) if < 4 hours since ingestion
- ☑ N-acetylcysteine (NAC) as soon as possible
- ☑ Consultation with transplant center

- Gastric decontamination with activated charcoal (1 g/kg, max 100 g) can be considered in patients who present early (< 4 hours) after ingestion and are protecting their airway.
- **Serum APAP level should be obtained at 4 hours after ingestion**, or at presentation if the timing of ingestion is unknown, and plotted on the nomogram *if the time of ingestion is known.*
  - ○ The nomogram starts at 4 hours post ingestion. Levels drawn prior to the 4-hour mark will generally not help guide treatment.
- ***N*-Acetylcysteine (NAC) is lifesaving, if given early enough, and should be administered for patients with:**
  - ○ APAP level above the treatment line of the Rumack-Matthew nomogram in the case of a single ingestion with known timing.
  - ○ History of APAP ingestion and *any* evidence of acute liver injury.
  - ○ Unknown ingestion time and initial APAP level > 10 mcg/mL.
  - ○ NAC has been shown to completely reverse the effects of an acetaminophen overdose if administered within 8 hours of the ingestion and may reduce morbidity up to 24 hours after ingestion.
- **If a patient presents at 8 hours or later after a suspected toxic ingestion, do not delay treatment while waiting for an acetaminophen level.**
- NAC can be given orally or intravenously (IV). Oral NAC may cause nausea and vomiting, while IV NAC is associated with hypersensitivity reactions in up to 10–20% of patients.
  - ○ If hypersensitivity develops, discontinue the infusion, provide standard management, such as antihistamines, steroids, and epinephrine if evidence of airway, breathing, or circulatory compromise.

Table 46.1 King's College Criteria

---

pH < 7.30 *or* all of the following:

INR > 6.5 (PT > 100 seconds)

Creatinine > 3.4 mg/dL

Grade III or IV hepatic encephalopathy

  ○ The IV route has not been shown to be superior to the oral regimen, but it is usually preferred.
- **Protocols for NAC dosing and duration vary by institution; thus, it is imperative to discuss with a local pharmacist.**
  ○ In the United States 150 mg/kg is the usual loading dose.
  ○ Therapy is discontinued once APAP metabolism is complete (level <10 mcg/mL) and liver injury is resolving (normal or near normal enzymes, absence of encephalopathy or coagulopathy).
- **Consultation with a transplant center** should occur for select high-risk patients according to the King's College Criteria (Table 46.1).

Sudden Deterioration

- Patients with APAP toxicity can develop multi-system organ failure, shock, AKI, and cerebral edema.
- Hypoglycemia is common, often requiring supplemental dextrose infusions.
- Hemodynamic support should be provided with intravenous fluids and a vasopressor (primarily norepinephrine).
- Respiratory support with supplemental oxygen, noninvasive ventilation, or invasive mechanical ventilation, should be instituted as required.
- Patients with evidence of AKI should have electrolytes monitored frequently and corrected. Renal replacement therapy may be required for electrolyte derangements, severe acidemia, or anuria, and should be initiated in consultation with a nephrologist.
  ○ NAC is cleared by dialysis, thus the infusion rate will need to be increased during renal replacement to maintain a therapeutic effect.

- Cerebral edema and imminent herniation should be managed with hyperosmolar therapy, mannitol or hypertonic saline, and potentially intracranial presure monitoring with subsequent cranial decompression if indicated.

Special Circumstances

- APAP crosses the placenta and has been associated with fetal demise, thus treatment with NAC should be pursued in pregnancy for the indications listed above.
- Large one-time ingestions of APAP producing serum levels > 300 mcg/mL should be managed in concert with a toxicologist, as these patients may require alternative NAC dosing regimens.

Salicylates

Overview

- Salicylates, the most common being aspirin (acetylsalicylic acid, ASA), are weak acids that are widely used in various commercially available preparations, including aspirin products, oil of wintergreen, Goody's Powder®, and Pepto-bismol®.
- ASA is rapidly absorbed in its uncharged, nonionized form, in the acidic environment of the stomach.
- At therapeutic doses, the majority of ASA is protein-bound and free molecules are largely ionized, preventing transport into tissue. In overdose, albumin becomes saturated and free ASA concentration increases.
- As acidemia worsens, nonionized ASA increases, promoting penetration into tissues, including the central nervous system (CNS).
- ASA is normally metabolized by the liver through conjugation, but in overdose these pathways become saturated and elimination is dependent on renal excretion, prolonging the half-life.

Presentation

Classic Presentation

- Tinnitus or impaired hearing are common, as are hyperventilation, nausea, vomiting, and vertigo.
- **Classic findings are: respiratory alkalosis (from direct stimulation of the medulla) and an anion gap metabolic acidosis (due to uncoupling of oxidative phosphorylation).**

Critical Presentation

- Cerebral edema resulting in altered mental status, coma, and convulsions
- Noncardiogenic pulmonary edema
- AKI
- Gastrointestinal (GI) hemorrhage and coagulopathy
- Severe acid–base disturbance

Diagnosis and Evaluation

- A thorough history is critical, including the amount of drug taken, drug preparation (i.e., enteric coated, chewable, liquid), the time of ingestion, and any co-ingestions.
- On examination the patient may be hyperthermic, tachycardic, hyperpneic, tachypneic, diaphoretic, and encephalopathic.
- An ASA level should be obtained promptly, although symptomatology and timing of ingestion may not perfectly correlate with the serum concentration.
- **Electrolytes should be assessed, with special attention to renal function and potassium level, as AKI will prevent elimination of salicylate, and hypokalemia will hinder urinary alkalinization, a cornerstone of treatment.**
- Arterial or venous blood gas to monitor serum pH and lactate concentration.
- **An acetaminophen level should be obtained in any suspected toxic overdose as co-ingestion is common.**

Critical Management

Critical Management Checklist

- ☑ Airway and ventilatory support as needed
- ☑ Activated charcoal (1 g/kg max 100 g) if < 4 hours since ingestion
- ☑ Consider renal replacement therapy (RRT)
- ☑ Urinary alkalinization (sodium bicarbonate)

- Aggressive fluid resuscitation, with balanced crystalloid, should be provided to patients with evidence of hypovolemia or hypotension.
- **Gastric decontamination with activated charcoal (1-2 g/kg, max of 100 g in adults, 50 g in pediatrics) should be provided to patients who can protect their airway and have no evidence of GI hemorrhage, especially in cases presenting < 2 hours after ingestion.**
- Whole bowel irrigation with polyethylene glycol (20–40 mL/kg/hr) can be considered in patients who have persistently elevated ASA levels, despite activated charcoal.
- **Urinary alkalinization, using a continuous infusion of sodium bicarbonate, is a cornerstone of therapy, titrating to a goal urine pH > 7.5.**
  - ○ Urinary alkalinization is achieved by administering a bolus of sodium bicarbonate bolus, 1–2 mEq/kg IV, followed by a continuous infusion at double the maintenance rate.
  - ○ **An infusion can be prepared by adding three ampules (50 mEq each) of sodium bicarbonate to 1 liter of D5 water (D5W) – do not use normal saline as this creates a very hypertonic solution.**
  - ○ Consider adding 40 mEq of potassium chloride to fluids, as hypokalemia will be exacerbated by alkalinization, impairing urinary alkalinization and thus ASA excretion.
  - ○ Alkalinization of serum relative to CSF will prevent transfer of salicylate into the brain and subsequent neurotoxicity.
- **Hemodialysis (iHD) serves as definitive treatment** for ASA intoxication due to the molecule's small size and low volume of distribution. **Renal replacement therapy (RRT), ideally with intermittent.**

- ○ Endotracheal intubation may be necessary for airway protection or respiratory muscle fatigue leading to worsening acidemia.
- ○ **Due to metabolic acidemia, intubation should be avoided if at all possible, and if required, should be performed in such a way as to minimize the duration of apnea.**
  - ▪ **Patients suffering salicylism should be considered physiologically difficult airways due to the risk of cardiac arrest in the peri-intubation period as a result of apnea worsening acidemia.**
  - ▪ Consider a bolus of 1–2 ampules of sodium bicarbonate (50–100 mEq) prior to intubation.
  - ▪ Intubation plan should focus on minimizing the apneic period, whether via rapid sequence intubation, ketamine-assisted intubation, or awake with topical anesthesia.
- ○ **Invasive mechanical ventilation is challenging in patients with ASA toxicity, as they will require a high minute ventilation to compensate for underlying metabolic acidosis.**
  - ▪ An arterial or venous blood gas should be drawn 10–15 minutes after intubation. The respiratory rate and tidal volume should be adjusted to maintain a pH > 7.20.
  - ▪ Higher tidal volumes may be required to maintain a safe pH.
  - ▪ Air trapping is common due to limited exhalation time – close attention should be paid to the flow waveforms to monitor for incomplete exhalation.
- ○ Serial ASA levels should be obtained to monitor therapy effects.
  - ▪ Continue therapy until the levels are at or below 30 mg/dL.
  - ▪ Concretions of ASA may exist in the GI tract, causing a delayed serum peak and prolonged toxicity.
- ○ Hemodialysis (iHD) serves as definitive treatment, removing the drug from the systemic circulation while also allowing for intensive management of volume status and acid-base disturbance.

Table 46.2 Indications for hemodialysis in salicylate toxicity

- End-organ damage such as altered mental status, acute lung injury, or coagulopathy
- AKI resulting in the inability to eliminate drug
- Inability to tolerate the necessary fluid load for alkalinization
- Refractory acidemia
- Absolute serum concentrations > 100 mg/dL in acute ingestion, or 60 mg/dL in chronic ingestion
- Clinical deterioration despite alkalinization and other supportive management

Sudden Deterioration

- Decline in mental status, coma, or seizure can be caused by **neuroglycopenia** or cerebral edema.
  - **Empiric dextrose (1 amp of D50) should be given prior to moving forward with intubation for airway protection, even if the serum glucose is normal.**
  - Any alteration in mental status should prompt consideration of iHD.
- Fluid overload can result in pulmonary edema and respiratory failure.
  - RRT should be initiated in patients that are unable to tolerate the fluid load necessary for urine alkalinization.
  - Respiratory support, in the form of non-invasive positive pressure or invasive mechanical ventilation, may be necessary and should be done early before the development of severe acidemia.
- **In patients on mechanical ventilation, sudden hypotension or desaturation should raise suspicion for critical air trapping or iatrogenic pneumothorax.**
  - Immediately disconnect the patient from the ventilator and ensure complete exhalation.
  - If hypotension persists, consider lung ultrasound or empiric needle or finger thoracostomy.
- Patients with ASA overdose are at risk of life-threatening GI bleeding. Blood products should be considered in patients with hematochezia, hematemesis, or unexplained hypotension.

Special Circumstances

- Chronic salicylism is a challenging diagnosis to make and may present with minimal or classic symptoms of ASA toxicity.
  - ASA levels may be in the therapeutic range.
  - iHD may be required in the case of suspected chronic toxicity, a detectable ASA level and any of the following:
    - AKI or severe acidemia, pulmonary edema, seizures, or coma.

Tricyclic Antidepressants

Overview

- Tricyclic antidepressants (TCAs) are commonly used in the management of neuropathic pain, mood disorders, insomnia, and migraine prophylaxis.
- TCAs are rapidly absorbed in the GI tract, are highly protein bound, and exhibit a long half-life due in part to a large volume of distribution.
- Toxicity primarily results from anticholinergic effects, alpha blockade, sodium channel blockade in cardiac tissue, and inhibition of norepinephrine reuptake at nerve terminals.
  - TCA bind fast sodium channels in the His-Purkinje system, prolonging absolute refractory period, similar to type Ia antiarrhythmic drugs (i.e., quinidine), producing a characteristic ECG pattern notable for a terminal R wave in aVR (Figure 46.2).
  - Anticholinergic effects include agitation, mydriasis, anhidrosis, hyperthermia, and tachycardia.
  - Alpha blockade may produce hypotension

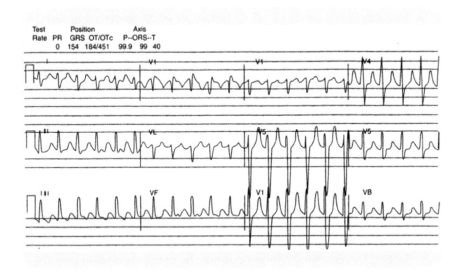

Figure 46.2 Classic ECG changes due to TCA overdose, including sinus tachycardia, QRS duration > 100 milliseconds, right axis deviation, terminal R wave in aVR (or S wave in I or aVL).

Presentation

Classic Presentation

- Anticholinergic toxidrome is usually present on initial presentation for clinically significant ingestions, including tachycardia, flushed skin with anhidrosis, and mydriasis.
- ECG with sinus tachycardia, widened QRS, and terminal r wave in aVR.
- Altered mental status, primarily diminished level of consciousness., confusion, or hallucinations, may be present.

Critical Presentation

- Ingestions between 10–20 mg/kg of a TCA may lead to life threatening toxicity.
- Wide complex tachydysrhythmia, ventricular arrhythmia.
- Seizures.
- Shock progressing to cardiovascular collapse.

Diagnosis and Evaluation

- The diagnosis is made based on history, physical examination, and classic ECG findings (Figure 46.2).
- The most important diagnostic investigation is the ECG. Common findings are sinus tachycardia and **right axis deviation**, and a **terminal R wave in aVR**. In addition to these findings, **QRS duration, in milliseconds (ms), can help predict clinical course**:
  - ○ < 100 ms – no significant toxicity.
  - ○ > 100 ms – 30% will have seizures.
  - ○ > 160 ms – 60% may have ventricular dysrhythmia.
- Venous or arterial blood gas may be obtained to identify potential acidemia.
- Assessment of serum electrolytes, including sodium and potassium, as well as renal function may help guide treatment.
- Testing for common co-ingestions may be useful depending on concerns for polysubstance ingestion.
- Serum or urine testing for TCA will be unlikely to change management in the acute setting.

Critical Management

Critical Management Checklist

☑ Airway and ventilatory support as needed
☑ Activated charcoal (1 g/kg max 100 g) if < 2 hours since ingestion
☑ if hypotensive or wide QRS, bicarbonate bolus (1-2 mEq/Kg IV) and drip (targeting pH 7.5-7.55.
☑ if severe shock, administer lipid emulsion therapy (1-1.5 ml/Kg up to 3 times)

- **Airway and ventilatory support as needed.**
- Hypotension should be managed with aggressive fluid resuscitation, sodium bicarbonate, and vasopressors as needed.
- GI decontamination if within 2 hours of ingestion (activated charcoal1 g/kg, maximum dose 50g).
- Early ECG is essential: **in the case of QRS prolongation or hypotension, sodium bicarbonate should be administered (up to 1–2 mEq/kg IV as a bolus) targeting a narrow QRS. An infusion should be started targeting serum pH 7.50–7.55.**
  - Increasing extracellular sodium reduces TCA interaction with sodium channels on cardiac myocytes, while increasing serum pH promotes non-ionized drug formation, thus inhibiting binding to sodium channels.
  - After the initial bolus, an infusion should be prepared by adding 150 mEq (3 amps) bicarbonate to a 1L bag of D5W (after removing 150 mL of D5W to create the appropriate concentration) and started at 250 mL/hour.
  - Additional boluses may be administered in the case of worsening hypotension or QRS widening despite the infusion.
  - **Hypertonic saline (3% sodium chloride) should be given in cases of refractory hypotension or when sodium bicarbonate is unavailable, in aliquots of 100 mL IV.** Repeat dosing can be considered, but more than 300 mL should not be given due to risks of hypernatremia.
- Seizures should be managed with benzodiazepines.
- **Cardiac arrest or severe shock should prompt initiation of intravenous lipid emulsion (Intralipid®) as a bolus of 1–1.5 mL/kg,**

which can be repeated three times if hemodynamics do not improve.

- ○ 1–1.5 mL/kg can be given as a bolus prior to starting an infusion at a rate of 0.25–0.5 mL/kg, until hemodynamic stability is achieved.
- ○ Lipid emulsion may sequester TCA, which are lipophilic, preventing interaction with alpha and sodium receptors, or serve as a direct inotrope and energy source for cardiac myocytes.
- Airway and ventilatory support as needed.
- **Although patients may exhibit significant anticholinergic features, physostigmine is contraindicated in TCA toxicity due to associations with bradyarrhythmia and cardiac arrest.**
- Hypotension is common in TCA toxicity due to alpha blockade and interaction with cardiac myocytes. Crystalloid should be utilized to optimize preload. Vasopressors should be initiated if hypotension persists despite an appropriate fluid challenge and alkalinization.
  - ○ Norepinephrine should be considered first-line given its alpha effects. Phenylephrine can be considered second-line.
- Seizures are usually brief and self-limited, but if persistent should be controlled with intravenous benzodiazepines.
  - ○ Phenobarbital or propofol can be used in cases of recurrent seizure.
  - ○ **Phenytoin and fosphenytoin should be avoided due to sodium channel blockade and increased risk of ventricular dysrhythmias.**
- Arrhythmias may occur due to interference with normal conduction, including ventricular tachycardia (VT) or ventricular fibrillation (VF).
  - ○ VT or VF should be managed in accordance with standard advanced cardiovascular life support (ACLS) measures, with few exceptions.
  - ○ Magnesium can be given in persistent arrhythmia as a dose of 1–2 g IV.
  - ○ **Class IA (quinidine, procainamide), and class IC (flecainide, propafenone) antiarrhythmics are contraindicated due to interactions with sodium channels in cardiac tissue.**
  - ○ Lidocaine has been cited as an option for refractory arrhythmia using traditional dosing (1–1.5 mg/kg IV, followed by an infusion of 1–4 mg/hour).
- Intensive care unit (ICU) admission for at least 12 hours of bicarbonate therapy should be considered for any patient with:

○ QRS > 100 ms, hypotension, dysrhythmia.
○ Altered mental status, respiratory depression, seizures.
- Patients who received GI decontamination and remain asymptomatic with normal vital signs and serial ECGs may be medically cleared after 6 hours of monitoring.

Beta-Blockers

Overview

- Beta-blockers are used in the management of coronary artery disease, essential hypertension, glaucoma, anxiety, and migraine prophylaxis.
- They are available as oral, intravenous, and ophthalmic preparations, and are rapidly absorbed with a rapid onset of action.
- Specific drugs vary in their degree of selectivity for different β receptors, with β1 activation increasing inotropy, chronotropy, and β2 binding promoting smooth muscle relaxation in the vasculature, bronchi, and glucose release.
- In overdose, selectivity is lost and β1 and β2 effects are seen.
- Some agents (e.g., labetalol, carvedilol) also have some alpha-adrenergic blockade.
- Observed toxicity depends on cardioselectivity, lipid solubility, and membrane stabilizing effect of the ingested medication:
  ○ Nonselective beta-blockers (e.g., propranolol) are associated with higher mortality than selective beta-blockers (e.g., metoprolol).
  ○ Highly lipid-soluble beta-blockers confer higher mortality due to CNS penetration and larger volumes of distribution.
  ○ Certain agents (e.g., propranolol) bind type Ia sodium channels, with resultant bradyarrhythmia and ventricular arrhythmias.
- **Propranolol accounts for the most fatalities of any beta-blocker.**

Presentation

See Table 46.2.

Table 46.2 Most common symptoms of beta-blocker overdose in order of frequency

Bradycardia
Hypotension
Unresponsiveness
Respiratory depression
Hypoglycemia
Seizures (with lipid-soluble agents)

Classic Presentation

- May be mild or even asymptomatic, especially in young healthy patients.
- Bradycardia due to sinus (SA) and atrioventricular (AV) nodal blockade.
- Hypoglycemia (more common in children).

Critical Presentation

- Symptomatic bradycardia, hypotension, cardiogenic shock.
- Respiratory depression (bronchospasm is less common).
- Seizures or coma.

Diagnosis and Evaluation

- Access to these agents in the appropriate clinical setting should raise suspicion for beta-blocker overdose – collateral information is essential.
- An ECG should be performed to assess for bradyarrhythmia and interval changes.
- Bedside fingerstick glucose testing will rule out hypoglycemia, which may be a cause of altered mental status in beta-blocker poisoning.
- While laboratory assessment may not aid in the initial diagnosis of toxicity, assessment of electrolytes, including calcium, and renal function can aid in management decisions.
- If concern for coingestion exists, acetaminophen and salicylate levels should be obtained.

Critical Management

Critical Management Checklist

- ☑ Airway and ventilatory support as needed
- ☑ Activated charcoal (1 g/kg max 100 g) if < 2 hours since ingestion
- ☑ Epinephrine for MAP support
- ☑ Glucagon 5 mg bolus & 5 mg/hr infusion
- ☑ Calcium gluconate/chloride bolus & infusion if improved hemodynamics
- ☑ High dose insuline euglycemia therapy (HIET): 1 unit/kg bolus & 0.5 unit/kg infusion with dextrose support
- ☑ if severe shock, administer lipid emulsion therapy (1-1.5 ml/Kg up to 3 times)

- **If patients present with concerns for significant beta-blocker toxicity, engage pharmacists early given multiple medications required to successfully treat this overdose and the required time for preparation.**
- Airway and ventilatory support as needed.
- GI decontamination if within 2 hours of ingestion (activated charcoal 1 g/kg, maximum dose 10 g).
- **Glucagon** (5 mg IV bolus and 5 mg/hour infusion) and atropine should be used as first-line for symptomatic bradycardia, although these agents rarely reverse toxicity completely.
  - ○ Nausea and vomiting are common adverse effects.
- **Calcium gluconate or calcium chloride** should be administered in bolus dosing, followed by an infusion if effective in improving hemodynamics.
  - ○ Administration of calcium, as calcium chloride (1 g IV push) or calcium gluconate (2 g IV push), may improve hypotension, although data regarding bradycardia resolution are not promising.
- Vasopressors should be utilized for shock while awaiting initiation of advanced therapies, with **epinephrine** being the initial agent of choice.
  - ○ Epinephrine (1–20 mcg/min) and norepinephrine (1–30 mcg/min) can be used to support the MAP, titrating to a goal of 65 mmHg.
  - ○ Inodilators (milrinone, dobutamine) should be avoided due to the vasodilation that can be seen in the peripheral vasculature, risking increasing hypotension.

- **High dose insulin euglycemia therapy (HIET) should be initiated on patients who present with signs of severe toxicity, including those presenting with hypotension.**
  - HIET, best studied in calcium channel blocker toxicity, may have benefit in beta-blocker poisoning and should be started at the onset of hypotension.
  - The mechanism of insulin in beta-blocker toxicity is not clear – changes in fatty acid metabolism, a direct inotropic effect, and increased uptake of glucose into cardiomyocytes may all play a role.
  - **HIET will take between 30–60 minutes after initiation to take effect; thus coadministration of the therapies above is recommended.**
  - Induction of therapy is accomplished with a bolus of 1 U/kg of insulin, along with 50 g of dextrose.
  - Infusions are as follows: insulin 1–10 U/kg/hour, dextrose 0.25–0.5 g/ kg/ hour, usually delivered in concentrations of d50 to d70.
  - The rate of infusion of insulin is dictated by hemodynamic improvement.
  - There is no consensus regarding methods of discontinuation of HIET – due to the half-life of insulin, hypoglycemia may persist long after discontinuation of the infusion.
  - **The initial bolus should be 1 unit/kg IV of regular insulin, followed by an infusion of 0.5 U/kg IV, titrating to resolution of hypotension – dextrose supplementation as a bolus (50 g IV) and infusion (0.5 g/kg/hour) are essential to avoid iatrogenic hypoglycemia.**
  - **Insulin causes potassium to shift toward the intracellular space, putting patients at significant risk of hypokalemia.**
  - Insulin infusion should not be started prior to achieving a potassium of at least 4.0–4.5 mmol/L. Scheduled potassium replacement may be required in order to tolerate the large insulin doses necessary to reverse beta blockade.
- Intravenous lipid emulsion should be given in patients who are at risk of cardiac arrest due to hemodynamic instability, or in patients who suffer cardiac arrest.
- Extracorporeal membrane oxygenation (ECMO) can be considered for certain patients who continue to be unstable despite standard therapies.

- ○ **Critically ill patients suffering from beta-blocker poisoning are at high risk of death, initially from profound shock, and later in their course, from ARDS due to the significant volumes administered from multiple infusions**.
- ○ Crystalloid should be used judiciously in the initial resuscitation.
- ○ Glucagon bypasses the beta receptor pathway, increasing intracellular calcium, contractility of cardiomyocytes, and subsequently chronotropy and inotropy.
- ○ Atropine may reduce bradycardia, although it is unlikely to resolve shock. It should be given in 0.5–1mg IV pushes, up to 3 mg.
- ○ Close coordination with pharmacy is essential due to the inherent complexities of managing the logistics of HIET. Ideally care should be delivered via an institutional protocol created with multidisciplinary input.
  - ▪ **Insulin causes potassium to shift toward the intracellular space, putting patients at significant risk of hypokalemia.**
  - ▪ Insulin infusion should not be started prior to achieving a potassium of at least 4.0–4.5 mmol/L. Scheduled potassium replacement may be required in order to tolerate the large insulin doses necessary to reverse beta blockade.
  - ▪ **Glucose needs to be monitored very closely; every 15–30 minutes while on the insulin infusion.**
- ○ Cardiac pacing, via transcutaneous or transvenous routes, can be initiated but is often ineffective secondary to failure to capture.
- ○ All symptomatic patients should be admitted to an ICU for close monitoring given the risk of hemodynamic collapse.

Sudden Deterioration

- Acute onset of arrhythmia after initiation of HIET should raise suspicion for critical hypokalemia. ECG changes consistent with hypokalemia include T wave inversions, ST depression, and U waves.
- Abrupt change in mental status, especially somnolence, or seizure after starting HIET should prompt evaluation for iatrogenic hypoglycemia.
- Extracorporeal life support in the form of venoarterial **ECMO** can be considered in patients who continue to be hypotensive despite initiation of HIET, intravenous lipid emulsion and vasopressor infusions.

Special Circumstances

- Hemodialysis can be considered in patients who present with toxicity after ingesting beta-blockers that are hydrophilic and poorly protein bound; these include **sotalol, nadolol,** and **atenolol.**

Calcium Channel Blockers

Overview

- Calcium channel blockers (CCB) are commonly used in the treatment of essential hypertension, atrial fibrillation, and migraine prophylaxis.
- CCB inhibit calcium channels in the myocardium, decreasing contractility, SA and AV node conduction; and in vascular smooth muscle, promoting coronary and peripheral vasodilation.
  - CCB interact with L-type calcium channels in the pancreas reducing insulin secretion and promoting hyperglycemia.
- Dihydropyridines (e.g., amlodopine, nicardipine) bind to smooth muscle calcium channels, while nondihydropyridines (e.g., verapamil, diltiazem), are more specific to myocardial tissue though selectivity is lost in overdose.
- Many CCB are highly protein bound with a high volume of distribution.
- **Verapamil and diltiazem are most often implicated in life-threating overdose, accounting for most fatalities.**

Presentation

Classic Presentation

- Hypotension with a relatively clear mental status.
- Reflex tachycardia may be present early in dihydropyridine overdose.
- **Hyperglycemia**, in patients without diabetes mellitus, is a classic finding.

Critical Presentation

- Symptomatic bradycardia, hypotension, and tissue ischemia.
- Pulmonary edema and cardiogenic shock.

Diagnosis and Evaluation

- Diagnosis requires a high degree of suspicion for ingestion in the appropriate clinical context, or collateral information suggesting significant ingestion.
  - If possible, identifying the formulation can be very helpful in guiding management, as extended release preparations are common and will require prolonged monitoring even if asymptomatic.
  - May be very challenging to distinguish from beta-blocker toxicity.
- ECG should be obtained to evaluate interval prolongation, although intervals are frequently normal in CCB toxicity.
- Serum electrolytes and markers of kidney function should be obtained, along with serum acetaminophen or salicylate levels if there are concerns for coingestion.
- Point of care blood glucose testing may show hyperglycemia, although absence of hyperglycemia does not rule out significant toxicity.

Critical Management

Critical Management Checklist

- ☑ Airway and ventilatory support as needed
- ☑ Activated charcoal (1 g/kg max 100 g) if < 2 hours since ingestion
- ☑ Epinephrine for MAP support
- ☑ Calcium gluconate/chloride bolus & infusion if improved hemodynamics
- ☑ High dose insuline euglycemia therapy (HIET): 1 unit/kg bolus & 0.5 unit/kg infusion with dextrose support
- ☑ Glucagon 5 mg bolus & 5 mg/hr infusion (though less likely to be effective as in beta blocker overdose)
- ☑ if severe shock, administer lipid emulsion therapy (1-1.5 ml/Kg up to 3 times)

Management is nearly identical to that of beta blocker overdoses (see page 493) with several exceptions

- Glucagon and atropine are often less effective than in beta-blocker toxicity but may be trialed for patients with mild symptoms

- Therapeutic Plasma exchange is an experimental option which may clear drug from the circulation by removing CCB plasma proteins
- Methylene blue, a nitric oxide scavenger and inhibitor of nitric oxide synthase in the endothelium, has been used as rescue therapy for some cases of CCB toxicity.
  - Administer as a bolus of 1–2 mg/kg.
  - If there is hemodynamic improvement with the bolus, an infusion can be initiated at 0.5–1 mg/kg/hour.

Sudden Deterioration

- Venoarterial ECMO has been described in case reports of massive overdoses of CCB, especially cardioselective agents such as verapamil and diltiazem. Consultation with the institutional ECMO team can be considered if patients are refractory to previously mentioned therapies and have no obvious exclusions (bleeding diathesis, devastating neurologic injury, significant trauma).
- Acute onset of arrhythmia after initiation of HIET should raise suspicion for critical hypokalemia. ECG changes consistent with hypokalemia include T wave inversions, ST depression, and U waves.
- Abrupt change in mental status, especially somnolence, or seizure after starting HIET should prompt evaluation for iatrogenic hypoglycemia.

Special Circumstances

- **Therapeutic plasma exchange (TPE) has been successful in case reports of amlodipine intoxication refractory to standard therapies and can be considered if patients remain moribund despite HIET and other supportive measures.**
  - TPE involves removal of patient plasma via a large bore dual lumen catheter and replacement with autologous plasma, albumin, or crystalloid.
  - **Amlodipine** is highly protein bound and thus may be successfully removed via TPE, while other CCBs may not.

○ Consultation with nephrology is essential. Serum levels of amlodipine may be useful in determining efficacy and the need for repeat sessions.

Digoxin

Overview

- Digoxin, a cardiac glycoside, is derived from the foxglove plant (*Digitalis purpurea*). Ouabain, lily of the valley, and oleander also contain cardiac glycosides, and thus act similarly in overdose.
- Common indications for digoxin include atrial fibrillation in the setting of congestive heart failure and left ventricular systolic dysfunction.
- Digoxin inhibits the sodium-potassium ATPase in cardiomyocytes, increasing intracellular calcium and subsequently myocardial contractility.
- Due to a narrow therapeutic index, toxicity is common in patients on digoxin, accounting for its relative decline in use over the past several decades.
- Digoxin has a relatively slow onset (1.5–6 hours), a very long half-life of up to 30 hours, and is cleared primarily by renal excretion.
- Toxicity may be acute or chronic, which have different characteristics (Table 46.3).
- Digoxin toxicity is potentiated by renal insufficiency, underlying cardiac disease, electrolyte abnormalities (e.g., hypokalemia, hypomagnesemia, hypercalcemia) and other cardioactive medications, including beta-blockers and calcium channel blockers.
- Drugs that slow digoxin clearance include quinidine, macrolides.

Table 46.3 Comparison of acute versus chronic digoxin overdose

Acute	Chronic
Lower mortality	Higher mortality
Bradyarrhythmia more common	Ventricular arrythmias more common
Younger patients	Older patients
Serum potassium high or normal	Serum potassium low or normal

Presentation

Classic Presentation

- Nonspecific symptoms are common, including nausea, anorexia, vomiting.
- CNS effects may be nonspecific, including headache, generalized weakness, and lethargy.
- Yellow-green chromatopsia (objects appearing yellow and green) is classic, but rarely seen in clinical practice. Blurry vision and other nonspecific visual disturbances are common.
- Premature ventricular contractions.

Critical Presentation

- Hyperkalemia is an ominous sign, suggestive of systemic blockade of Na-K ATPase.
- Ventricular arrhythmia including ventricular tachycardia, torsades de pointes, and ventricular fibrillation.
- **Bidirectional ventricular tachycardia is pathognomonic for digoxin toxicity.**
- Delirium, hallucinations, and seizures.

Diagnosis and Evaluation

- **Clinicians should be suspicious of toxicity in any patient taking digoxin who presents with nonspecific symptoms or new/ worsening arrhythmia.**
- The diagnosis is challenging to confirm in the absence of known ingestion, given the litany of nonspecific symptoms that are often present early in the patient's course.
- **Timing of the ingestion is particularly key, as levels drawn within 6 hours of ingestion may be falsely elevated, as the drug has not yet redistributed.**
- Inciting events that may tip patients into toxicity include new renal failure or initiation of medications that change metabolism of digoxin, including **amiodarone, macrolides, itraconazole, verapamil,** and others.

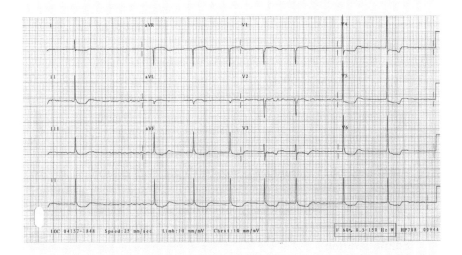

Figure 46.3 Digoxin effect seen on ECG.

- An ECG should be obtained if there is suspicion for digoxin intoxication. See Figure 46.3.
  - The classic digitalis effect – scooped, downsloping ST depressions, described as the "Salvador Dali mustache" - is not a sign of toxicity per se.
  - Digoxin toxicity can produce a wide variety of arrhythmias, but the most characteristic are non-paroxysmal atrial tachycardia with AV block, new onset Mobitz type I, and bidirectional VT.
- Serum electrolytes, including magnesium, and measures of kidney function should be obtained on arrival, and 6 hours post-ingestion, to guide management.
- If there is suspicion for coingestion, serum acetaminophen and salicylate levels should be measured.
- **Serum digoxin levels should be obtained promptly, as they can help suggest the diagnosis but they are not diagnostic of toxicity in isolation.**
  - Patients may be toxic at therapeutic levels, especially in the setting of hypokalemia, or asymptomatic at supratherapeutic levels.

Critical Management

- Airway and ventilatory support as needed.
- Unstable bradycardia should be temporized with traditional therapies, including pacing, atropine, epinephrine, or dopamine.
  - GI decontamination if within 2 hours of ingestion (activated charcoal 1 g/kg, maximum dose 50 g).
- Hypokalemia on presentation must be corrected prior to administration of antidigoxin Fab, with a goal of 4.0–5.0 mmol/L.
- **Antidigoxin Fab should be given to all patients exhibiting severe toxicity. In cases where the amount of drug ingested is unknown, 10 vials are given empirically. In cardiac arrest, 20 vials are given and ACLS should be continued for up to 30 minutes after administration.**
  - Patients presenting with a history of significant GI losses should receive appropriate crystalloid resuscitation to optimize renal perfusion.
  - Unstable bradycardia may develop in patients with digoxin toxicity, and while antidigoxin Fab is the antidote, it is unlikely to be readily available when the patient presents.
    - While awaiting antidigoxin Fab, atropine (0.5 mg IV push) or epinephrine (5–10 mcg IV push) can be given for unstable bradycardia.
    - Life-threatening arrythmias should be treated in accordance with ACLS protocols, with lidocaine having a preferential role in the management of VT.
  - **Prior to administering antidigoxin Fab, hypokalemia must be corrected.**
    - Hyperkalemia in the setting of digoxin intoxication is reflective of global poisoning of Na-K ATPase throughout the body.
    - Antidote administration results in a rapid correction of Na-K ATPase dysfunction (approximately 90 minutes) and subsequently a rapid drop in serum potassium.
    - Clinicians should strive to achieve a serum potassium of 4.0–5.0 mmol/L to serve as a buffer prior to antidigoxin Fab.
    - For similar reasons, hyperkalemia prior to giving the antidote should be tolerated unless potassium is markedly elevated or believed to be responsible for arrhythmia, which is generally rare.

- Digoxin-associated hyperkalemia with ECG changes should receive antidigoxin Fab, but calcium administration is controversial due to high intracellular calcium levels.
- If a patient with a digoxin overdose has life-threatening hyperkalemia with QRS widening or hemodynamic collapse, calcium gluconate or chloride is likely safe as an adjunctive therapy.
- Insulin (5–10 U regular IV, depending on renal function) and dextrose (50 g IV) can be given to temporize hyperkalemia until antidote is available, though priority should be given to the antidote and potassium levels should be followed closely after treatment.

○ **Generally agreed-upon indications for antidigoxin Fab include:**
- **Life-threatening arrhythmia, including unstable bradycardia, high-grade AV block, and any ventricular arrhythmia**
- **Acute kidney injury**
- **Acute encephalopathy**
- **Hyperkalemia**
- **Cardiac arrest**
- Some sources recommend antidogixin Fab for a single ingestion of > 10 grams in adults, or a level of > 10 ng/mL at least 6 hours post ingestion.

○ The required dose of antidigoxin Fab is calculated with the knowledge that 10 vials will neutralize 0.5 mg of drug. When determining the dose required for a given ingestion:
- In the case of a known ingestion, the dose can be calculated as follows: number of vials $= {}^{(\text{mg of digoxin ingested} \times 0.8)}/_{0.5}$
- In the case of a known steady state concentration of digoxin (i.e., a value obtained at least 6 hours after the last known ingestion), the dose is calculated as follows: number of vials $= {}^{\text{dixogin level} \times \text{weight (kg)}}/_{100}$

○ Digoxin serum assays are unable to distinguish between free drug and drug-antidigoxin Fab complexes for up to 3 weeks after antidote administration; thus treatment after initial management is guided by symptoms rather than digoxin levels.

○ All symptomatic patients should be admitted for cardiac monitoring, while patients receiving antidigoxin Fab for unstable arrhythmia, cardiac arrest, acute encephalopathy, or significant renal failure should be observed in an ICU setting.

Sudden Deterioration

- Patients who suffer cardiac arrest as a result of digoxin intoxication should undergo **ACLS for at least 30 minutes after antidigoxin Fab administration**. These patients should receive 20 vials of antidigoxin Fab.
- Consider potassium chloride administration in patients who have a borderline serum level prior to giving antidigoxin Fab and become newly unstable after the antidote is administered.
- Rapid onset of hypotension after antidigoxin Fab infusion should raise concern for anaphylaxis, which occurs in up to 1% of cases. Management should focus on close assessment for airway edema, early epinephrine administration (0.3 mg IM), and provision of antihistamines.

Special Circumstances

- Patients treated with antidigoxin Fab can rarely have recrudescence of digoxin toxicity, usually within 24 hours of administration (normal kidney function) up to 72 hours in renal injury. As such, patients with digoxin-associated renal injury should be monitored inpatient for at least 72 hours.
- Patients with implanted pacemakers are especially challenging to diagnose with digoxin toxicity, as pacemaker activity can mask ECG changes.
  - These patients should be treated if there is evidence of hyperkalemia (K > 5.5 mmol/L), AKI, or progressive encephalopathy.

BIBLIOGRAPHY

Boehnert MT, & Lovejoy FH. Value of the QRS duration versus the serum drug level in predicting seizures and ventricular dysrhythmias after an acute overdose of tricyclic antidepressants. *N Engl J Med* 1985;313:474–479.

Levine M, Nikkanen H, & Pallin DJ. The effects of intravenous calcium in patients with digoxin toxicity. *J Emerg Med* 2011;40:41–46.

Marx JA, Hockberger RS, Walls RM, et al., eds. *Rosen's Emergency Medicine: Concepts and Clinical Practice*, 7th ed. Philadelphia, PA: Mosby Elsevier, 2010.

Nelson L, Lewin NA, Howland MA, et al., eds. *Goldfrank's Toxicologic Emergencies*. New York, NY: McGraw-Hill Medical, 2010.

Rumack BH, & Matthew H. Acetaminophen poisoning and toxicity. *Pediatrics.* 1975;55:871–876.

Smilkstein MJ, Knapp GL, Kulig KW, et al. Efficacy of oral *N*-acetylcysteine in the treatment of acetaminophen overdose. Analysis of the national multicenter study (1976 to 1985). *N Engl J Med* 1988;319:1557–1562.

Tintinalli JE, Stapczynski JS, Cline DM, et al. eds. *Emergency Medicine: A Comprehensive Study Guide.* New York, NY: McGraw-Hill Medical, 2011.

SECTION 11

Trauma

JULIE WINKLE

47

· · · · · · · ·

General Trauma Principles

BENJAMIN SCHNAPP

Introduction

- Optimal initial management of the trauma patient during the first several hours after injury offers the best chance of a good outcome.
- Patient management consists of rapid primary survey, resuscitation of vital functions, a more detailed secondary assessment, diagnostic tests to ascertain the extent of traumatic injury, and finally, the initiation of definitive care.

Diagnosis and Evaluation

Primary Survey

The primary survey should be completed promptly in a consistent and thorough manner for every trauma patient. *For each of the subsequent chapters in this section on trauma, the critical management sections assume primary survey reassessment (i.e., ABCs) as the first step prior to further critical management actions.*

Airway

- Voice changes or other abnormal sounds can indicate upper airway obstruction or tracheobronchial tree injury.
- Rapid sequence intubation is the preferred method of securing the airway.
- Cervical spine immobilization should be prioritized when intubating the undifferentiated trauma patient.
- The sympathetic response to pain may deceivingly maintain blood pressure; induction agents may drop blood pressure. **Consider dose reduction of induction agents to maintain hemodynamic stability**.
- Distribution of drugs may take longer in cases of poor perfusion. **Consider a larger than usual dose of paralytic.**
- Airway adjuncts are particularly valuable in endotracheal intubation for trauma patients. Consider the gum elastic bougie, supraglottic airway devices, hyperangulated geometry laryngoscope blades, video laryngoscopes, or fiberoptic scopes. A cricothyrotomy kit should be readily available for endotracheal intubation attempts that result in a "cannot intubate, cannot oxygenate" scenario.

Indications for early intubation in trauma

| Head injury with GCS $\leq$ 8 |
| Penetrating neck trauma |
| Inhalation burns |
| Increased respiratory effort |
| Significant chest trauma |
| Agitation/uncooperativeness |

Breathing

- Visualize chest rise; auscultate breath sounds; palpate the chest wall for crepitus or flail segments and assure the trachea is midline.
- **A surgical chest tube (28–32F) should be placed immediately if there is concern for tension pneumothorax** (severe shortness of breath, unilateral decreased breath sounds, jugular venous distension [JVD], hypotension).

- **If there is delay in tube thoracostomy, decompress the lung with a needle thoracostomy in the fourth intercostal space (approximately nipple level), anterior axillary line or a finger thoracostomy.** This is an updated recommendation per the ATLS tenth edition.
- The extended FAST (eFAST) examination can be used for rapid detection of a pneumothorax. Interrogation of the pleural line with the linear ultrasound probe may be used to find a lung point (the junction between sliding lung and absent lung [high specificity for pneumothorax]) or the absence of lung sliding (high specificity and sensitivity for pneumothorax).

Circulation

- The primary circulation survey includes establishment of vascular access, assessment and control of bleeding, and judicious fluid resuscitation.
- Examine the patient for signs of hemorrhage, including all compartments that can hold life-threatening amounts of blood. If there are obvious sources of ongoing hemorrhage, apply direct pressure or a tourniquet if needed.

Sources of Hypotension in Trauma

Bleeding	Nonbleeding
Chest	Tension pneumothorax
Abdomen	Pericardial tamponade
Pelvis (retroperitoneal)	Spinal cord injury (neurogenic shock)
Long bones (femur fracture)	Cardiac dysfunction (infarction, arrhythmia)
Street (external)	Toxic ingestion

- Look for other signs of poor perfusion, such as cool extremities, duskiness, pulseless extremity, and slow capillary refill.
- Place **two large-bore (18-gauge or larger) peripheral IVs**; if access proves to be difficult, consider placement of an intraosseous line or large bore central venous catheter (e.g., introducer).
- **Assess pelvis stability by squeezing in** firmly from the sides of the pelvis with both hands. If there is movement, maintain inward pressure

and notify the team that the pelvis is unstable; there should be no more examinations of the unstable pelvis, and a pelvic binder or bedsheet should be immediately placed to prevent the possibility of worsened pelvic bleeding.

Disability

- Evaluation for disability in the primary survey should include GCS, neurological examination to evaluate for neurological deficit, and pupil examination for signs of intracranial injury.
- Most patients should be assumed to have cervical spine injury until demonstrated otherwise. Cervical spine immobilization should be maintained until clinical or radiographic clearance is obtained.
- Penetrating trauma to the neck with no clear signs of neurological injury does not require cervical spine immobilization. If a cervical collar was placed by EMS in a penetrating trauma, and there are no signs of neurological deficit, it should be removed.
- **For patients being emergently intubated, attempt to obtain a baseline neurological examination so the patient's deficits can be followed over time.**

Exposure

- Remove all clothing from the patient to look for any injuries that may be otherwise missed.
- Cover the patient and keep them warm as much as possible to avoid hypothermia.

EMS

- **Emergency medical services (EMS) can provide invaluable information on a trauma patient**
- Important aspects of the scene history include mechanism of injury, vital signs, mental status, IV access, or any changes or interventions en route.
- Attempt to obtain more details (e.g., amount of damage to the vehicle, size of knife, family members to contact etc.) once the patient is stabilized. If necessary, appoint one of your team members to gather the prehospital history.

Imaging

- The screening AP chest radiograph in the trauma bay generally remains routine for patients sustaining significant blunt or penetrating trauma.
- Patients who are hemodynamically stable and have no clinical suggestion of an unstable pelvic fracture and who will undergo abdominopelvic imaging with CT scan, may forego a screening pelvic radiograph.
- Perform an eFAST examination to assess for free fluid in the abdomen, thorax and in the pericardium as well as for pneumothorax. **If the patient is unstable with a positive abdominal FAST, then the patient should be brought immediately to the operating room.**
- If the patient with a positive FAST is hemodynamically stable, further imaging with CT scan may be obtained to guide further management.
- A combination of mechanism of injury, vital signs, reliability and findings of the physical examination, clinical appearance of the patient, age and existing comorbidities all contribute to the extent of imaging required.

Secondary Survey

- **Examine and palpate the entire patient in detail**, beginning at the head and proceeding towards the feet.
- Do not forget easily missed areas such as the axilla, perineum, back of the patient, the ears, and the nose. These can hide significant injuries.
- **Most trauma patients do not require a rectal exam**, as the yield for actionable findings is low. Exceptions include penetrating injuries near the pelvis, pelvic fractures and spinal injuries.

Blood Tests

- Obtain a baseline set of laboratory tests, including lactate, complete blood count, coagulation studies, basic metabolic panel, and most importantly, a type and screen.
- The **initial hematocrit is of little value** for evaluating for significant hemorrhage. It may be falsely reassuring (i.e., elevated) since the body has not had time to equilibrate to its losses.

- Elevated lactate levels may indicate inadequate tissue oxygenation and suggest the need for further resuscitation. Levels above 2 mmol/L are correlated with longer ICU and hospital stays. Serial lactate levels may be helpful in guiding the need for further resuscitation.
- Viscoelastic testing (i.e., thromboelastography [TEG] and rotational thromboelastometry [ROTEM]) is used in many centers to functionally assess coagulopathy and guide resuscitation.
- Other baseline labs, such as an alcohol level, serum tox screen and liver function tests, may be drawn but are generally not helpful in the immediate management of a trauma patient.

Critical Management

Early hemorrhage control should be one of the initial priorities in the resuscitation of a trauma patient. This can be accomplished with a variety of techniques such as torniqueting, pressure bandages or operative control.

Classes of Shock

	Class I	Class II	Class III	Class IV
Blood loss	< 15%	15–30%	31–40%	>40%
Pulse	–	- or ↑	↑	↑↑
Blood pressure	–	–	- or ↓	↓
Respirations	–	-	↑	↑↑
Mental status	Normal/mild	Anxious	Anxious/mild	Lethargic/significant
	Anxiety		Confusion	Confusion
Base excess	0 to −2 mEq/L	−2 to −6 mEq/L	−6 to −10 mEq/L	−10 or lower mEq/L

- Many patients with hemorrhage may initially show no evidence of blood loss (class I shock) or little evidence of blood loss, such as isolated tachycardia (class II shock). **Only when the patient has lost over 30% of their blood volume do they begin to manifest the classic signs of**

shock, such as low blood pressure (class III shock), and altered mental status (class IV shock).

- The goal in trauma resuscitation should be to prevent the "trauma triad of death" – hypothermia, acidosis and coagulopathy.
- Patients demonstrating traumatic hemorrhagic shock should have resuscitation based on several key tenets, termed *damage control resuscitation*:
  - ○ Early hemorrhage control
  - ○ Hemostatic resuscitation
  - ○ Permissive hypotension

Hemostatic Resuscitation

- The term hemostatic resuscitation refers to the goal of replacing lost blood with volume that resembles the composition of whole blood, aiming to avoid dilutional coagulopathy.
- If the patient demonstrates evidence of shock, initiate rapid **volume replacement with packed red blood cells or whole blood**.
- Uncrossmatched type O+ should be used for men and uncrossmatched type O- should be used for women because of the risk of Rh sensitization.
- Crystalloid should be used judiciously in trauma resuscitation as risks include: dilution of coagulation factors, hypothermia, and increased intravascular pressure risking clot dislodgement and bleeding.
- **If you suspect large volume blood loss, initiate your massive transfusion protocol.**
- Massive transfusion protocol should bring packed red blood cells (PRBC), fresh frozen plasma (FFP), and platelets to be given in as close to a **1:1:1** ratio as possible.
- If FFP is not available, or will be delayed, prothrombin complex concentrate (PCC) can be considered as it can be given rapidly without the need to thaw.
- In patients receiving large volume resuscitation, ionized Ca2+ is likely to be low due to dilution and chelation effects by preservatives in transfused blood. Calcium chloride or calcium gluconate 1–2 g can be given for repletion and may have positive effects on inotropy and the clotting cascade with little risk to the patient.

- Tranexamic acid (TXA) may be indicated for patients with suspected major hemorrhage (CRASH-2 trial). The dose is 1 g, administered within 3 hours of the onset of bleeding.

Permissive Hypotension

- **Also referred to as "hypotensive resuscitation" (colloquially, "don't pop the clot"), this strategy delays or limits fluids or blood products to the bleeding trauma patient in order to target a lower-than-normal blood pressure** (i.e., systolic blood pressure [SBP > 90 mmHg]).
- Organ perfusion is adequate at these pressures and aiming for higher pressures appears to increase the possibility of dislodging a clot that may be controlling bleeding without conferring any advantages.
- Patients with suspected head injury are not appropriate for this strategy and goal systolic blood pressure should be normal (> 110–120 mmHg).
- Current clinical guidelines recommend permissive hypotension, particularly for patients with penetrating trauma. However, definitive evidence for improved outcomes is lacking.
- There is no role for vasopressor agents in the acutely bleeding trauma patient. They have been shown to increase hemorrhage and do not appear to increase end organ perfusion. If the patient's blood pressure is low, they likely need additional blood products until source control is obtained unless a medical cause of trauma is suspected.

Disposition

- Ultimately, **a bleeding trauma patient needs their source of bleeding controlled**. This often occurs in the OR but may also occur in the interventional radiology suite.
- With increasing nonoperative management of trauma (especially solid organ injuries), patients are often managed outside of the operating room.
- If your patient is suspected to have injuries that will require a higher level of care than your facility provides, transfer should be initiated immediately and should not be delayed for imaging.

Sudden Deterioration

Repeat primary survey

Massive transfusion as necessary

Shock workup (likely hemorrhagic)

- **Any clinical deterioration should prompt reassessment of the primary survey (i.e., ABCs).** Repeated evaluation of the ABCs should be performed with any clinical change.
- Worsening hypotension in trauma should be assumed to be hemorrhagic shock until proven otherwise.
- Check access and ensure products are rapidly infusing; shorter/larger lines are preferred for ability to provide higher infusion rates
- Patients who transiently respond to fluid or blood administration are at high risk for deterioration. Initial improvement with resuscitation followed by recurrent hypotension is concerning for ongoing or recurrent hemorrhage.

48

· · · · · · · ·

Severe Traumatic Brain Injury

JACOB D. ISSERMAN

Introduction

- Severe traumatic brain injury (TBI) is usually defined as a Glasgow Coma Scale (GCS) < 9.
- The goals of early resuscitation should focus on identifying and treating the primary injuries and limiting the negative cascade of secondary injuries such as hypotension and hypoxia.
- All patients with suspected severe TBI need an emergent computed tomography (CT) scan of the brain to identify hemorrhage immediately following initial stabilization.
- 10% of severe TBI patients have concomitant c-spine injury.
- See Table 48.1 for common patterns of TBI.

Table 48.1 Common traumatic brain injury patterns

Diagnosis	Classic findings	Images/ management considerations
Traumatic SAH	CT imaging: localized bleeding in superficial sulci, adjacent skull fracture, and cerebral contusion as well as external evidence of traumatic injury	
Epidural	Classically transient LOC, then lucid interval, followed by deterioration CT imaging: bright, lens-shaped collection because spread is contained by dural attachments at the cranial sutures	
Subdural hematoma	CT imaging: bright, crescent shaped collection along the hemispheric convexity, collection crosses suture lines	

Table 48.1 (cont.)

Diagnosis	Classic findings	Images/management considerations
Intraparenchymal hemorrhage	CT imaging: hyperdense areas, surrounded by hypodense rings of edema	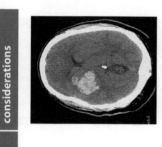
DAI (diffuse axonal injury)	CT imaging: acutely may be normal, later edema, atrophy, loss of grey-white differentiation	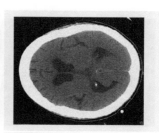 Medical: (1) ICP precautions and monitoring (2) Avoid causes of secondary brain injury: hypotension, hypoxia, fever, hyperglycemia, and seizures

Basilar skull
fracture

Clinical:

(1) Battle sign
(2) Raccoon eyes
(3) Hemotympanum
(4) CNS otorrhea/rhinorrhea

Depressed skull fracture

Medical:

(1) Steroids for delayed cranial nerve palsies
(2) Admission for observation
(3) Antibiotics for immunocompromised

Clinical: palpable deformity on exam, either with or without overlying laceration

Neurosurgical debridement recommended if:

(1) Dural penetration
(2) Significant intracranial hematoma
(3) Frontal sinus involvement
(4) Cosmetic deformity
(5) Wound infection or contamination
(6) Pneumocephalus

Presentation

- Severe TBI should be considered in the unconscious or altered patient with GCS $\leq$ 8 following head trauma with:
  - Significant mechanism of injury (fall from height, high speed MVC), or
  - Significant physical examination findings (depressed skull fracture, facial trauma, scalp lacerations).
  - Elderly patients or patients on therapeutic anticoagulation with signs of minimal or minor head trauma.

Diagnosis and Evaluation

Physical Examination

- Glasgow Coma Scale.
- Pupillary reflex examination.
- Neurologic status should be reevaluated frequently.

Glasgow Coma Scale (GCS)

Score	Eyes	Verbal response	Motor response
1	Closed	None	No response to painful stimuli
2	Open to pain	Incomprehensible sounds	Decerebrate (extension) to painful stimuli
3	Open to voice	Inappropriate words	Decorticate (flexion) to painful stimuli
4	Open spontaneously	Disoriented, confused speech	Withdraws to painful stimuli
5		Oriented, normal speech	Localizes painful stimuli
6			Follows commands

Add the total of each column.

Neuroimaging

- Obtain non-contrast head CT as quickly as possible.
- Subsequent MRI or angiography studies usually in consultation with neurosurgery and driven by clinical scenario.

Critical Management

- ☑ Airway management.
- ☑ Prioritize cerebral perfusion pressure.
- ☑ Consider TXA in appropriate population.

Rapid Sequence Intubation (RSI)

- The cerebral perfusion of severe TBI patients is tenuous, and first pass successful intubation is critical.
- The RSI medications should include a sedative and a paralytic agent with these objectives:
  - Maintenance of hemodynamic stability and CNS perfusion.
  - Maintenance of adequate oxygenation.
  - Prevention of increases in intracranial pressure.
  - Prevention of vomiting and aspiration.

Induction Agents

- Etomidate (0.3 mg/kg) has been demonstrated to be hemodynamically stable and not increase ICP.
- Ketamine (1.5 mg/kg) should be considered if hypotensive or normotensive (avoid if the patient is already hypertensive).

Paralytic Agents

- Rocuronium (RSI dose 1.2 mg/kg), onset of action 45–60 seconds.
  - Succinylcholine (1.5 mg/kg IV), onset of action 45–60 seconds (avoid in patients with crush injuries or hyperkalemia).
- Vecuronium (0.1–0.2 mg/kg), onset of action 60–90 seconds.

Breathing

- Avoid hypoxemia that may worsen cerebral ischemia (goal pulse oximeter of 95% or $PO_2 > 60$ mmHg).
- Maintain $PaCO_2$ levels of 35–40 mmHg. Avoid hypercarbia as it may result in increased ICP.
- Hyperventilation resulting in hypocarbia may cause cerebral vasoconstriction and ultimately worsen cerebral blood flow.
- Monitor ventilation closely with continuous quantitative end-tidal $PaCO_2$.

Circulation

- The goal is to maintain cerebral blood flow (CPP). Targets vary by age, but generally target CPP > 60 mmHg.
  - CPP = MAP − ICP.
  - Systemic hypotension causes a decrease in CPP and must be avoided. A patient with increased ICP needs a higher blood pressure to maintain cerebral perfusion.
- Judicious use of isotonic crystalloid, followed by PRBC transfusion should be given to maintain SBP > 90.
- Viscoelastic tests (thromboelastography [TEG] and rotational thromboelastometry [ROTEM]) and coagulation studies should be ordered to assess for coagulation status.

Intracranial Pressure

- Intracranial pressure is normally ≤ 15 mmHg.
  - Traumatic causes of increased ICP:
    - Intracranial mass lesions (hematomas).
    - Cerebral edema (acute hypoxic ischemic encephalopathy, large cerebral infarction, severe traumatic brain injury).
    - Obstructive hydrocephalus.
- See the box below for clinical signs of increased ICP and impending herniation.

Clinical signs of increased ICP and impending herniation

Unilateral or bilateral fixed and dilated pupil(s)

Decorticate or decerebrate posturing

Cushing reflex: bradycardia, hypertension, and/or respiratory depression Decrease in GCS > 2

- **Ocular ultrasound**
  - Can assist in detection of ICP by measuring the optic nerve sheath diameter.
  - Measure transverse diameter of nerve approximately 3 mm posterior to globe.
  - The average of two measurements > 5 mm is suspicious for increased ICP.
- **Management of increased ICP**
  - The goal is to maintain cerebral perfusion pressure > 60 mmHg.
  - Treatment is aimed at decreasing ICP first, then increasing MAP.

Decrease Intracranial Pressure

- Mechanical:
  - Elevate head of bed to 30 °.
  - Optimize venous drainage by keeping the neck in neutral position and loosening neck braces if too tight.
- Osmotic therapy:
  - Mannitol 20% (0.25–1 g/kg) over 5 minutes, works in the short term as a temporizing measure. May cause hypotension, so avoid in patients with SBP < 90.
  - Hypertonic saline (3%) 150–250 mL through a peripheral line. This is preferable if the patient is hypotensive.
  - Hypertonic saline (23.4%) 30 mL over 2–10 minutes via central line (often referred to as hypertonic 30 mL "bullet").
- Hyperventilation:
  - Decreasing P_aCO_2 causes cerebral vasoconstriction, resulting in a decrease in cerebral blood flow and temporary decrease in ICP. This technique should be avoided in the vast majority of cases; it should be used as a temporary therapy only in the setting of impending herniation.

- If an external ventricular drain (EVD) is in place, CSF can be removed at 1–2 mL/minute (pause drainage every 2–3 minutes). Continue until ICP is < 20 or fluid is not easily withdrawn.

Increase Mean Arterial Pressure (if MAP < 80)

- Isotonic crystalloid boluses.
- Vasopressors to maintain CPP > 60 (consider phenylephrine or norepinephrine).
- Packed red blood cells if active hemorrhage or hemoglobin < 7–8 g. There is no accepted optimal hemoglobin level or RBC transfusion threshold for patients with traumatic brain injury.

Tranexamic Acid (TXA)

- Could consider 1g TXA over 10 minutes followed by 1 g infusion over 8 hours for mild–moderate TBI (GCS 9–15) presenting within 3 hours, but not for severe TBI.

Neurosurgical Issues

- All severe TBI patients with intracranial bleeding should have a neurosurgical evaluation early in their ED course.
- Seizure prophylaxis with Levetiracetam (Keppra) or other anti-epileptic medication is usually indicated.
- Invasive ICP monitoring (external ventricular drain or intraparenchymal monitor) is indicated for severe TBI and a CT showing hematomas, contusions, swelling, herniation, or compressed basal cisterns.
  - The goal is to reduce cerebral activity and oxygen demand.
  - These agents cause hypotension and decreased CPP and should only be initiated with neurosurgical input.

Sudden Deterioration

- Prioritize cerebral perfusion pressure/osmotic agents for acute lowering ICP.
- Consider shock workup.

- Neurosurgery consult.
- Repeat imaging.
- Acutely worsening neurologic status is generally concerning for decreased CPP. Temporary efforts should be made to counter the increased ICP via raising the MAP (with vasopressors) while enlisting neurosurgical consultants for subsequent imaging and workup.
- Hemodynamic changes should prompt echocardiography as stress cardiomyopathy has been described with traumatic brain injury.
- Can slow-push 23.4% hypertonic saline bullet (institutional protocols vary) for concern for herniation.
- Repeat head imaging is essential with clinical changes in neurological exam. CT is likely the most readily available imaging study; however, consultation with neurosurgical colleagues will drive imaging exam of choice for given pathology.

Special Circumstances

- Anticoagulation
- Warfarin:
  - Reverse if INR > 1.5 (goal is INR ≤ 1.4).
  - Vitamin K 10 mg IV over 10 minutes.
  - Prothrombin complex concentrate (PCC) 25–50 U/kg
  - Recheck INR 1 hour after infusion.
- Antiplatelet agents (aspirin, clopidogrel, ticagrelor, prasugrel):
  - Check platelet function test, treat if abnormal
  - Desmopressin (DDAVP) 0.3 microgram/kg (~20 micrograms in 50 mL NS) over 15–30 minutes.
  - Platelet transfusion if surgical intervention is imminent.
- Direct Thrombin Inhibitor (Dabigatran):
  - If PTT is in normal range, it is unlikely that a significant drug effect is present.
  - Reversal agent – idarucizumab 5 mg IV.
  - Activated charcoal will adsorb if given within 2 hours of last dose.
  - Can potentially be dialyzed and ~60% will be removed within 2–3 hours.
- Direct Xa inhibitors (Rivaroxaban, Apixaban, Edoxaban):
  - Check anti-Xa level
  - Activated charcoal will adsorb if given within 2 hours of last dose.

- ○ Prothrombin complex concentrate (PCC) 25 U/kg
- Liver failure with known coagulopathy or elevated PT or INR > 1.5:
  - ○ Vitamin K 10 mg IV over 10 minutes (monitor for hypotension/anaphylaxis).
  - ○ FFP 15 mL/kg IV or PCC 50 U/kg IV.
- The use of TEG has not been found to be reliable to guide therapy in the setting of patients with therapeutic anticoagulation.

BIBLIOGRAPHY

Al-Rawi PG, Tseng MY, Richards HK, et al. Hypertonic saline in patients with poor-grade subarachnoid hemorrhage improves cerebral blood flow, brain tissue oxygen, and pH. *Stroke.* 2010;41:122–128.

Blaivas M, Theodoro D, Sierzenski PR. Elevated intracranial pressure detected by bedside emergency ultrasonography of the optic nerve sheath. *Acad Emerg Med* 2003;10:376–381.

Bourgoin A, Albanèse J, Léone M, et al. Effects of sufentanil or ketamine administered in target-controlled infusion on the cerebral hemodynamics of severely brain-injured patients. *Crit Care Med* 2005;33:1109–1113.

Brain Trauma Foundation; American Association of Neurological Surgeons; Congress of Neurological Surgeons; Joint Section on Neurotrauma and Critical Care, AANS/CNS, Bratton SL, Chestnut RM, Ghajar J, et al. Guidelines for the management of severe traumatic brain injury. *J Neurotrauma* 2007;24 Suppl 1:S1–106.

Bullock M, Chesnut R, Ghajar J, et al. Guidelines for the surgical management of traumatic brain injury. *Neurosurgery* 2006;58(3) Supplement:S2–47–S2–55.

Crashingpatient.com [homepage on the Internet]. New York, NY: Scott Weingart; ©2006–2012 [updated 2012; cited August 1, 2012]. Available from: www.crashingpatient.com/ [last accessed February 17, 2023].

Eisenberg HM, Frankowski RF, Contant CF, et al. High-dose barbiturate control of elevated intracranial pressure in patients with severe head injury. *J Neurosurg* 1988;69:15–23.

Emcrit.org [home page on the Internet]. New York, NY: Scott Weingart; c2008–2012 [updated 2012; cited 2012 Aug 1]. Available from: www.emcrit.org/ [last accessed February 17, 2023].

Fredriksson K, Norrving B, Strömblad LG. Emergency reversal of anticoagulation after intracerebral hemorrhage. *Stroke* 1992;23:972–977.

Kelly DF, Goodale DB, Williams J, et al. Propofol in the treatment of moderate and severe head injury: a randomized, prospective double-blinded pilot trial. *J Neurosurg* 1999;90:1042–1052.

Kerr ME, Sereika SM, Orndoff P, et al. Effect of neuromuscular blockers and opiates on the cerebrovascular response to endotracheal suctioning in adults with severe head injuries. *Am J Crit Care* 1998;7:205–217.

Samama CM. Prothrombin complex concentrates: a brief review. *Eur J Anaesthesiol* 2008;25:784–789.

Swadron SP, Leroux P, Smith WS, et al.. Emergency neurological life support: traumatic brain injury. *Neurocrit Care* 2012;17 Suppl 1: 112–121.

Vigué B. Bench-to-bedside review: optimising emergency reversal of vitamin K antagonists in severe haemorrhage – from theory to practice. *Crit Care* 2009;13:209.

49

. . . .

Neck Trauma

VISHAL DEMLA

Penetrating Neck Trauma

Introduction

- The incidence of penetrating neck trauma is reported to be approximately 1–5% of all traumatic injuries.
- Innocuous-appearing neck injuries have the potential to cause either immediate or delayed life-threatening injuries and complications.
- Penetrating neck injuries are generally described according to the zones of the neck (see Table 49.1). This helps to define the potentially injured structures and allows for a common nomenclature.

Presentation

- In **penetrating injuries**, it is important to look for hard and soft signs of injury (see Table 49.2).
- Hard signs are associated with a high rate of major/vascular injury and should have operative evaluation

Table 49.1 Zones of the neck

Zones	Landmarks	Structures/considerations
I	Defined inferiorly by clavicles and superiorly by the cricoid cartilage	In addition to neck structures (e.g., trachea, esophagus, neck vessels), consider injuries to thoracic structures, i.e., lung, subclavian vessels, common carotid artery, thoracic duct
II	Extends from the cricoid cartilage inferiorly to the angle of the mandible superiorly	Easily accessible surgically with ability to obtain proximal and distal control of bleeding. Includes carotid vessels, internal jugular veins, pharynx, esophagus
III	Includes the area superior to the angle of the mandible to the base of the skull	In addition to neurovascular injury (e.g., distal carotid, vertebral artery, cranial nerves), consider as a head injury

Diagnosis and Evaluation

- High-resolution CT-angiography (CTA) is the initial diagnostic study of choice in the stable patient with penetrating neck trauma.
  - CTA can be the initial diagnostic study of choice regardless of zone of injury.
  - CTA is particularly useful for zone I and III penetrating injuries, which are more difficult to evaluate by physical examination or operative exploration.
  - Historically, stable, symptomatic patients with zone II penetrating injury required mandatory surgical exploration. However, with the diagnostic capabilities of CTA, there has been a paradigm shift and selective exploration is recommended.
- Injuries can be categorized into laryngotracheal (airway), pharyngoesophageal (digestive tract), and vascular.
  1. Laryngotracheal:
     - Symptoms include hoarseness, dyspnea, stridor, subcutaneous air, hemoptysis, and tenderness of the laryngeal area.
     - Plain radiographs may be used as an initial screening tool but are not definitive to rule out injuries.

Table 49.2 Hard and soft signs of injury

Hard signs	Soft signs
Expanding hematoma	Hemoptysis/hematemesis
Severe active bleeding	Oropharyngeal blood
Shock not responding to fluids	Dyspnea
Decreased/absent extremity pulse	Dysphonia/dysphagia
Vascular bruit/thrill	Subcutaneous/mediastinal air
Cerebral ischemia	Chest tube leak
Airway obstruction, stridor	Nonexpanding hematoma
Air bubbling through wound	Focal neurological deficit (contralateral side)
	Carotid: <u>sensory</u> or motor deficits, ipsilateral Horner syndrome
	Vertebral: ataxia, vertigo, emesis, or visual field deficit; Carotid – cavernous sinus fistula: orbital pain, decreased vision, diplopia, proptosis, seizures, epistaxis Cervicothoracic seat belt sign

- ☐ May show extraluminal air, edema, or fracture of laryngeal structures.
  - Direct laryngoscopy or flexible nasopharyngoscopy should be performed to evaluate for laryngeal injury if CTA is positive or inconclusive.
    - ☐ Usually indicated in stable patients with penetrating injuries to zone I.

2. Pharyngoesophageal:
   - Symptoms include dysphagia, odynophagia, hematemesis, and blood in nasogastric tube or orogastric tube. However, even patients with significant injuries may present with no clinical signs.
   - Esophageal injuries are the leading cause of delayed mortality, especially if there is a delay in diagnosis > 24 hours.
   - Broad-spectrum antibiotics are recommended for esophageal injuries.
   - Similar to laryngotracheal injuries, plain radiographs may be used as an initial screening tool. These can demonstrate subcutaneous emphysema, retropharyngeal air, or pneumomediastinum if a perforation is present.

- Esophagoscopy or esophagography is the gold standard for diagnosing esophageal injury and should be used when there is high suspicion of injury and negative CT. Indicated in stable but symptomatic patients with penetrating zone I injury and blunt neck injury.

3. Vascular:
   - Symptoms include shock, evidence of cerebral stroke, vascular bruit, upper extremity ischemia, expanding hematoma, pulsatile hematoma, or large hemothorax.
   - Angiography/four-vessel cerebrovascular angiography (FVCA) is still considered the gold standard for any vascular injury. It should be considered when CTA is positive, inconclusive, or more information is needed (e.g., occasionally requested by surgeons for preoperative planning).

Critical Management

- Unstable patients with penetrating neck injuries require immediate surgical consultation and exploration in the OR.
- Unstable patients include those patients with hard signs: clear airway injury (air bubbling through wound), hemodynamic instability despite resuscitation, uncontrolled bleeding (including expanding hematoma), or evolving neurological deficit.

Airway

- Penetrating trauma can cause significant disruption to neck anatomy and may make airway management difficult (Figure 49.1).
- Indications for immediate airway management in the context of neck trauma include stridor, respiratory distress, shock, and rapidly expanding hematoma.
- Airway protection should be considered in patients who demonstrate progressive neck symptoms such as worsening swelling, voice change, dysphagia, or subcutaneous emphysema.
- Rapid sequence intubation (RSI) has a very high success rate and should be initiated early in the appropriate circumstances.
- The presence of neck trauma, by itself, is not a contraindication to RSI.
- Consider RSI if patient is not difficult to bag and there is no anatomical disruption.

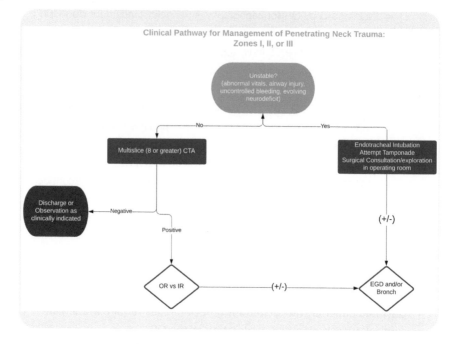

Figure 49.1 Clinical pathway for management of penetrating neck trauma.

- If oral rapid sequence intubation is planned it should be under a double setup with preparations and personnel in place to perform immediate surgical cricothyrotomy if oral endotracheal intubation is not possible.
- Consider an awake intubation if difficulty is anticipated in bagging or with suspected tracheal disruption. Awake intubation is preferably done with a fiberoptic scope, if available, which allows better visualization if anatomy is distorted.
- Consider direct tracheal intubation for open tracheal injuries, but be wary of potentially causing complete transection of the trachea.

Breathing

- Patients with zone I injury are especially prone to pneumothoraces and hemothoraces.
- Tension pneumothorax should be considered in a patient with hypotension, respiratory distress and decreased breath sounds.

- Prompt needle decompression and open thoracostomy should be performed (recent data favor the fifth intercostal space at the anterior axillary line).

Circulation

- Bleeding should be managed by direct compression.
- If central venous access is necessary, place a large-bore single lumen catheter through the subclavian (on opposite side of injury) or femoral vein.
- If the patient is unstable or hard/soft signs are present, the patient needs emergent surgical consultation and should proceed to the OR regardless of zone of injury.

Special Considerations

- Cervical spine immobilization is not always necessary in penetrating neck trauma – unless there is an overt neurological deficit or an adequate physical examination cannot be performed.
- Cervical spine injuries are rare in penetrating neck trauma. There is an abundance of literature (but no randomized trials) corroborating the safety of removing the cervical collar for penetrating neck trauma in patients with no signs of spinal cord injury. Removal of the collar facilitates the physical examination and is highly recommended to evaluate for penetrating injuries to the posterior neck.

Blunt Neck Trauma

Introduction

- Most blunt trauma is due to motor vehicle collisions, followed by falls from height and motorcycle crashes.
- The most common injuries to the neck from blunt trauma are cervical spine injuries and blunt cerebrovascular injuries (BCVI).

- Near hanging or strangulation is also a cause of neck injury and can result in significant bony and vascular injury.
- Injuries to the laryngotracheal and pharyngoesophageal structures of the neck are much less common than in penetrating trauma. However, laryngeal fractures may result from crush injuries or direct blow to the neck.
- Missed or delayed diagnosis of cervical spine injuries and BCVI can have devastating neurologic consequences. The consistent use of decision rules and screening criteria to identify these injuries can decrease the rate of missed injuries.

Presentation

- Patients with blunt neck trauma have a wide range of clinical presentations. Significant injury should be suspected in all multi-trauma patients, particularly those with associated craniofacial trauma and traumatic brain injury.
- The most common finding on physical exam is tenderness to palpation of the midline. The presence of focal neurologic deficits, including weakness, paresthesias or incoordination of the extremities should prompt full evaluation for cervical spine and BCVI.
- Patients with intoxication or altered mental status cannot reliably be ruled out for injury based on clinical exam.
- Any suspicion for neck injury after blunt trauma warrants cervical spine immobilization with cervical collar until full evaluation can be completed.

Diagnosis and Evaluation

- Clinical decision rules, such as the NEXUS criteria or the Canadian C-spine Rules should be utilized to determine which patients meet criteria for cervical spine imaging.
- NEXUS criteria should not be used in patients > 60 years old.
- For patients that meet criteria for c-spine imaging, CT scan shows improved sensitivity and negative predictive value over plain films for the diagnosis of cervical spine injury and is the preferred imaging modality.

Table 49.3 The American College of Surgeons Trauma Quality Improvement Program (TQIP) Best Practices Guideline

Criteria categories	Signs and findings present
Clinical signs and symptoms of BCVI	• Arterial hemorrhage • Cervical bruit • Expanding cervical hematoma • Focal neurological deficit • Neurologic findings unexplained by intracranial findings • Ischemic stroke on secondary CT scan
Clinical risk factors that mandate radiologic screening for BCVI	• High energy mechanism • Horner's syndrome • Neck soft tissue injury • Near hanging • Direct blow to the neck
Injuries of concern associated with possible BCVI	• LeForte II or III fracture • Cervical spine fractures • Basilar skull fracture with or without carotid canal involvement • Diffuse axonal injury

Table 49.4 Denver Grading Scale of blunt cerebrovascular injury

Grade	Description
I	Luminal irregularity or dissection with < 25% luminal narrowing
II	Dissection or intramural hematoma with > 25% luminal narrowing, intraluminal thrombus, or raised intimal flap
III	Pseudoaneurysm
IV	Occlusion
V	Transection with free extravasation

• Evidence-based screening protocols based on the Expanded Denver Criteria (Table 49.4) and the American College of Surgeons Trauma QI Program are recommended for the detection of BCVI in adult patients (Table 49.3).

Critical Management

Airway

- Blunt neck trauma has a lower incidence of airway compromise and obstruction than penetrating, however, assessment for airway compromise is imperative.
- Maintenance of cervical spine immobilization during RSI is important in all undifferentiated trauma patients, but particularly patients with suspected or known cervical spine injury.
- Videolaryngoscopy (VL) may be preferred to direct laryngoscopy (DL) in patients with cervical spine injury as it can provide better first pass success and causes less cervical spine motion during intubation.

Circulation

- In the setting of an unstable cervical spine injury, neurogenic shock (loss of sympathetic tone from cervical or thoracic injury) and spinal shock (loss of cord function below specific level) should be a consideration in a patient with persistent hypotension after other causes of shock have been assessed.
- Once a patient has undergone adequate fluid resuscitation, vasopressor therapy should be initiated to maintain adequate end organ perfusion. Either norepinephrine or phenylephrine are usually recommended.
- There is some support that augmented MAP goals of 85–90 should be maintained for 5–7 days after injury for spinal cord perfusion to stabilize and improve neurologic outcomes.

Disability

- Frequent neurologic assessment is important to quickly recognize any potentially worsening injury or cerebral ischemia.
- BCVI injuries most commonly require either therapeutic anticoagulation or antiplatelet therapy to avoid thromboembolic events and subsequent stroke, so timely diagnosis of other injuries and assessing safety of anticoagulation is a priority.

Sudden Deterioration

- In addition to airway management and surgical consultation, Zone II injuries may need balloon tamponade of vascular injury if direct pressure is insufficient.
- High grade injuries (Table 49.4. Denver Grading Scale of BCVI) are greatest risk of deterioration or stroke. These injuries may require therapeutic anticoagulation or interventions such as stent or embolization. Immediate neurosurgery or interventional radiology consultation is indicated.

BIBLIOGRAPHY

Bromberg WJ, Collier B, Diebel L, et al. Blunt cerebrovascular injury practice management guidelines: East Practice Management Guidelines Committee. *J Trauma* 2010;68;471–477.

Demla V, Shah K. Neck trauma: current guidelines for emergency physicians. *Emerg Med Pract Guidelines Update* 2012;4(3):1–9.

Navsaria P, Thoma M, & Nicol A. Foley catheter balloon tamponade for life-threatening hemorrhage in penetrating neck trauma. *World J Surg* 2006;30**:**1265–1268. https://doi.org/10.1007/s00268-005-0538-3

Newton K. Neck. In: Marx JA, Hockberger RS, Walls RM, et al., eds. *Rosen's Emergency Medicine: Concepts and Clinical Practice*, 7th ed. Philadelphia, PA: Mosby Elsevier, 2010.

Schaider J, & Bailitz J. Neck trauma: don't put your neck on the line. *Emerg Med Pract* 2003;5(7):1–28.

Sutijono D. Blunt neck trauma. In: Shah K, ed. *Essential Emergency Trauma*. Philadelphia, PA: Lippincott Williams & Wilkins, 2011.

Tisherman AT, Bokhari F, Collier B, et al. Clinical practice guidelines: penetrating neck trauma. *J Trauma* 2008;64:1392–1405.

Walls RM, Vissers RJ. The traumatized airway. In: Hagberg CA., ed. *Benumof's Airway Management*. Philadelphia, PA: Mosby Elsevier, 2007.

50

Thoracic Trauma

LAUREN BECKER

Introduction

- Trauma to the thorax is often categorized as penetrating (i.e., gunshot wound, stab wound) or blunt (i.e., motor vehicle collision, fall).
- Bedside ultrasound is useful in the initial assessment of the patient with chest trauma to rapidly evaluate for pneumothorax and pericardial effusion, as part of the extended focused assessment with sonography in trauma (eFAST).
- Penetrating injuries to "the box" (the area defined by the clavicles superiorly, nipple lines laterally, and costal margins inferiorly) are of particular concern because of the high likelihood of injury to the heart and mediastinal structures.
- The diaphragm may elevate as high as the fourth intercostal space on exhalation, so concurrent abdominal injury must be considered when penetrating trauma is located at or below the fourth intercostal space.

Pneumothorax

- Pneumothorax occurs when air enters the pleural space, causing the lung to collapse.

- Tension pneumothorax results from increasing air collection in the pleural space, causing high intrathoracic pressures and impeding venous return to the heart, which results in hypotension and hemodynamic collapse.

Presentation

Classic Presentation

- Patient with traumatic pneumothorax may present with complaints of pleuritic chest pain and/or dyspnea.
- Physical examination findings in pneumothorax include decreased or absent breath sounds, hyperresonance to percussion, and crepitus on the side of the injury.

Critical Presentation

- Tension pneumothorax presents with hypotension, tachypnea, tachycardia, distended neck veins, diminished or absent breath sounds on the affected side, and tracheal deviation away from the side of injury.

Diagnosis and Evaluation

- Tension pneumothorax is a clinical diagnosis.
- Though chest radiography is insensitive for pneumothorax, it is often the first imaging test performed in trauma patients. Detection of pneumothorax by supine chest radiography is particularly insensitive as air in the pleural space tends to accumulate anteriorly. If a patient is able to sit upright, an upright PA film is preferred.
- Because of the poor sensitivity of chest radiography for pneumothorax, there should be a low threshold to pursue further imaging with CT scan.
- Ultrasound performed by a trained provider looking for lung sliding and comet tails has superior sensitivity and specificity to supine chest radiography and similar sensitivity to chest CT in detecting pneumothorax.
- Of patients with minor penetrating chest trauma with an initial chest radiograph negative for pneumothorax, 12% will develop a delayed pneumothorax requiring intervention. These patients should be

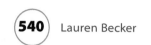

monitored and undergo repeat chest radiography at 3–6 hours or undergo evaluation with ultrasound or CT.

Critical Management

- Needle decompression/chest tube.
- Tension pneumothorax needle decompression classically consists of a 14-gauge angiocatheter inserted at the second intercostal space at the midclavicular line. Recent data (and in the obese patient) show increased success at the fourth intercostal space mid-axillary line, followed by tube thoracostomy. If tube thoracostomy can be performed immediately, this may be preferable.
- Tube thoracostomy is also indicated for any patient with pneumothorax who has dyspnea, hypoxia, or chest pain, when the pneumothorax is > 15% of the chest cavity.
- Classic teaching recommends that a large chest tube (36 French or greater) should be used in traumatic pneumothorax given potential concurrent hemothorax; however, more recent data suggests that smaller tubes may be equally effective.
- Prophylactic antibiotics after tube thoracostomy are controversial.
- Asymptomatic patients with an occult or small pneumothorax may be observed with subsequent tube thoracostomy available with clinical decompensation.

Sudden Deterioration

- Evaluate for tension pneumothorax.
- Sudden deterioration in a patient with known or suspected pneumothorax must raise concern for the development of tension physiology.
- Positive-pressure ventilation can convert a simple pneumothorax to a tension pneumothorax. The trauma patient who decompensates after intubation must be evaluated for pneumothorax.

Hemothorax

- Hemothorax results when injury to thoracic, mediastinal, chest wall, or abdominal structures causes blood to collect in the pleural cavity.
- The hemithorax can hold 40% of the blood volume, making this a potential space for exsanguination.

Presentation

Classic Presentation

- Physical examination findings include decreased breath sounds and dullness to percussion on the affected side. In addition, evidence of rib fractures or chest wall ecchymosis increases concern for hemothorax.

Critical Presentation

- Massive hemothorax is defined as hemothorax of > 1500 mL and may cause hypoxia secondary to lung collapse, as well as hypotension secondary to hypovolemia and impedance of venous return (tension hemothorax).

Diagnosis and Evaluation

- A hemothorax must be 400–500 mL in volume to be visible on an upright chest radiograph.
- Hemothorax will appear on a supine chest radiograph as opacification of the affected hemithorax (not as a fluid level); for this reason, even a substantial hemothorax can be missed on a supine radiograph.
- Bedside ultrasonography can reveal fluid in the pleural space and has a sensitivity of 100% for effusions greater than 100 mL, making it more sensitive than portable chest X-ray for detection of hemothorax.
- CT scan has the highest sensitivity and specificity for detection of hemothorax.

Critical Management

- Large bore chest tube
- Consider surgical management
- Hemothorax should be drained with a large (36 French or greater) chest tube; retained hemothorax can consolidate and result in infection and fibrosis.
- Initial drainage of > 1500 mL or continued drainage of > 200 mL/hour should prompt consideration of surgical management.
- Retained hemothorax following tube thoracostomy is a risk factor for infection and should generally prompt early video-assisted thorascopic surgery (VATS); however, recent data indicate that small retained hemothoraces < 300 mL may be considered for observation.

Sudden Deterioration

- Consider hemorrhagic shock.
- Consider surgical management.
- The development of massive hemothorax can cause sudden hemodynamic instability. If this is suspected, immediate tube thoracostomy must be performed to drain the hemothorax.
- Hemorrhagic shock should be treated with resuscitation using crystalloids and blood products. Surgical intervention is recommended for the indications described above and should be considered in any patient who shows signs of continuous bleeding or persistent hemodynamic instability.

Cardiac Tamponade

- Cardiac tamponade is the accumulation of fluid in the pericardial space causing pressure on the chambers of the heart, leading to impaired filling/preload and subsequent decrease in cardiac output.

Presentation

Classic Presentation

- Beck's triad (hypotension, distant heart sounds, jugular venous distension) describes the classic presentation of cardiac tamponade.

- Pulsus paradoxus (a systolic blood pressure fall of 10 mmHg or more during inspiration) may be present reflecting ventricular interdependence.

Critical Presentation

- Tamponade can impede cardiac output to the point of cardiac arrest and should be considered as a reversible cause in all PEA arrests.

Diagnosis and Evaluation

- Pericardial effusion may be diagnosed on FAST examination with the finding of fluid surrounding the heart.
- Chest radiography may show an enlarged cardiac silhouette.
- Most specifically, cardiac tamponade is identified on ultrasound by diastolic collapse of the right ventricle.

Critical Management

- Consider ED versus surgical thoracotomy.
- Traumatic pericardial tamponade must be treated with immediate surgical thoracotomy to address the cause of the bleeding into the pericardium.
- Emergency department thoracotomy is indicated in the patient with traumatic arrest due to penetrating chest trauma with recent signs of life (such as spontaneous ventilation, palpable pulse, measurable blood pressure, or cardiac electrical activity). This procedure allows the physician to perform pericardiotomy to release tamponade, repair cardiac lacerations, cross-clamp the aorta to prevent exsanguination from abdominal injuries and perform internal cardiac massage and defibrillation.
- Factors that predict survival after ED thoracotomy include penetrating injury (8.8% survival), particularly stab wounds (16.8% survival), and signs of life on arrival at the hospital (11.5% survival).
- Survival is extremely low in patients with blunt trauma, multiple injuries, and those with no signs of life in the field (1–2%).

Sudden Deterioration

- Consider ED thoracotomy
- Consider pericardiocentesis
- In-hospital cardiac arrest due to pericardial tamponade is an indication for ED thoracotomy.
- Pericardiocentesis or pericardial window in traumatic pericardial tamponade may briefly stabilize the patient if surgical management is not immediately possible; however, it will not fix the underlying cause of the tamponade and surgical thoracotomy must follow.

Aortic Injury

- Blunt aortic injury carries a very high mortality and 75–90% of patients with this condition die immediately at the scene of the accident.
- Injuries include aortic dissection, pseudoaneurysm, and rupture, the latter of which is almost universally fatal.
- Patients with blunt aortic injury who survive transport to the emergency department will often be hemodynamically stable initially, so the clinician must be alert to the possibility of this critical injury in the stable patient with a concerning mechanism.

Presentation

Classic Presentation

- The classic mechanism for blunt aortic injury is sudden deceleration (such as a fall from > 3 m or high-speed head-on motor vehicle collision).
- However, lower-speed collisions may account for many cases of traumatic aortic rupture, especially in patients over 60 years old and in cases of lateral impact.
- Patients may complain of chest pain, back pain, and dyspnea and will frequently have multiple associated injuries.
- Steering wheel or seat belt contusion on the chest, flail chest, unequal extremity pulses, hoarseness, and paraplegia raise concern for aortic injury; however, physical examination is not sensitive in the evaluation of aortic injury and the physician must have a low threshold to pursue diagnostic imaging.

Critical Presentation

- The critical patient with aortic injury who survives transport to the emergency department has a high probability of aortic rupture resulting in complete hemodynamic collapse and death if not quickly diagnosed and treated.

Diagnosis and Evaluation

- See Figure 50.1 below for an example of blunt aortic injury on plain film and CT.

Chest radiography findings concerning for blunt aortic injury
Widened mediastinum (> 8 cm on supine or > 6 cm on upright film)
Obscured aortic knob
Left apical cap (blood above apex of lung)
Large left hemothorax
Rightward deviation of nasogastric tube
Rightward deviation of trachea or downward deviation of right mainstem bronchus Wide left paravertebral stripe

- CT scan of the chest with contrast should be performed if any of these findings are present on chest radiography.
- A negative chest radiograph is not sufficient to exclude aortic injury, and CT scan should be performed if there is any clinical suspicion for this injury.
- Transesophageal echocardiography by a skilled operator can accurately identify aortic injury and may be performed if a patient is unable to undergo CT scan.

Critical Management

- Consider surgical management
- Impulse control via negative inotrope
- Immediate surgical repair is necessary in patients who are unstable due to traumatic aortic injury.
- Medical management of the stable traumatic aortic injury is with impulse control or the reduction of systolic pressure changes per unit time. Use a

short-acting beta-blocker, such as esmolol, to reduce inotropy and heart rate to a goal of 60 bpm, followed by an arterial vasodilator such as nicardipine or sodium nitroprusside to reduce blood pressure to 100–120 mmHg. These measures minimize risk of rupture prior to repair and can allow delay of repair while other more critical injuries are managed.

Sudden Deterioration

- Consider hemorrhagic shock versus obstructive shock (in the scenario of retrograde aortic dissection causing tamponade).
- The patient with traumatic aortic injury is at extremely high risk for deterioration.
- Rapid surgical consultation at the first suspicion of traumatic aortic injury must be obtained to expedite repair.

(a)

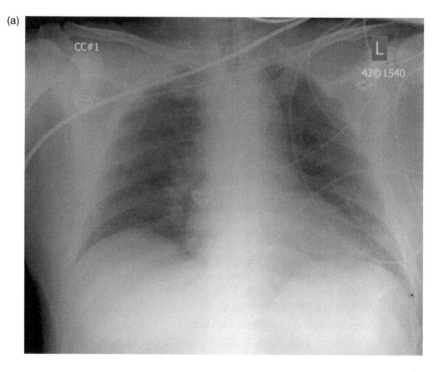

Figure 50.1 Image (a) demonstrates a wide mediastinum suspicious for blunt aortic injury on portable chest radiograph. The diagnosis is confirmed on CT (b).
(Image courtesy of Michael A. Gibbs, MD.)

Tracheobronchial Injury

- Injury to the tracheobronchial tree is relatively uncommon, accounting for 1–2% of injuries to the pulmonary system in blunt thoracic trauma. However, mortality remains approximately 10%.

Presentation

Classic Presentation

- May present with dyspnea, subcutaneous emphysema, sternal tenderness, and Hamman's sign (a "crunching" sound heard on auscultation of the precordium due to mediastinal emphysema).
- Tracheobronchial injury should be suspected in the presence of a large air leak from a chest tube, or a rapidly reaccumulating pneumothorax or pneumomediastinum.

(b)

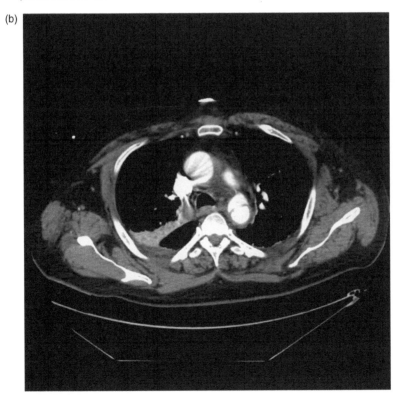

Figure 50.1 (*cont.*)

Critical Presentation

- Tracheal transection is usually associated with multiple other severe injuries and is generally fatal.
- Missed tracheobronchial injury can result in mediastinitis, bronchial stenosis, and recurrent pulmonary infections.

Diagnosis and Evaluation

- Definitive diagnosis may be established by bronchoscopy or operative evaluation.
- High-quality CT scan may also diagnose tracheobronchial injury.

Critical Management

- Observation versus surgical management.
- Most tracheobronchial injuries should be surgically repaired; however, observation may be considered in hemodynamically stable patients in whom ventilation is not compromised, there is no accumulating subcutaneous or mediastinal emphysema, and there is no involvement of the esophagus.

Sudden Deterioration

- Evaluation for pneumothorax/tension pneumothorax or hemothorax (if penetrating trauma mechanism).
- Definitive airway management (if not already performed).
- Bronchoscopy.
- Prompt CXR or lung POCUS can evaluate for pneumothorax/hemothorax.
- After definitive airway management, bronchoscopy can aid in the workup for worsening tracheobronchial injury or air leak on ventilator.

Flail Chest

- Flail chest occurs when three or more ribs are each fractured in two or more places resulting in a "floating" segment of the rib cage. The floating segment paradoxically moves inward with inhalation and outward with exhalation and can greatly increase work of breathing.

Presentation

Classic Presentation

- The patient with flail chest may present with pain, dyspnea, tachypnea, chest wall tenderness and crepitus, and visible flail segment on observation of breathing.

Critical Presentation

- Patients with a significant flail chest, especially older patients or those with underlying lung disease or multiple other injuries, may present with respiratory distress or failure.

Diagnosis and Evaluation

- Chest radiograph shows multiple rib fractures.
- Patients who present with flail chest should receive CT of the chest to evaluate for other injuries including blunt aortic injuries, pulmonary contusions and pneumothorax.

Critical Management

- Airway management
- Analgesia/regional anesthesia
- External stabilization of the flail segment restricts chest expansion and is not recommended.
- Positive-pressure ventilation, either invasive or noninvasive, may be used in patients with hypoxia, hypercapnea, or respiratory distress.

- As with all chest wall injuries, pain management is critical to prevent splinting and the development of atelectasis or pneumonia. An epidural catheter or regional nerve blocks are preferred for pain control in severe chest injury.
- Elderly trauma patients who sustain blunt chest trauma with rib fractures have twice the mortality and morbidity of younger patients with similar injuries. For each additional rib fracture in the elderly, mortality increases by 19% and the risk of pneumonia by 27%. Aggressive pain control with epidural catheter placement is recommended in these patients.
- Surgical fixation of rib or sternal fractures may be considered.

Sudden Deterioration

- Definitive airway management
- Patients with flail chest can deteriorate rapidly to the point of respiratory failure due to increased work of breathing combined with hypoxia caused by underlying lung contusion.
- Endotracheal intubation and mechanical ventilation is indicated for the decompensating patient with flail chest.

BIBLIOGRAPHY

Ayoub F, Quirke M, Frith D. Use of prophylactic antibiotic in preventing complications for blunt and penetrating chest trauma requiring chest drain insertion: a systematic review and meta-analysis. *Trauma Surg Acute Care Open* 2019;4(1):e000246. https://doi.org/10.1136/tsaco-2018-000246

Ball CG, Kirkpatrick AW, Laupland KB, et al. Factors related to the failure of radiographic recognition of occult posttraumatic pneumothoraces. *Am J Surg* 2005;189:541–546; discussion 546.

Bosman A, de Jong MB, Debeij J, et al. Systematic review and meta-analysis of antibiotic prophylaxis to prevent infections from chest drains in blunt and penetrating thoracic injuries. *Br J Surg* 2012;99:506–513.

DuBose J, Inaba K, Demetriades D, et al. Management of post-traumatic retained hemothorax: a prospective, observational, multicenter AAST study. *J Trauma Acute Care Surg* 2012;72:11–22; discussion 22–4; quiz 316.

Fabian TC, Davis KA, Gavant ML, et al. Prospective study of blunt aortic injury: helical CT is diagnostic and antihypertensive therapy reduces rupture. *Ann Surg* 1998;227:666–676; discussion 676–677.

Fabian TC, Richardson JD, Croce MA, et al. Prospective study of blunt aortic injury: Multicenter Trial of the American Association for the Surgery of Trauma. *J Trauma* 1997;42:374–380; discussion 380–383.

Leigh-Smith S, & Harris T. Tension pneumothorax – time for a re-think? *Emerg Med J* 2005;22:8–16.

Moore EE, Knudson MM, Burlew CC, et al. Defining the limits of resuscitative emergency department thoracotomy: a contemporary Western Trauma Association perspective. *J Trauma* 2011;70:334–339.

Moore F, Duane TM, Hu CK, et al. Presumptive antibiotic use in tube thoracostomy for traumatic hemopneumothorax: an Eastern Association for the Surgery of Trauma practice management guideline. *J Trauma Acute Care Surg* 2012;73:S341–344.

Mowery NT, Gunter OL, Collier BR, et al. Practice management guidelines for management of hemothorax and occult pneumothorax. *J Trauma* 2011;70:510–518.

Neff MA, Monk JS, Jr., Peters K, et al. Detection of occult pneumothoraces on abdominal computed tomographic scans in trauma patients. *J Trauma* 2000;49:281–285.

Ordog GJ, Wasserberger J, Balasubramanium S, et al. Asymptomatic stab wounds of the chest. *J Trauma* 1994;36:680–684.

Rhee PM, Acosta J, Bridgeman A, et al. Survival after emergency department thoracotomy: review of published data from the past 25 years. *J Am Coll Surg* 2000;190:288–298.

Rowan KR, Kirkpatrick AW, Liu D, et al. Traumatic pneumothorax detection with thoracic US: correlation with chest radiography and CT – initial experience. *Radiology* 2002;225:210–214.

Sastry P, Field M, Cuerden R, et al. Low-impact scenarios may account for two-thirds of blunt traumatic aortic rupture. *Emerg Med J* 2010;27:341–344.

Simon B, Ebert J, Bokhari F, et al. Management of pulmonary contusion and flail chest: an Eastern Association for the Surgery of Trauma practice management guideline. *J Trauma Acute Care Surg* 2012;73:S351–361.

Soni NJ, Franco R, Velez MI, et al. Ultrasound in the diagnosis and management of pleural effusions. *J Hosp Med* 2015;10(12):811–816. https://doi.org/10.1002/jhm.2434

Spodick DH. Acute cardiac tamponade. *N Engl J Med* 2003;349:684–690.

51

Solid Organ Abdominal Trauma

JAYARAM CHELLURI

Introduction

- Injuries are generally classified based on mechanism into either blunt or penetrating. Each has a different method of evaluation and treatment.
- *Blunt injuries*
  - Solid organs are commonly injured with acceleration/deceleration injuries (i.e., motor vehicle collisions [MVC], falls from height) and crush injuries.
  - Blunt injuries are associated with greater mortality than penetrating ones.
  - The spleen is the most commonly injured solid organ followed by the liver.
- *Penetrating injuries*
  - Stab wounds:
    - Stab wounds are less likely to cause intra-abdominal injury and penetrate the peritoneum requiring surgical intervention when compared to projectile wounds.

- The small and large bowel are the most common organs injured, and the liver is the most commonly injured solid organ given its surface area in the abdominal cavity.
  - Projectile wounds or gunshot wounds (GSW):
    - Degree of injury is correlated to velocity of projectile
      - Medium- and high-velocity projectiles create explosive type injuries and create a secondary zone of injury through tissue.
    - GSWs are associated with greater mortality than stab wounds.

Presentation

- In both blunt and penetrating trauma, patients may have extensive intra-abdominal injuries with seemingly insignificant signs of external trauma.
- The ability to adequately identify injuries on physical examination may be compromised by concomitant injuries (i.e., head trauma) or confounding factors (i.e., intoxication).
- **Common symptoms are abdominal, back or flank pain, nausea, vomiting, confusion, or dizziness.**
- **Common signs are tenderness to palpation, abdominal distension, and ecchymosis (e.g., seat-belt sign) but they are not universally present.**

Diagnosis and Evaluation

- The initial evaluation should be aimed at determining which patients need immediate operating room laparotomy versus those that are stable for further diagnostic workup.
- Indications for emergent surgical intervention may include:
  - Hemodynamic instability
  - Peritonitis on exam
  - Visible evisceration of intra-abdominal contents
  - Blood on rectal examination
- **Primary survey**
  - Regardless of the mechanism of injury, the primary survey (i.e. "ABCs") should focus on identifying and addressing immediate life-threatening causes of injury.

- Fully undress all patients to assess for injuries that may not be initially visible, with particular attention to the groin, axilla, perineum or skin folds.
- **Adjuncts to the primary survey**
  - All patients after significant trauma, both blunt and penetrating, should receive screening AP chest radiography.
  - Screening pelvis X-ray may be used selectively in blunt trauma patients with concern for unstable pelvic fractures or in penetrating trauma patients to assess missile trajectory or fracture.
  - *Extended Focused Assessment with Sonography for Trauma (eFAST)* – Sensitivities between 85–96% and specificity exceeding 98% to assess for hemoperitoneum.
  - Primarily assessing for either pneumothorax or intraperitoneal hemorrhage, the eFAST consists of ultrasound evaluation of lungs, heart, right upper quadrant, left upper quadrant, and suprapubic areas. Increase sensitivity by performing upper quadrant scans in Trendelenburg.
  - In hypotensive trauma patients, sensitivities approach 100%.
  - Any hypotensive trauma patient with a positive eFAST should go directly to the operating room for emergent laparotomy.
  - Positive eFAST examination in a hemodynamically stable patient will still need abdominal CT imaging to identify the location and severity of injury. Non-operative management may still be an option.
  - A positive eFAST in penetrating abdominal trauma is a strong predictor of injury and patients should proceed directly to laparotomy. If negative, additional diagnostic studies should be performed to rule out injury.
- **Laboratory tests**
  - Sending a blood type and screen is essential in the setting of trauma.
  - Complete blood count may not reflect blood loss initially and clinical scenario should take precedence.
  - Lactate level is nonspecific but is a useful marker of severity of illness.
  - Pancreatic enzymes, liver function tests and chemistry are unreliable in the setting of trauma.
  - Hematuria on urinalysis may be useful to evaluate for possible renal injury.
  - Coagulation studies, thromboelastography (TEG), may assist in targeting resuscitation.

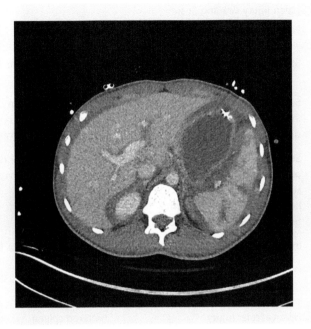

Figure 51.1 Grade 5 splenic injury with active extravasation of contrast.

- **Computed tomography (CT)**
  - ○ Has become the main diagnostic modality for patients with abdominal trauma.
  - ○ Is indicated in any patient with concerning abdominal pain, tenderness to palpation, visible seat belt sign, or an unreliable physical examination.
  - ○ CT is very accurate for identification of solid visceral organ injuries and can identify retroperitoneal bleeding.
  - ○ Active bleeding from the liver/spleen can be visualized by extravasation of IV contrast (often called a "blush"). See Figure 51.1.
  - ○ CT can guide nonoperative management by aiding in grading of lacerations and contusions (see Tables 51.1, 51.2 and 51.3).
  - ○ Oral contrast is not necessary and does not significantly increase sensitivity in detecting traumatic injuries
  - ○ Administering rectal contrast is recommended to identify rectal or large bowel injury in penetrating trauma.

Table 51.1 Spleen Injury Grading Scale

Grade	Hematoma	Laceration
I	Subcapsular, < 10% surface area	Capsular tear, < 1 cm parenchymal depth
II	Subcapsular, 10–50% surface area; intraparenchymal < 5 cm in diameter	Capsular tear, 1–3 cm parenchymal depth that does not involve a trabecular vessel
III	Subcapsular, > 50% surface area or expanding; ruptured subcapsular or parenchymal hematoma; intraparenchymal hematoma 5 cm or expanding	> 3 cm parenchymal depth or involving trabecular vessels
IV	Involves the hilum	Involves segmental or hilar vessels leading to devascularization > 25% of spleen
V	Hilar vascular injury devascularizing spleen	Shattered spleen

- **Local wound exploration**
  - ○ Useful in determining the depth of a wound and to determine whether the wound has penetrated the peritoneum.
- **Diagnostic peritoneal lavage (DPL)**
  - ○ Is useful for determination of intra-abdominal bleeding when the patient is unstable and unable to obtain CT, FAST is negative or inconclusive, and source of hemorrhage is unclear.
- **Serial abdominal examination**
  - ○ In patients who are hemodynamically stable and have a reliable physical examination, serial abdominal exams are safe and reliable after both blunt trauma and stab wounds to the abdomen.
  - ○ They should occur at least every 6 hours for a duration of 12 to 24 hours.
  - ○ **Magnetic resonance Imaging (MRI)** is generally not helpful in the acute management of solid organ abdominal trauma.

The following tables demonstrate grading systems for blunt injuries to various solid abdominal organs (adapted from the American Association of Surgery for Trauma).

Table 51.2 Liver Injury Grading Scale

Grade	Hematoma	Laceration
I	Subcapsular < 10% surface area	Capsular tear, < 1 cm parenchymal depth
II	Subcapsular 10–50% surface area; intraparenchymal < 10 cm in diameter	Capsular tear, 1–3 cm parenchymal depth, < 10 cm in length
III	Subcapsular, > 50% surface area of ruptured subcapsular or parenchymal hematoma; intraparenchymal hematoma > 10 cm or expanding	> 3 cm parenchymal depth
IV	Involves segmental or hilar vessels leading to devascularization > 25% of liver	Parenchymal disruption involving 25–75% hepatic lobe or 1–3 Couinaud's segments
V	Hilar vascular injury devascularizing liver	Parenchymal disruption involving > 75% of hepatic lobe or > 3 Couinaud's segments within a single lobe; vascular injury – juxtaheptatic venous injuries

Critical Management

Critical Management Checklist

- ☑ Primary and secondary surveys
- ☑ Large bore IV access
- ☑ eFAST
- ☑ Hemostasis/damage control resuscitation/REBOA if available

Primary survey: assessment of airway, breathing, and circulation.

Secondary survey: head-to-toe evaluation by systems to identify further life- or limb-threatening injury.

eFAST: as described above, ultrasound evaluation of lung/pleura, pericardium, pelvis and upper quadrants of the abdomen.

- • **Resuscitation**
  - ○ The goal of resuscitation in patients with hemorrhagic shock is arresting hemorrhage, reversing shock and preventing coagulopathy, termed Damage Control Resuscitation.

Table 51.3 Kidney Injury Grading Scale

Grade	Characteristics
I	Contusion: microscopic or gross hematuria, urological studies normal; Subcapsular hematoma: nonexpanding without parenchymal lacerations
II	Nonexpanding perirenal hematoma confined to renal retroperitoneum; Laceration < 1 cm parenchymal depth of renal cortex without urinary extravasation
III	> 1 cm parenchymal depth of renal cortex without collecting system rupture or urinary extravasation
IV	Parenchymal laceration extending through renal cortex, medulla, collecting system; vascular – main renal artery or vein injury with contained hemorrhage
V	Completely shattered kidney; Vascular – Avulsion of renal hilum which devascularizes kidney

- ○ **Hemostatic resuscitation** involves administration of fluid and blood products that comes as close as possible to whole blood transfusion.
  - ▪ Limit crystalloid infusion.
  - ▪ Transfusion of RBC:FFP:PLT in as close to 1:1:1 ratio as possible.
  - ▪ Use of whole blood transfusion when possible.
- ○ **Permissive Hypotension** – also termed hypotensive resuscitation (colloquially, "don't pop the clot"), limits the amount of fluids or blood products in order to target a lower-than-normal blood pressure.
  - ▪ Goal SBP 80–90 until major bleeding has been stopped.
  - ▪ Targeting a lower SBP or MAP goal and limiting fluid resuscitation likely has mortality benefit, as well as lower risks of multi-organ dysfunction and ARDS.
  - ▪ Data is most supportive for patients with penetrating abdominal trauma.
  - ▪ Not appropriate in patients with concomitant head injury.
- • **Non-operative management**
  - ○ Patients who do not require exploratory laparotomy are candidates for non-operative management, which can include observation or angiography with or without embolization.

- **Angiography and embolization**
  - Is a useful modality in management of bleeding, particularly in splenic, liver and renal injuries. Indicated in:
    - Higher grades of injury
    - Active extravasation of contrast
    - Presence of pseudoaneurysm and
    - Significant hemoperitoneum
- **Resuscitative Endovascular Balloon Occlusion (REBOA)**
  - For patients in profound hemorrhagic shock, REBOA is a minimally invasive technique that serves as an alternative to thoracotomy and aortic cross clamping for hemorrhage control in non-compressible sites, such as the abdomen or pelvis.
  - There is no evidence that REBOA has improved survival compared with standard treatment for severe hemorrhage.
  - Zones of the aorta: zone 1 (~20 cm long) extends from left subclavian artery to celiac (approx. xiphoid process); zone 2 (~3 cm long) extends from celiac artery to caudal renal artery; and zone 3 (~10 cm long) extends from caudal renal artery to the aortic bifurcation (approx. superior to umbilicus). Approximate insertion distances are listed in placement depth image (Figure 51.2).
  - Avoid placement of REBOA in zone 2.

Sudden Deterioration

- Reassess vital signs and look for signs of hypovolemia, poor organ perfusion, and shock.
- Repeat abdominal examination and eFAST (perform in Trendelenburg position to enhance sensitivity) to assess for change.
- **The most likely reason for sudden deterioration in a trauma patient with solid organ injury is hemorrhagic shock. Continue aggressive resuscitation (massive transfusion protocol, if necessary) and facilitate the process to get patient to the OR for laparotomy.**

Figure 51.2 The aorta is divided into zones with approximate depths to estimate balloon placement.

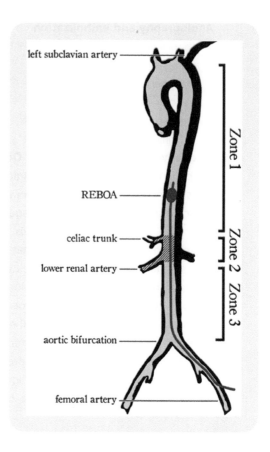

left subclavian artery

Zone 1

REBOA

celiac trunk

lower renal artery

Zone 2

Zone 3

aortic bifurcation

femoral artery

BIBLIOGRAPHY

American Association for the Surgery of Trauma. *Trauma Source:* Injury scoring scale. Chicago, IL: American Association for the Surgery of Trauma, 2013. Available from: www.aast.org/resources-detail/injury-scoring-scaleCannon JW, Khan MA, Raja AS, et al. Damage control resuscitation in patients with severe traumatic hemorrhage. *J Trauma* 2017;82(3):605–617.

Owattanapanich N, Chittawatanarat K, Benyakorn T, et al. Risks and benefits of hypotensive resuscitation in patients with traumatic hemorrhagic shock: a meta-analysis. *Scand J Trauma Resusc Emerg Med* 2018;26(1):107. (Meta-analysis; 30 studies)

Stassen NA, Indermeet B, Cheng JD, et al. Selective non operative management of blunt splenic injury: an Eastern Association for the Surgery of Trauma practice management guideline. *Trauma Acute Care Surg* 2012;73:S294–300.

52

Severe Pelvic Trauma

JEFFREY PEPIN

Introduction

- Severe pelvic fractures are a major cause of morbidity and mortality in trauma patients.
- As hemorrhage is the main cause of mortality in pelvic trauma, it is critical to assess hemodynamic stability and identify ongoing bleeding in the chest, abdomen, and long bones. **If no clear source of hemorrhage is identified and a patient remains unstable, suspicion for primary pelvic hemorrhage should be high.**
- Suspect pelvic fracture in all cases of serious or multi-system trauma patients.
- In pelvic trauma, there is a high incidence of associated injuries; therefore, special attention should be paid to the rectal and urogenital examinations.
- *Classification:* The most commonly used classification system for pelvic fractures is the Young–Burgess system (Table 52.1; Figure 52.1). This system categorizes injuries on the basis of mechanism of injury and can be used to predict the risk of blood loss.

Table 52.1 Young–Burgess classification system for pelvic fractures

Mechanism and type	Characteristics	Hemi-pelvis displacement	Stability
APC-I	Pubic diastasis < 2.5 cm	External rotation	Stable
APC-II	Pubic diastasis > 2.5 cm, anterior sacroiliac joint disruption	External rotation	Rotationally unstable, vertically stable
APC-III	Type II plus posterior sacroiliac joint disruption	External rotation	Rotationally unstable, vertically unstable
LC-I	Ipsilateral sacral buckle fractures, ipsilateral horizontal pubic rami fractures (or disruption of symphysis with overlapping pubic bones)	Internal rotation	Stable
LC-II	Type I plus ipsilateral iliac wing fracture or posterior sacroiliac joint disruption	Internal rotation	Rotationally unstable, vertically stable
LC-III	Type II plus contralateral anterior sacroiliac joint disruption (APC)	Internal rotation	Rotationally unstable, vertically unstable
Vertical shear	Vertical pubic rami fractures, sacroiliac joint disruption ± adjacent fractures	Vertical (cranial)	Rotationally unstable, vertically unstable

Presentation

Classic Presentation

- Severe pelvic trauma may present with pain at the fracture site, low back, abdominal, or hip.
- They are frequently hypotensive and require rapid fluid resuscitation.
- It is important to keep pelvic fractures high in the differential diagnosis when evaluating any patient with multiple injuries or hypotension.

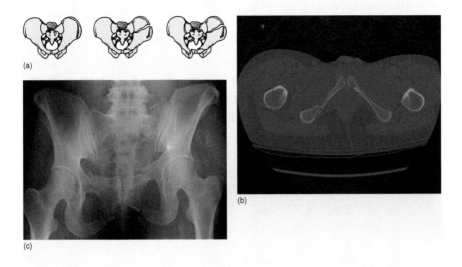

Figure 52.1 (a) Young–Burgess lateral compression (LC) pelvic fracture classifications; (b) computed tomography (CT) of LCI fracture pattern; (c) radiograph of LCI fracture pattern.

(Reprinted with permission from Hammel J. Pelvic fracture. In: Legone, E, Shockley, L, Traum, W. A Comprehensive Emergency Medicine Approach. Cambridge University Press, 2011.)

Critical Presentation

- Severely injured patients are often hypotensive and require aggressive resuscitation and pelvic binding as subsequently detailed.

Diagnosis and Evaluation

- **Signs of pelvic trauma**
  - Ecchymosis, abrasions, or hematomas
  - Pelvic and leg deformity or asymmetry
  - Bony tenderness to palpation
  - Instability with gentle lateral pressure on the iliac wings
  - Peripheral neurovascular deficit
  - Difficulty with active and passive range of motion of the hip
  - Blood at urethral meatus
  - Rectal bleeding and poor sphincter tone

- **Diagnostic tests**
  - ○ *eFAST examination*
    - ▪ All trauma patients should have an extended focused assessment with sonography for trauma to investigate for internal bleeding and pneumothorax.
    - ▪ **eFAST examinations are not sensitive or specific for retroperitoneal injuries but they are highly sensitive in detecting clinically significant hemoperitoneum.**
  - ○ *Chest radiography*
    - ▪ Portable chest radiography is complementary to the e-FAST to determine the presence and extent of chest injuries.
  - ○ *Pelvic radiography*
    - ▪ Anteroposterior (AP) pelvic radiography is the initial imaging modality of choice; it identifies up to 90% of fractures.
    - ▪ Posterior sacroiliac ligament disruption may be difficult to diagnose with plain films.
    - ▪ In the past, inlet and outlet pelvic views (taken with beam 45° caudally or cephalad, respectively) were used to demonstrate posterior dislocation of pelvic ring and opening of pubic symphysis; these views are now replaced by CT imaging.
  - ○ *Abdominal/pelvic CT*
    - ▪ Provides optimal imaging for evaluation of bony pelvic anatomy, while also providing information on pelvic, retroperitoneal, and intra-abdominal bleeding.
    - ▪ In patients with a significant mechanism of injury, CT of the abdomen/pelvis is often performed.
    - ▪ Intravenous contrast is necessary to highlight active hemorrhage.
    - ▪ CT scan can also confirm hip dislocation associated with an acetabular fracture.

Critical Management

- ☑ Examine the pelvis
- ☑ Correct hemodynamic instability
- ☑ eFAST examination and pelvic radiograph
- ☑ Hemorrhage control/pelvic binding, if indicated
- ☑ Avoid hypothermia
- ☑ Invasive/operative management

- **Examine the pelvis**
  - Lateral compression of the ala to assess for gross movement of the pelvic structure.
  - DO NOT ROCK THE PELVIS OR APPLY LATERAL DISTRACTION!
  - Vaginal exam in women and rectal exam in all patients should be performed to assess for occult open pelvic fracture.
- **Correct hemodynamic instability**
  - Intravenous access should be obtained above the diaphragm.
  - In hypotensive patients, IV crystalloids should be limited and quickly replaced with blood products as soon as they are available.
  - Consider initiation of massive transfusion protocols as hemodynamically unstable patients may require high volumes of blood products.
- **eFAST examination and pelvic radiograph**
  - Evidence of intra-abdominal free fluid is an indication of coexisting intra-abdominal injury. Depending on a patient's hemodynamic stability, this may be an indication for emergent laparotomy prior to pelvic repair.
  - Always obtain an AP radiograph of the pelvis when history/ mechanism suggests pelvic injury or in an unconscious trauma patient.
  - Pelvic radiographs should not delay pelvic binding.
- **Hemorrhage control/pelvic binding**
  - The primary goal is early reduction of pelvic volume, which decreases venous hemorrhage through tamponade and clot formation, thereby improving mortality.
  - Noninvasive methods are preferred initially.
  - Circumferential wrapping of the pelvis with a sheet is an easy and inexpensive option. Commercially available pelvic binders are also an option.
  - Other methods of stabilization, more complicated and less commonly used, include military anti-shock trousers (MAST), spica casting, applications of a posterior C-clamp, or external fixation.
  - Early binding should be a priority in the prehospital setting (if local protocols allow) when injury of the pelvis is suspected.
  - Radiographic Young–Burgess indications for binding:
    - AP compressions, type II: pubic diastasis > 2.5 cm, anterior SI joint disruption (OPEN BOOK).

- Lateral compression, type II: Type I plus ipsilateral iliac wing fracture or posterior SI joint disruption.
- Lateral compression, type III: Type I or type II on ipsilateral pelvic and external rotation injury on contralateral pelvis with pubic rami fracture or disruption of the sacrotuberous and/or sacrospinous ligaments.
- AP compression, type III: Type II plus posterior SI joint disruption, Pubic diastasis > 4cm.
- Vertical shear: Vertical pubic rami fractures, SI joint disruption +/- adjacent fractures.
- **Avoid hypothermia**
  - Use warm fluids and keep warm sheets/blankets on the patient.
- **Invasive/operative management. There are four accepted strategies for controlling pelvic bleeding:**
  - Angiography with selective arterial embolization.
  - Mechanical stabilization via external fixation.
  - Surgical pre-peritoneal packing.
  - REBOA (retrograde endovascular balloon occlusion of the aorta) in patients with severe hemorrhagic shock.

Sudden Deterioration

Consider pelvic binder if not already implemented.

Consult interventional radiology for emergent embolization.

- **Hypotension**
- If pelvic binding and resuscitative efforts seem to be failing, pelvic bleeding is likely ongoing.
- **Suspicion for arterial bleeding should prompt activation of the interventional radiology suite to initiate arterial embolization via angiography.**
- Suspicion should be higher for venous bleeding and should initiate operative management for pre-peritoneal packing to tamponade venous bleeding that cannot be addressed via angiography. In many cases, patients need both modalities.

53

Soft Tissue Injury

Crush Injury, Compartment Syndrome, and Open Fractures

KATRINA HARPER-KIRKSEY

Crush Injury

- Severe crush injury can result in sequelae such as significant bony fractures, rhabdomyolysis, extremity compartment syndrome, or crush syndrome.
- Crush syndrome comprises the systemic manifestations that arise as a result of a crush injury followed by reperfusion. From the rupture of muscle cells, substances such as myoglobin, potassium, phosphorus, and creatinine phosphokinase are released into the bloodstream. The patient can subsequently develop hyperkalemia, hypocalcemia, hypovolemia, shock, compartment syndrome, lactic acidosis, or renal failure from traumatic rhabdomyolysis (seen in up to 40% of patients with crush injury).

Presentation

Classic Presentation

- Following extrication, crush injury may manifest as neurologic deficiency such as flaccid paralysis and sensory loss. Gross edema commonly follows. Distal pulses remain present, and if lost, a concurrent vascular injury or compartment syndrome should be suspected.
- Crush syndrome may present with hypotension due to third spacing, acute renal failure, and metabolic abnormalities.

Diagnosis and Evaluation

- **Physical exam**
  - Initial physical examination should clearly document extent of soft tissue injury, sensation and motor function, and presence or absence of distal pulses or Doppler signals.
- **Laboratory evaluation**
  - Evaluate for electrolyte abnormalities such as hypocalcemia, hyperkalemia, and hyperphosphatemia that result from massive cellular damage. Stress-related hyperglycemia may also be seen.
  - *Venous (or arterial) blood* gas will reveal metabolic acidosis.
  - *Creatine phosphokinase (CPK),* as the surrogate marker to assess the extent of muscle damage. CPK 5x normal indicates rhabdomyolysis.
  - Serum lactate and uric acid.
  - *Urinalysis and urine myoglobin* will determine the presence of myoglobin indirectly. Myoglobin in the urine will be detected as "blood" on the urine dipstick but there will be no red blood cells noted on the urine analysis. Urinalysis will also give a measurement of urine pH.
- **Obtain an ECG to evaluate for signs of hyperkalemia.**
  - The increase in serum potassium is most severe in the first 12–36 hours after muscle injury. Initially, there may be peaked T waves and prolonged PR interval. At levels between 7–8 mEq/L, the ECG may reveal a widened QRS and flattened P waves. For potassium levels > 8 mEq/L, the ECG may degenerate into a sine wave pattern (see Figure 53.1), followed by ventricular fibrillation and cardiac arrest.

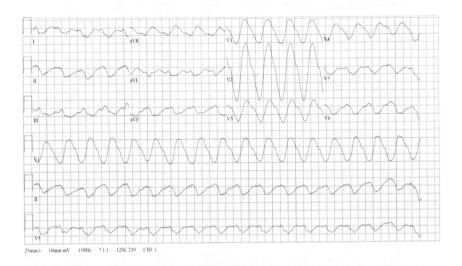

Figure 53.1 Severe hyperkalemia on ECG.

Critical Management

- **Treatment of crush injury should be aimed at preventing crush syndrome.**
- **Intravenous fluid resuscitation**
  - Aggressive fluid resuscitation with isotonic crystalloid should be initiated as soon as possible, even prior to extrication.
  - The majority of metabolic derangements can be addressed with intravenous fluid hydration as this will reduce lactic acidosis and flush out the myoglobin and CPK.
  - No specific fluid regimen is recommended, but it is reasonable to give isotonic saline at 2.5 mL/kg/hour, up to 500–1000 mL/hour for a goal of 3–12 L/day in an otherwise healthy adult patient.
  - If rhabdomyolysis develops, early hydration is the key to prevent or lessen the severity of acute renal failure. Urine output should be maintained at 200–300 mL/hour until myoglobinuria resolves and CPK values return to normal.
  - Consider *placement of a Foley catheter* to monitor urine output carefully. Low urine output suggests ongoing hypovolemia or acute renal failure.

- ○ *Alkalinization of urine* with sodium bicarbonate is controversial. Some experts recommend administering bicarbonate-containing fluid until urine pH reaches 6.5 to prevent uric acid deposition in the kidneys. However, there is no clear evidence to demonstrate added benefit of bicarbonate infusion versus normal saline.
  - ○ Though there is no current consensus on **mannitol** administration, if urinary output is < 50 mL/hour, 1–2 g/kg of mannitol may be considered provided this results in further increased urine output (described as at least 30–50 mL/hour above baseline). Loop diuretics may be harmful by increasing the risk of cast formation; however, its use may be justified in volume-overloaded patients.
- **Correction of metabolic derangements**
  - ○ Most metabolic abnormalities will improve with appropriate and aggressive crystalloid administration. Frequent monitoring of acidosis and electrolytes is imperative.
  - ○ Only treat symptomatic hypocalcemia, otherwise calcium can precipitate in muscles and lead to hypercalcemia during recovery.
  - ○ *Dialysis* should be initiated in the case of acute renal failure with hyperkalemia, acidosis or fluid overload.
- **Wound management**
  - ○ Debridement should be considered only in open crush injury in an attempt to avoid infection of the injured limb.
  - ○ Fasciotomies are generally not indicated in crush injury unless compartment syndrome is suspected.
  - ○ Splint joints in a functional position and allow active and passive movement once analgesia achieved

Sudden Deterioration

- **Hypovolemic shock** is a manifestation of **crush syndrome**. Placement of two large-bore IVs and aggressive volume resuscitation is necessary in the hypotensive individual.
- **Cardiac arrhythmias and cardiac arrest** contribute to a large percentage of early deaths in **crush injury** patients with crush syndrome due to life-threatening hyperkalemia. It should be addressed quickly and aggressively.

- Calcium administration to stabilize the cardiac membranes is first-line treatment for severe hyperkalemia defined either with ECG changes or serum potassium > 7 mEq/L.
- Temporary reduction in potassium can be achieved with intravenous insulin with glucose, intravenous sodium bicarbonate, and inhaled beta-2 agonists; all of which act to drive extracellular potassium into the intracellular compartment. Consider potassium binding resins and dialysis for prevention and treatment of hyperkalemia.

Compartment Syndrome

- Extremity compartment syndrome is a rare but serious complication of trauma, surgery, repetitive muscle use, or other conditions in which increased pressure within a fascial compartment ultimately results in decreased perfusion.
- As compartmental pressure increases, tissue pressure exceeds the venous pressure and impairs blood outflow, leading to further increases in pressure. Once compartmental pressure exceeds perfusion pressure, circulation is compromised, resulting in tissue hypoxia and loss of viability of nerve and muscle tissue.
- The lower leg is the most common area affected, but it can also affect the arms, hands, feet, and buttocks.

Presentation

Classic Presentation

- The hallmark presentation in compartment syndrome is pain that is out of proportion to injury or findings. Patients can describe the pain as "deep," "burning," and "unrelenting" with difficulty in localization. Pain with passive stretching of the muscle groups or tightness of the compartment is also common.
- Compartment syndrome can occur when the compartment is seemingly open, such as open fractures and stab wounds.
- In trauma, the anterior compartment of the leg is the most common location of compartment syndrome; however, it is possible for it to occur in any extremity compartment.

- Symptoms commonly arise within 2 hours of injury but can also present up to 6 days later.

Critical Presentation

- In addition to pain, the findings of paresthesias, paralysis, poikilothermia, and pulselessness in compartment syndrome are late findings and should not be relied upon in the initial evaluation.
- It is estimated that muscles and nerves can tolerate ischemia for 4–6 hours without significant sequelae. After this, there is risk of permanent nerve damage, myonecrosis and muscle contractures. After 8 hours, necrosis of tissue and a nonfunctional limb is likely.
- Rarely, rhabdomyolysis, renal failure, and disseminated intravascular coagulation (DIC) can result from tissue necrosis secondary to the failure to relieve compartmental pressure.
- Delay in diagnosis correlates directly with worse outcomes.

Diagnosis and Evaluation

- **Physical examination** is paramount as the physician must rely on clinical judgment for diagnosis. See Table 53.1 for lower leg compartment syndrome findings.
  - General findings
    - Pain out of proportion to injury
    - Analgesia use out of proportion to injury
  - Anterior compartment
    - Weakness of toe extension
    - Pain on passive toe flexion
    - Diminished sensation in the first web space
  - Deep posterior compartment
    - Weakness of ankle inversion and toe flexion
    - Pain on passive toe extension referred to the posterior leg
    - Diminished sensation over medial sole of foot
- **Measurement of compartmental pressures**
  - Commercially available devices exist (e.g., Stryker) that easily and accurately measure pressures.

Table 53.1 Mangled Extremity Severity Score (MESS)

Points	Component
Skeletal and soft tissue injury	
1	Low energy (stab, simple fracture, civilian gunshot wound)
2	Medium energy (open or multiplex fractures, dislocation)
3	High energy (close-range shotgun/military gunshot wound; crush injury)
4	Very high energy (same as above plus gross contamination, soft tissue avulsion)
Limb ischemia (doubled if > 6 hours)	
1	Pulse reduced or absent but perfusion normal
2	Pulseless, paresthesias, diminished capillary refill
3	Cool, paralyzed, insensate, numb
Shock	
0	Systolic blood pressure always > 90 mmHg
1	Hypotensive transiently
2	Persistent hypotension
Age (years)	
0	< 30
1	30–50
2	> 50

- Compartmental pressures > 30 mmHg or compartmental pressures within 10–30 of patient's diastolic pressure (delta-P) should prompt emergent consideration for intervention.
- Doppler ultrasound is not indicated because arterial blood flow can appear normal in cases of clear compartment syndrome.
- There is no blood test to diagnose compartment syndrome although a creatinine phosphokinase of 1000–5000 and the presence of myoglobinuria can support the diagnosis. Necrotic muscle tissue will produce lactic acid but these are late and non-specific findings.

Critical Management

- The treatment of compartment syndrome is immediate relief of the pressure. This starts with removing any constricting devices, bandages or casts.
- Surgical intervention is the definitive treatment in which complete fasciotomy of all involved compartments is performed.
- Neutral elevation is the preferred position. Raising the limb above the heart decreases perfusion without decreasing compartment pressures.
- In addition to a rapid diagnosis and facilitating emergent fasciotomy, the emergency physician should administer timely prophylactic antibiotics and analgesia.

Sudden Deterioration

- Any patient with significant trauma, crush injury, or vascular injury to an extremity should be continually monitored for the development of compartment syndrome as the onset may be insidious and the diagnosis may be difficult to recognize.
- Patients are at risk for hyperkalemia, hyperphosphatemia, lactic acidosis, and arrhythmias if there is necrotic tissue present at the time of compartment release.
- Patients suffering from late/unrecognized compartment syndrome can rarely progress to DIC, which can lead to acute worsening of their clinical status.

Open Fractures

- **Open fractures** are complex injuries of not only bone but the surrounding neurovascular and soft tissue structures. The communication with the outside world results in contamination, and gross deformity may result in compromised vascular supply. This combination places the wound at very high risk of infection and wound healing complications.
- Appropriate classification of open fractures determines choice of antibiotics and predicts risk of surgical wound infection.

Presentation

Classic Presentation

- **Open fractures** typically demonstrate obvious physical exam findings with disruption of the original anatomy and visible bony structures.
- The main concerns are arterial injury compromising the viability of the extremity and deep tissue and joint space contamination that can lead to long-term infectious complications, such as osteomyelitis.

Critical Presentation

- The Mangled Extremity Severity Score (MESS) is the most widely validated classification system of the lower extremity when evaluating the severity of **open fractures**. A score of 6 or less predicts limb viability while a score of 7 or higher predicts the need for amputation. MESS has high specificity but low sensitivity.

Diagnosis and Evaluation

- Obtain radiographs to better understand the internal disruption and identify fractures which may not be obvious on physical examination.
- Wounds in the vicinity of a fracture should be considered an "open fracture" until proven otherwise. Wound cultures prior to debridement are not necessary.
- A thorough sensory and motor examination is necessary to identify a peripheral nerve injury. Evaluate capillary refill time, temperature and color of skin, and presence or absence of distal pulses.

Critical Management

- Dislocations with concern of arterial injury should be reduced immediately.
- The simplest method to reduce hemorrhage from a long bone deformity is to apply traction and splint the extremity.
- Intravenous analgesia with narcotics is often necessary.
- **Prophylactic IV antibiotics** should be administered in the ED as soon as possible. The Gustilo-Anderson classification (see Table 53.2) has

Table 53.2 Gustilo-Anderson open fracture classification system

Grade	Injury
I	Wound < 1 cm with low energy, minimal contamination
II	Wound 1–10 cm long, low energy, without gross contamination or soft tissue damage
IIIA	Wound > 10 cm with adequate soft tissue coverage, or any high energy trauma with or without gross contamination
IIIB	Extensive soft tissue loss with periosteal stripping and bone exposure. Flap coverage required
IIIC	Arterial injury requiring repair

been used to guide antibiotic therapy, as different types of open fractures have varying rates of infection.
- Administration of cephalosporins has been shown to decrease rates of infection significantly, especially when given in the first 1–2 hours.
    - Type I and II fractures are adequately covered with **Cefazolin 2 g IV q8 hr**
    - Type III fractures are recommended **ceftriaxone 2 g IV or Cefazolin 2 g IV Q8 hr + Gentamycin 5 mg/kg IV q24 hr**
- Many authors recommend the addition of metronidazole or penicillin to cover *Clostridium* for any fracture with suspected soil or fecal contamination.
- Duration of prophylactic antibiotics is usually 24–48 hours.
- Tetanus toxoid is the standard treatment for patients who have completed the primary tetanus immunization series. Those who have not received the series or particularly tetanus-prone wounds should receive the tetanus immune globulin in addition to the toxoid.

Sudden Deterioration

- **Hypovolemic shock** should prompt high suspicion for concurrent vascular injury. Proceed with immediate fracture reduction, volume resuscitation, as well as emergent trauma/vascular surgery consultation. In patients with arterial injury, consider early administration of uncrossmatched blood and instituting massive transfusion protocol.

BIBLIOGRAPHY

Frykberg ER, Dennis JW, Bishop K, et al. The reliability of physical examination in the evaluation of penetrating extremity trauma for vascular injury: results at one year. *J Trauma* 1991;31(4):502–511.

Garner MR, Sethuraman SA, Schade MA, et al. Antibiotic prophylaxis in open fractures: evidence, evolving issues and recommendations. *J Amer Acad Ortho Surg* 2020;28(8):309–315.

Gonzalez D. Crush syndrome. *Crit Care Med* 2005;33:S34–41.

McQueen MM, Duckworth AD. The diagnosis of acute compartment syndrome: a review. *Eur J Trauma Emerg Surg* 2014;40(5):521–528.

Moshe Michaelson MD. Crush injury and crush syndrome. *World J Surgery* 1992;16:899–903.

Sever MS & Vanholder R. Recommendations for the management of crush victims in mass disasters. *Nephrol Dial Transplant* 2012;27(1):i1–i67.

54

· · · · · · · ·

Burn Resuscitation

AARON SURREY

Introduction

- ○ Two-thirds of reported burn cases admitted to burn centers affect less than 10% of total body surface area (TBSA) and require a relatively short hospitalization.
- ○ The majority of patients with major burn injury or significant physiological derangements survive.
- ○ Improvement in mortality rates is related to advances in resuscitation, infection control, modulation of the hypermetabolic response to traumatic injury, and early excision and grafting.
- ○ Traditional classification of burns of first, second, third, and fourth degree have been replaced by a more descriptive explanation of injury depth:

Superficial (formerly classified as first degree)
a. Extent of injury: epidermis
b. Sensitivity: hyperalgesic
c. Appearance: erythema

Partial thickness (formerly classified as superficial and deep second degree)
a. Extent of injury: epidermis and partial dermis
b. Sensitivity: hyperalgesic
c. Appearance: blisters, pink, moist (blanching with pressure)

Full thickness (formerly classified as third degree)
a. Extent of injury: epidermis and dermis
b. Sensitivity: insensate
c. Appearance: opaque, white, black, leathery

Muscle/fascia involvement (formerly classified as fourth degree)
a. Extent of injury: epidermis and dermis as well as subcutaneous tissue, muscle, and/or bone
b. Sensitivity: insensate
c. Appearance: disfiguring, black, leathery

- Presentation
  - Flame and scald burns are the most common cause of burn injuries.
    - Examples of flame injuries include house fires and automobile crashes, while examples for scald burns include hot oil or liquid burns.
  - Contact burns from grasping hot objects are the most common cause of burn injuries in children.
  - Electrical burns (unpredictable flow of energy [i.e., entry/exit]) can occur from exposure to electrical current in the home or at work, or rarely from lightning injuries.
  - Chemical burns typically result from acidic or alkali chemical exposure.

Diagnosis and Evaluation

  - A complete set of vital signs including height and weight should be obtained on all burn victims. Large burn injuries (total body surface area (TBSA) >20%) require continuous monitoring.
  - Laboratory tests

- It is reasonable to obtain a complete metabolic panel (CMP) and complete blood count (CBC) in most patients with significant burn injury.
- A Creatine kinase (CK) may be useful to assess for muscle injury and evaluate for rhabdomyolysis, while a urinalysis can evaluate for myoglobinuria.
- Obtain a carboxyhemoglobin (COHb) if there is concern for carbon monoxide (CO) poisoning.
- A blood gas may show signs of hypercarbia, hypoxia, and acidosis.
- Obtain a lactate to evaluate for evidence of hypoperfusion in the setting of significant burn injuries or hemodynamic instability.

- Imaging
  - Obtain a chest X-ray in patients suspected of inhalational injury and/or have been intubated.
  - Perform further imaging such as CT scans if traumatic mechanism is suspected.
- EKG
  - EKG should be obtained in all electrical injuries, patients with pre-existing cardiac disease, and otherwise at the provider's discretion.

Critical Management

☑ Systematic trauma principles as applicable
☑ Primary survey with particular attention to signs of inhalational injury, respiratory insufficiency, and, circumferential burns,
☑ Fluid resuscitation formulas

- Safety
  - Providers caring for burn victims should don protective equipment to limit potential exposures from body fluids or chemical contamination and to reduce the risk of early nosocomial infections.
  - Utilize in-line cervical immobilization in patients with associated trauma or altered mental status.
- Access
  - Establish early intravenous access. Since delayed resuscitation may increase mortality, early intraosseous or central access should be considered if providers are unable to obtain peripheral access.

- If necessary, access can be obtained through thermally injured areas that have been properly prepped with an aseptic technique. Early thermal injuries are not infected or colonized with bacteria.
- Perform a primary survey on arrival for all significant burn injuries.
  - Airway
    - Asses the airway immediately. Inhalation injury puts patients at risk for early airway compromise due to a progressive edematous state.
      - Normal oxygen and chest X-ray does not exclude inhalation injury.
    - Maximum airway edema from thermal injury occurs at 24 hours; clinical signs of deterioration should be managed with early controlled intubation.
    - Perform endoscopic visualization of the posterior oropharynx for all patients at risk for upper airway injury to determine need for early intubation.
      - Clinical signs and symptoms include stridor, dysphonia, dysphagia, neck edema, carbonaceous sputum, singed facial hair, facial burns, and mucosal burns.
    - Consider early intubation if upper airway patency is threatened, gas exchange or lung mechanics is inadequate, or airway protection is compromised by mental status.
      - Succinylcholine can be used in the first 24 hours after injury, after which the risk of clinically significant hyperkalemia increases.
      - If possible, intubate using a 7.5 endotracheal tube or larger to facilitate future bronchoscopy (therapeutic scope requires at least 7.5 ETT).
  - Breathing
    - Respiratory insufficiency or failure may result from both mechanical and physiological mechanisms following a thermal injury.
    - Circumferential burn injuries to the torso may reduce chest wall compliance, resulting in ineffective ventilation.
      - Treatment includes early recognition and endotracheal intubation.
      - Escharotomies at the bilateral mid-axillary lines can be performed for circumferential torso burns if there are clinical signs of ineffective ventilation such as increased peak airway pressures, insufficient tidal volumes, or hypercarbia.
      - Secondary escharotomies along the subcostal margin are occasionally necessary to complete chest cavity decompression.
    - Physiological failure is typically associated with chemical burns causing pneumonitis, and less commonly due to direct thermal injury.
      - Treatment is early recognition and supportive care.

- Avoid ventilator-associated injury by using lung protective ventilation including low tidal volumes, avoidance of excessive plateau pressures, and prevention of atelectasis.
- **Circulation**
  - **Hypotension and shock may be observed in patients with severe burn injuries.**
    - Both plasma extravasation through burn injuries and third spacing from increased capillary permeability contribute to a hypovolemic state.
    - Correcting intravascular volume deficits is a crucial component of burn management.
    - Lactated ringer's (LR) is the preferred fluid for initial fluid resuscitation.
      - Recommended pre-hospital and initial fluid rates until TBSA can be calculated during the secondary survey as follows:
        - < 5 years old: 125 mL/hour
        - 6–13 years old: 250 mL/hour
        - > 13 years old: 500 mL/hour
    - Increased capillary permeability can result in a reduced vascular tone, which may warrant vasopressors. However, this should be considered only if the patient has been adequately fluid resuscitated.
    - While less common, cardiac insufficiency has been observed following major thermal injuries and should be addressed with inotropic support if appropriate.
    - Circumferential burns are at risk for reduced distal circulation.
      - Escharotomies should be performed for signs of compromised distal perfusion, diminished or absent pulses, or elevated compartment pressure.
  - **Disability/neurological deficits**
    - Patients are typically alert and oriented. If altered, consider conditions including but not limited to CO poisoning, cyanide (CN) poisoning, hypercarbia, or substance abuse. Additionally, patients who present after burn injury may have other traumatic injuries.
    - CO poisoning is the most frequent immediate cause of death following inhalation injury.
      - Symptoms of CO poisoning are nonspecific and include headache, altered mental status, chest pain, dyspnea, and vomiting.
      - The classic cherry-red skin is a late finding typically seen post-mortem.
    - Patients with high or presumed high COHb should receive 100% oxygen until COHb normalizes.

- While hyperbaric oxygen therapy (HBO) may be considered in a subset of patients with CO toxicity, do not delay transfer to a burn facility to initiate HBO.
  - **CN poisoning is difficult to detect and results in high morbidity and mortality.**
    - Produced by combustion of numerous household products such as plastics and wool.
    - Inhaled CN can be rapidly fatal after even a few breaths. Signs and symptoms include headache, altered mental status, syncope, cyanosis, and hemodynamic instability.
    - CN toxicity causes a high anion gap metabolic acidosis and an elevated serum lactate.
    - CN levels are unreliable and are rarely readily available.
    - Patients with suspected CN poisoning should be treated presumptively using hydroxycobalamin or cyanide antidote kit.
- Exposure/environmental
  - **Stop the burning process by removing clothing, shoes, jewelry, etc.**
    - Cool material adhering to burns and cut around/remove as much as of it as possible.
  - **Remove contact lenses if present.**
  - **Avoid hypothermia.**
    - Provide a warm environment.
    - Cover exposed burns with sterile dressings to prevent heat loss.
- Secondary survey
  - **The secondary survey of a burn patient should follow a systematic approach similar to that of a trauma patient. This includes obtaining further history and a head-to-toe exam to assess TBSA as well as to evaluate for other injuries.**
  - **TBSA estimation (do not include superficial burns).**
    - "Rule of Nines":
      - Adults: head 9%, torso 18% each for anterior and posterior, each arm 9%, each leg 18%, genitals 1%.
      - Children: head 18%, torso 16% each for anterior and posterior, arm 10%, leg 14%.
    - "Rule of Palms" or "1% rule":
      - The size of the patient's hand including the fingers is approximately 1% of TBSA.
      - This may be more useful for scattered burns.

- Lund-Browder Charts may be available for more accurate TBSA estimations.
  - ○ Fluid rate should be adjusted based off the TBSA.
    - Fluid resuscitation is aimed at maintaining organ perfusion while avoiding excessive fluids. This requires frequent re-evaluations and fluid rate adjustments as needed.
      - ☐ Over-resuscitation can result in acute respiratory distress syndrome (ARDS) and abdominal compartment syndrome. It also increases the risk of pneumonia, bacteremia, multiorgan failure, and death.
      - ☐ Under-resuscitation can result in hemodynamic instability as well as organ dysfunction or failure (most commonly acute kidney injury).
  - ○ While numerous burn fluid resuscitation formulae exist, the modified Brooke and the Parkland are the most commonly utilized.
  - ○ Modified Brooke (or Parkland) formula estimates fluid requirements during the initial 24 hours as 2 mL (or 4 mL in case of Parkland) TBSA (%) ideal body weight (IBW) (kg) for all burns > 20% TBSA.
    - The first half is administered in the first 8 hours after injury (not after presentation), with the second half given over the subsequent 16 hours.
    - Advanced Burn Life Support (ABLS) 2018 guidelines recommend 2 mL ✕ TBSA ✕ IBW if greater than 14 years old, 3 mL ✕ TBSA ✕ IBW if less than 14 years old, and 4 mL ✕ TBSA ✕ IBW for all electrical injuries.
      - ☐ For infants and young children, add a D_5LR maintenance rate.
    - Using 4 mL ✕ TBSA ✕ IBW for all burn injuries may result in over-resuscitation.
    - Adjust for fluid resuscitation given prehospital/during initial phase if necessary.

Example: Modified Brooke Formula Calculation
Patient: Age 50 years; IBW 70 kg
~10% TBSA superficial
~50% TBSA partial and full thickness
2 mL × 50% × 70 kg = 7.0 liters
Half is administered over the first 8 hours:
Total volume: 7.0 L/2 = 3.5 L
Hourly rate: 3.5 L/8 hours = 438 mL/hour
Half is administered over the remaining 16 hours:

Total volume: 3.5 L/16 hours

Hourly rate: 219 mL/hour

○ It is important to note that these formulae are estimations only. Adjustments to initial volume resuscitation should be based on the patient's physiological response.

- Maintain urine output goal of 0.5 mL/kg/hour (or 1 mg/kg/hour for children < 30 kg).
  - Adjust fluid rates by no greater than one-third at a time.
  - If oliguric, rule out other causes such as foley malposition or abdominal compartment syndrome to avoid over-resuscitation.
- Other parameters to consider trending include serum lactate, base deficit, and pH.

Sudden Deterioration

○ Early airway management.
○ Consider concomitant cyanide toxicity and treat accordingly.
○ Escharotomy if indicated for restrictive physiology/tension from circumferential scar formation.
○ Mixed shock workup.
● Special considerations
   ○ Up to 5.8% of burns are complicated by major trauma. Delayed diagnosis of associated injuries may increase morbidity, mortality, and length of stay.
   ○ Tdap booster should be administered in all superficial partial thickness or greater burns if not administered in the past 5 years.
   ○ Prophylactic antibiotics are not indicated in the initial management of burn injury.
   ○ Bronchoscopy should be performed to confirm inhalational injury and stage severity, but should not delay transfer to definitive care.
   ○ The American Burn Association has determined criteria for patients who would benefit from transfer to a burn center:

Partial thickness burns > 10% TBSA.

Any full thickness burn.

Burns involving the face, hands, feet, genitalia, perineum, or major joints.

Chemical or electrical burns, including lightning injury.

Inhalation injury.

Burn patients with preexisting medical conditions that may complicate management, prolong recovery, or affect mortality.

Patients with burns and concomitant trauma if the burn poses the greatest immediate risk of morbidity or mortality. If the trauma poses the greater immediate risk, the patient may be initially stabilized in a trauma center before transfer to a burn center. In such situations, physician judgment in concert with the regional medical control plan and triage protocols is necessary.

Children with burns in a hospital without qualified personnel or equipment for the care of children.

Burn injury in patients who will require special social, emotional, or rehabilitative intervention.

- Sudden Deterioration
  - Acute deterioration may be caused by numerous etiologies in the setting of a burn patient, including:
    - Shock, caused by any combination of hypovolemic, distributive, and cardiogenic shock; ultrasound can assist in the differential.
    - Abdominal compartment syndrome from increased permeability and/or volume over-resuscitation. This can cause low cardiac output and hypotension from reduced preload due to IVC compression, difficulty ventilating, renal dysfunction/oliguria, and bowel ischemia.
    - ARDS related to vascular permeability and/or over-resuscitation.

BIBLIOGRAPHY

American Burn Association. Burn incidence and treatment in the United States: 2016. Chicago, Il: American Burn Association, 2016.

Advanced Burn Life Support (ABLS) Provider Manual: 2018 Update. Chicago, Il: American Burn Association, 2018.

Barajas-Nava LA, Lopez-Alcalde J, Roquei Figuls M, et al. Antibiotic prophylaxis for preventing burn wound infection. *Cochrane Database Syst Rev* 2013;(6):CD008738.

Boyd JH, Sirounis D, Maizel J, et al. Echocardiography as a guide for fluid management. *Crit Care* 2016;20(1):274.

Chung KK, Wolf SE, Cancio LC, et al. Resuscitation of severely burned military casualties: fluid begets more fluid. *J Trauma* 2009;67(2):231–237.

Herndon DL. *Total Burn Care*, 5th ed. Philadelphia, PA: Elsevier Saunders, 2017.

Klein MB, Hayden D, Elson C, et al. The association between fluid administration and outcome following major burn: a multicenter study. *Ann Surg* 2007;245(4):622–628.

Liang JL, Tiwari T, Moro P, et al. Prevention of pertussis, tetanus, and diphtheria with vaccines in the United States: recommendations of the Advisory Committee of Immunization Practices (ACIP). *MMWR Recomm Rep* 2018;67(2):1.

Martyn JA, & Ritchtsfeld M. Succinylcholine-induced hyperkalemia in acquired pathologic states: etiologic factors and molecular mechanisms. *Anesthesiology* 2006;104(1):158–169.

Orgill DP, & Piccolo N. Escharotomy and decompressive therapies in burns. *BCR* 2009;30:759–768.

Rehberg S, Maybauer MO, Ekhbaatar P, et al. Pathophysiology, management, and treatment of smoke inhalation injury. *Expert Rev Respir Med* 2009;3(3):283.

Santaniello JM, Luchette FA, Esposito TJ, et al. Ten-year experience of burn, trauma, and combined burn/trauma injuries comparing outcomes. *J Trauma* 20014;57(4):696.

SECTION 12

End of Life

ASHLEY SHREVES

55

Care of the Dying Patient

ASHLEY SHREVES

Introduction

- Palliative medicine focuses on maximizing the quality of life of patients with serious illnesses.
- For many patients in the critical care setting, the best medical treatments and technologies are unable to reverse advanced disease processes, as evidenced by the fact that 20% of Americans died in or after ICU care.
- Even when treatments can prolong life, they may not ultimately allow patients to achieve a quality of life acceptable to them. Functional and cognitive independence are highly valued by patients and yet most chronically, critically ill patients never live independently again.
- Honest, transparent, empathetic communication is the cornerstone of determining how to deliver effective, patient-centered medical care in this setting.
- When critical care interventions are no longer able to achieve the stated goals of the patient and family, transitioning away from life-prolonging care often makes the most sense, especially because these treatments can be burdensome and contribute to patient suffering.

- The "withdrawal" of life-sustaining treatments like ventilatory support and hemodialysis often signify to the medical staff and family that the patient has entered the dying process.
- Care of the dying patient is complex as patients and families have intense emotional, spiritual, psychosocial, and medical needs.
- While optimizing comfort through effective symptom-based therapies is essential, high-quality end-of-life care typically extends beyond these measures, involving an interdisciplinary team to tend to a wide range of needs that patients and families manifest.

Presentation

Classic Presentation

- At the end-of-life, there are two classically described trajectories of dying:
  - *Easy road:* Decreased functionality marked by increasing time spent in bed and sleeping, with the patient eventually becoming comatose, followed by death.
  - *Difficult road:* Functional loss occurs but end-of-life symptoms are also pronounced, particularly terminal delirium, dyspnea, and pain.

Critical Presentation

- Dying in the critical care setting most often follows the withholding or withdrawal of life-sustaining treatments and therefore has its own unique trajectory.
- Symptom burden and the dying trajectory vary widely depending on a multitude of factors such as the underlying disease process, the severity of illness, and types of life-sustaining intervention being withdrawn.
- **While the prevalence of distressing symptoms such as pain, discomfort, thirst, anxiety, and dyspnea are high in critically ill patients, high rates of comfort have been reported in those undergoing withdrawal of life-sustaining therapies.**

Diagnosis and Evaluation

- When critical care is no longer achieving patient-centered goals and/or the patient is dying despite aggressive use of life-sustaining therapy, a meeting should be held to determine the "goals of care."
- Many dying patients are sedated, comatose, or delirious and can no longer participate in medical decision-making; therefore, legally appropriate surrogate decision-makers should be identified.
- Previously completed advance directives, including the designation of a health care proxy, should be reviewed.
- Efforts should be made to gather all the important decision-makers in the patient's family and hold a meeting with the treatment team, ideally with members of the palliative care service present.
- Clear, compassionate, culturally sensitive language should be used to communicate the patient's overall prognosis and elicit previously expressed values, goals, and preferences.
- Many departments have protocolized this "goal-setting conference" (Table 55.1).
- If all agree that life-sustaining treatment is no longer able to achieve the patient's goals, an ideal plan often includes a transition to care that maximizes comfort and dignity while not prolonging the patient's dying process.

Critical Management

Critical Management Checklist

- ☑ Prepare
- ☑ Premedicate
- ☑ Procedure (withdrawal of respiratory support)
- ☑ Prognosis

- **Withdrawal of ventilator support** or "liberation from the ventilator": a common step preceding death in the ICU.
  - *Preparation:*
    - Ensure that "Do not resuscitate" (DNR)/"Do not intubate" (DNI) orders and paperwork are completed.
    - Ensure that the spiritual needs of patient and family are met, which may include completion of important religious rituals.

Table 55.1 The goal-setting conference

Ten-step guide	Tips/examples
Establish a proper setting	Quiet, appropriate parties invited, pagers/phones turned off.
Introductions	"Can you tell me something about your mom?"
Assess patient/family understanding	"What have the doctors told you about your mom's condition?"
Medical review/ summary	Start with a warning shot. Give small pieces of information. Avoid jargon. "I'm afraid I have some bad news. Your mom is dying."
Silence/reactions	"I wish we had better treatments for her disease." "I can only imagine how disappointed you must be." "You've been so devoted and loving to your mom."
Discuss prognosis	Assess the amount of information desired. Present prognostic data using ranges.
Assess goals	Not prolonging the dying process, a peaceful death, being surrounded by family? "If your mom could talk to us right now, what would she tell us is most important to her?"
Present broad options	"Based on what we've discussed and what you've told me about your mom, *I recommend* that we refocus our efforts on maximizing her comfort and not prolong her dying process."
Translate goals into care plan	"Maintaining your mom on life support does not seem consistent with what her wishes would be, therefore I'm recommending that we liberate her from the machine and allow her to have a natural death."
Document	Write DNR orders, discontinue and add appropriate therapies, give a new care plan.

Source: Adapted from Weissman DE. "The Family Goal Setting Conference" and "Communication Phrases Near the End of Life" pocket cards from Medical College of Wisconsin.

- Chaplaincy or even physician instruction regarding end-of-life communication that expresses gratitude and forgiveness can be a helpful tool in allowing patients and families to achieve peace and closure (Table 55.2).

Table 55.2 Six things to say before you die

1. I love you
2. Thank you
3. Please forgive me
4. I forgive you
5. Good-bye
6. I'm going to be okay

- Discontinue unnecessary laboratory testing and therapies that are not supporting goals, such as artificial nutrition and hydration, vasopressors, and antibiotics.
- **Consider simulation of extubation, which would include placing patient on pressure support while on ventilator, to anticipate degree of respiratory distress and extent of opiate need.**
  - *Premedication:*
    - Glycopyrrolate 0.2 mg every 6 hours to minimize respiratory secretions.
    - **Morphine 2–6 mg IV, depending on size of patient, opiate tolerance, simulation.**
  - *Procedure:*
    - Turn off monitors as alarms will be distracting and the patient's visible signs of discomfort, rather than vital signs, should guide management.
    - The ETT can be easily removed after cuff deflation.
    - **Adequate analgesia and sedative medications should be available, either through continuous drips that can be titrated for symptom control or in prefilled syringes that can be delivered as IV pushes at the bedside.**
    - *Dosing instructions:* for patients already on opiate and benzodiazepine infusions, bolus doses used for dyspnea should be approximately double the hourly infusion rate (i.e., if fentanyl is infusing at 100 micrograms/hour, the patient should receive 200-microgram boluses every 10–15 minutes until comfort is achieved).
    - Oxygen does not need to be administered as it might prolong the patient's dying process, and opiates can adequately palliate dyspnea.
    - *Goal:* no signs of respiratory distress and/or dyspnea, which would include gasping, accessory muscle use, or labored breathing.
  - *Prognosis:*
    - If desired, families should be informed regarding the estimated survival time once ventilator support is discontinued, as this allows for adequate

preparation and planning. Prognostic estimates should be communicated as time frames: minutes to hours, hours to days, or days to weeks.

  ▪ Once ventilator support is removed, the median time to survival is just under an hour, though some patients may survive for days. Predictors of shorter survival include such variables as multi-organ failure, use of vasopressors, and brain death.

- **Other symptom considerations**
  ○ *Terminal delirium:*
    ▪ This is common and easily treatable with antipsychotics.
    ▪ Haldol 0.5–2 mg IV every 6 hours is an adequate dosing regimen for most patients.
  ○ *Pain:*
    ▪ Pain is common in critically ill patients.
    ▪ Dying patients are often sedated and/or unable to communicate, so nonverbal cues such as grimacing, moaning, and restlessness should be used.
    ▪ Opiates are the mainstay treatment. Hydromorphone is preferred over morphine in patients with renal or liver failure.

- **Other considerations**
  ○ *Transferring patients to the palliative care unit or inpatient hospice:*
    ▪ Hospitals are increasingly incorporating palliative care and hospice units into their institutions. These can be ideal settings for transitions from LST to comfort-focused care.
  ○ *Improving the family's experience:*
    ▪ **Families rate factors such as "preparation for death"; timely, compassionate communication; care maintaining comfort, dignity, and personhood; open access and proximity of the family to the patient; interdisciplinary care; and bereavement support as highly important in the setting of a dying patient.**
    ▪ Surprisingly, families of patients who have died rather than survived in the ICU show higher satisfaction with the care delivered.

Special Circumstances

- **Young children**
  ○ Family members of dying patients may include young children. Depending on their age and maturity, children will have varying

abilities to process death and dying. Child life specialists and social workers can be incredibly valuable resources in facilitating communication and coping in this group.

- **Organ** donation
  - ○ The local organ donor network should be contacted early and often for patients in whom the withdrawal of life-sustaining treatments is planned. Assumptions should never be made regarding the patient's suitability as a donor and/or the family's preferences regarding this option.

A Helpful Resource

The Center to Advance Palliative Care has created a website called **IPAL-ICU** (www.capc.org/toolkits/integrating-palliative-care-practices-in-the-icu/) that is an invaluable resource for clinicians hoping to improve the practice of palliative care within the ICU setting.

BIBLIOGRAPHY

Angus DC, & Barnato AE. Use of intensive care at the end of life in the United States: an epidemiologic study. *Crit Care Med* 2004;32:638–643.

Camhi SL, & Mercado AF. Deciding in the dark: advance directives and continuation of treatment in chronic critical illness. *Crit Care Med* 2009;37:919–925.

Cooke CR, & Hotchkin DL. Predictors of time to death after terminal withdrawal of mechanical ventilation in the ICU. *Chest* 2010;138:289–297.

Kompanje EJ, & van der Hoven B. Anticipation of distress after discontinuation of mechanical ventilation in the ICU at the end of life. *Intensive Care Med* 2008;34:1593–1599.

Mularski RA, & Heine CE. Quality of dying in the ICU: ratings by family members. *Chest* 2005;128:280–282.

Nelson JE, & Puntillo KA. In their own words: patients and families define high-quality palliative care in the intensive care unit. *Crit Care Med* 2010;38:808–818.

Prendergast TJ, & Claessens MT. A national survey of end-of-life care for critically ill patients. *Am J Respir Crit Care Med* 1998;158:1163–1167.

Rocker GM, & Heyland DK. Most critically ill patients are perceived to die in comfort during withdrawal of life support: a Canadian multicentre study. *Can J Anaesth* 2004;51:623–630.

Wall RJ, & Curtis JR. Family satisfaction in the ICU: differences between families of survivors and nonsurvivors. *Chest* 2007;132:1425–1433.

Index